EXERCISE AND FITNESS TRAINING AFTER STROKE

Commissioning Editor: Rita Demetriou-Swanwick
Development Editor: Catherine Jackson
Project Manager: Sukanthi Sukumar
Designer: Mark Rogers
Illustration Manager: Jennifer Rose
Illustrator: Antbits Ltd
Photos in Chapter 10: Forth Photography

EXERCISE AND FITNESS TRAINING AFTER STROKE

A HANDBOOK FOR EVIDENCE-BASED PRACTICE

Edited by

Gillian Mead MB BChir MA MD FRCP
Professor of Stroke and Elderly Care Medicine
University of Edinburgh
Edinburgh

Frederike van Wijck PhD MSc BSc MCSP FHEA
Reader in Neurological Rehabilitation
Institute for Applied Health Research and
School of Health and Life Sciences
Glasgow Caledonian University
Glasgow

Foreword by

Peter Langhorne
Professor of Stroke Care, Academic Section of Geriatric Medicine,
Glasgow Royal Infirmary, Glasgow, United Kingdom

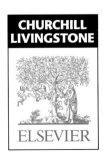

CHURCHILL
LIVINGSTONE

ELSEVIER

Edinburgh   London   New York   Oxford   Philadelphia   St Louis   Sydney   Toronto   2013

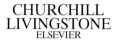

ISBN 978 0 7020 4338 3

British Library Cataloguing in Publication Data
A catalogue record for this book is available from the British Library

Library of Congress Cataloging in Publication Data
A catalog record for this book is available from the Library of Congress

Notices

Knowledge and best practice in this field are constantly changing. As new research and experience broaden our understanding, changes in research methods, professional practices, or medical treatment may become necessary.

Practitioners and researchers must always rely on their own experience and knowledge in evaluating and using any information, methods, compounds, or experiments described herein. In using such information or methods they should be mindful of their own safety and the safety of others, including parties for whom they have a professional responsibility.

With respect to any drug or pharmaceutical products identified, readers are advised to check the most current information provided (i) on procedures featured or (ii) by the manufacturer of each product to be administered, to verify the recommended dose or formula, the method and duration of administration, and contraindications. It is the responsibility of practitioners, relying on their own experience and knowledge of their patients, to make diagnoses, to determine dosages and the best treatment for each individual patient, and to take all appropriate safety precautions.

To the fullest extent of the law, neither the Publisher nor the authors, contributors, or editors, assume any liability for any injury and/or damage to persons or property as a matter of products liability, negligence or otherwise, or from any use or operation of any methods, products, instructions, or ideas contained in the material herein.

 your source for books, journals and multimedia in the health sciences

www.elsevierhealth.com

Working together to grow libraries in developing countries

www.elsevier.com | www.bookaid.org | www.sabre.org

ELSEVIER   BOOK AID International   Sabre Foundation

The Publisher's policy is to use paper manufactured from sustainable forests

Printed in China

CONTENTS

FOREWORD

Peter Langhorne
Professor of Stroke Care
University of Glasgow

The last twenty years have seen dramatic changes in the way in which stroke patients are managed and the nihilism that previously surrounded stroke care has been replaced with a much more optimistic and proactive approach. Stroke has become to be seen as a medical emergency with a rapid increase in the number of drugs now available, particularly in the area of stroke prevention. The provision of multidisciplinary stroke unit care has moved from being an occasional service development to a recognised national quality standard.

These changes in management have also reflected a change in the philosophy of rehabilitation, from promoting compensation for impairments to restoration of recovery through active learning and training. We have also recognised that recovery is better with the active participation of patients; there has been a move away from patients being seen as passive recipients of care to being active participants in recovery. Finally, stroke is recognised as a chronic disease in which long-term lifestyle management is very important.

This book, *Exercise and Fitness Training After Stroke: A Handbook for Evidence-based Practice*, exemplifies these changes very clearly. It is the first book dedicated to exercise and fitness training after stroke. After reviewing the evidence base (randomised trials and systematic reviews) demonstrating that exercise improves fitness after stroke, it then focuses on the implementation of this evidence including the design of models for the delivery of exercise services. Among the many features to commend it are the expert multidisciplinary authorship, the focus on a multidisciplinary audience of physiotherapists, occupational therapists, exercise professionals and students. Also its advice is shaped by expert experience but grounded in reliable clinical evidence. What is particularly striking is the clear mission to enable stroke survivors to benefit from exercise and fitness training that is embedded in their normal lifestyle routines. This book will be a milestone in the development of services for stroke survivors and for promoting long-term recovery after stroke.

PREFACE

Stroke is the leading cause of adult disability in the USA and Europe and is the second most common cause of death worldwide. With recent advances in the management of acute stroke, more and more people are surviving the immediate effects of a stroke, and, more recently, the focus of much research and service development is turning to the longer-term needs of stroke survivors. There is an increasing body of evidence that exercise and fitness training after stroke will improve stroke survivors' physical function and is likely to have other benefits such as a reduction in the risk of recurrent stroke and heart attacks, as well as reduced fatigue and improved mood.

In this book, we will use the American College of Sports Medicine definition of exercise, i.e. exercise is defined as planned, structured, repetitive bodily movement done to improve one or more components of physical fitness. During stroke rehabilitation, specific exercises will be given as part of therapeutic interventions, with the aim to improve passive and active movement, normalise tone, and facilitate the recovery of functions such as balance, gait, transfers and arm function. What differentiates Exercise after Stroke, as interpreted in this book, from exercises in the context of therapeutic interventions is that the aim of 'exercise' is to improve physical fitness.

WHAT IS THE PURPOSE OF THIS BOOK?

This book is unique because it aims to provide exercise professionals and other suitably qualified practitioners with the necessary information to design and evaluate exercise programmes for people after stroke that are safe and effective, based on current evidence and aligned with national clinical guidelines and service frameworks. The book goes beyond stroke rehabilitation and aims to encourage a healthy lifestyle through regular physical activity to enhance health and wellbeing.

FOR WHOM IS THIS BOOK INTENDED?

While this book is designed primarily for exercise professionals, it will also be highly relevant to health professionals involved in the care of stroke survivors, as they will increasingly collaborate with exercise professionals to develop pathways into community Exercise after Stroke services. Students of all these disciplines will also find this book highly relevant to their future practice. Sports scientists wishing to develop novel research in this area will find this book invaluable as it provides a review of the current state of knowledge. We hope that stroke survivors and their carers may also be able to find relevant information about their condition, and the opportunities offered by exercise training, in this book.

WHY DO EXERCISE PROFESSIONALS AND OTHER SUITABLY QUALIFIED PRACTITIONERS NEED TO BE KNOWLEDGEABLE ABOUT EXERCISE AFTER STROKE?

Exercise and fitness training for stroke survivors should be delivered by exercise professionals with current knowledge about the long-term physical and psychological consequences of stroke and about the benefits of exercise after stroke. They need to know how to design, adapt and tailor exercise programmes to stroke survivors, and they need to be familiar with the roles and responsibilities of exercise and health professionals involved. Whilst this book cannot be a substitute for practical training, it provides the knowledge required for working with stroke survivors in practice. Health professionals need to understand how exercise can facilitate ongoing recovery from stroke, after formal rehabilitation has ended, and how to work with exercise professionals to develop pathways into exercise after stroke. Health professionals may wish to consider how to incorporate exercise training into the early rehabilitation of stroke survivors, in order to reduce the physical deconditioning that occurs early after stroke.

WHAT WILL I LEARN BY READING THIS BOOK?

The book is in four parts.

Part 1 provides essential background knowledge about: the clinical manifestations of stroke; how stroke is managed within hospital and community settings and the long-term problems after stroke, focusing on those problems that are particularly relevant to the delivery of exercise. This part will provide the reader with a wider understanding of the complexities of stroke and the investigations and treatment approaches currently advocated. The importance of teamwork in stroke care is emphasised by discussing the complementary roles of each health professional and how they work together as a team.

Part 2 focuses on the evidence base for exercise and fitness training after stroke. It opens by discussing the evidence that physical fitness is impaired after stroke, then moves on to explore the benefits of exercise after stroke by describing the findings from rigorous clinical trials. It also covers concepts of exercise behaviour and communication to facilitate the engagement of stroke survivors in exercise and fitness training. It finishes by describing one stroke survivor's recovery – and the role that exercise has played in this.

Part 3 is more practical and describes how to prepare for exercise after stroke, and then how to design, implement and evaluate an exercise and fitness training programme. This part will emphasise the importance of safety through robust referral procedures, as well as the design and delivery of exercise programmes that are adapted to stroke in general and tailored to the individual with their unique interests, goals and constellation of impairments and activity limitations.

Part 4 takes a broader view and describes existing models of community exercise after stroke services, and provides best practice guidance on how to develop these services to a high standard. Throughout this section, the close working relationship between health and exercise professionals, as well as service users, is emphasised. The conclusion summarises the key points from the book. It also looks to the future, identifying where further research is needed, and how this might help shape exercise after stroke services of the future.

Although there are many textbooks about stroke and stroke rehabilitation, none of these is dedicated to exercise and fitness training after stroke. At the time of writing, this is – to our knowledge – the only textbook on this subject. The editors and authors have brought this book together driven by their own passion for the subject and their commitment to achieving the vision of 'more people after stroke, more active more often, exercising safely and effectively'.

Gillian Mead and Frederike van Wijck

ACKNOWLEDGEMENTS

First of all, we would like to thank all of the authors for the specialist knowledge and experience that they bring to the book. The editors and authors have been working with each other for several years, initially performing original research to explore the feasibility and benefits of exercise after stroke, and then developing and delivering the first UK validated specialist course on stroke for exercise professionals entitled 'Exercise after Stroke: Specialist Instructor Training Course'. It was from this work that the concepts and content of this book emerged. Whilst we are indebted to all contributors in this book, special thanks goes to Mr John M.A. Dennis for the role he has played in developing and delivering exercise services for stroke survivors in Scotland and his invaluable, continuous advice and contribution to a substantive part of this book. We are also indebted to Dr Susie Dinan-Young whose links with the Department of Health England, SkillsActive and Register of Exercise Professionals ensured that the body of knowledge within the book was regularly disseminated and reviewed by relevant stakeholders. We are grateful to Thavapriya Sugavanam for her invaluable review of the section on goal setting in the book. Professor Marie Donaghy provided expert advice and guidance about how to bring together the knowledge of our author team in order to create this book, for which we are most grateful. We would also like to thank our publishers, who have guided the production of this book and 'Forth Photography' for taking photos for Chapter 10 and the front cover of this book.

We would like to express our thanks to Chest Heart & Stroke Scotland, Edinburgh Leisure, NHS Greater Glasgow and Clyde and the Scottish Government for providing the funding to develop and deliver the 'Exercise after Stroke: Specialist Instructor Training Course'. Subsequent funding from the Scottish Government's National Advisory Committee on Stroke enabled us to map the provision of exercise services in Scotland, and to develop best practice guidance for community Exercise after Stroke services.

We are indebted to our Reference Group, a multidisciplinary group comprising more than 30 individuals including consultants in stroke medicine and geriatrics, stroke clinical specialists and academics in physiotherapy, occupational therapy, speech and language therapy, nursing, exercise physiology and exercise science, patient and carer representatives, representatives from stroke charities (i.e. Different Strokes, The Stroke Association and Chest Heart & Stroke Scotland), the Register for Exercise Professionals and SkillsActive, health promotion officers and representatives from Edinburgh Leisure and Glasgow Leisure, as well as the Scottish Government. The expert input from this group has been invaluable in the design of our course and we would like to thank them for their commitment, support and invaluable expertise.

We are grateful to Later Life Training, which is now providing the 'Exercise after Stroke: Specialist Instructor Training Course' across the UK. Our thanks are extended to the University of Edinburgh and Queen Margaret University, both of which supported our work. The four stroke charities in the UK – The Stroke Association, Chest Heart & Stroke Scotland, Different Strokes and Northern Ireland Chest Heart and Stroke – have also supported our work on exercise after stroke.

We would like to thank the students who joined our course, for their curiosity, enthusiasm and input in shaping the course, as well as their commitment to serving stroke survivors.

We thank the stroke survivors with whom we have had the privilege and pleasure to work over the years, for their ideas, support and inspiration – and for teaching us that exercise after stroke should above all be enjoyable. We are especially grateful to Mr Alan Robertson and Mr Les Gardiner, for kindly allowing us to photograph them for Chapter 10, and to Mr John Brown, who shared with us his moving account of how stroke affected his life and the role that exercise played in his recovery.

We thank all our collaborators for joining us in our collective vision of enabling stroke survivors to lead a more active and healthy life through physical activity.

Finally, we would like to express our sincere thanks to Mark Beeston and Chris Eilbeck, who have provided unending support whilst we have produced this book.

Gillian Mead and Frederike van Wijck

ACKNOWLEDGEMENTS

CONTRIBUTORS

Catherine S. Best, PhD, BSc
Researcher, University of Stirling, Stirling

Sheena Borthwick, BSc, CertMRCSLT
Speech and Language Therapist, Clinical Specialist in Stroke, NHS Lothian

John Brown
Stroke Survivor

John M.A. Dennis, BSc (Eng), BSc (CNAA), MCSP, SRP
Physiotherapy Team Lead, NHS Greater Glasgow and Clyde

Susie Dinan-Young, PhD, PGDip, BEd
Honorary Senior Research Fellow, Department of Primary Care and
Population Health, University College Medical School, London

Marie Donaghy, PhD, BA (Hons), FCSP, FHEA
Emeritus Professor, School of Health Sciences, Queen Margaret University,
Edinburgh

Carolyn A. Greig, PhD
Senior Research Fellow, Geriatric Medicine, Royal Infirmary, Edinburgh

Pauline Halliday, BSc
Occupational Therapist (Clinical Specialist in Stroke), Royal Infirmary
of Edinburgh, Edinburgh

Gillian Mead, MB, BChir, MA, MD, FRCP
Professor of Stroke and Elderly Care Medicine, University of Edinburgh,
Edinburgh

David H. Saunders, PhD, MPhil, BSc
Lecturer in Exercise Physiology, Institute of Sport, PE and Health Science,
University of Edinburgh, Edinburgh

Mark Smith, MPhil, BSc (Hons), GradDipPhys, MCSP
Consultant Physiotherapist in Stroke Rehabilitation, NHS Lothian

Bex Townley
L4 Exercise Specialist (including Exercise and Fitness After Stroke), Health and Activity Co-ordinator, Older Adults, Carmarthenshire County Council; Later Life Training Senior Tutor and EfS Lead

Frederike van Wijck, PhD, MSc, BSc, MCSP, FHEA
Reader in Neurological Rehabilitation, Institute for Applied Health Research and School of Health and Life Sciences, Glasgow Caledonian University, Glasgow

Sara Wicebloom-Paul, MSc
Gym Instructor, Exercise to Music Instructor, Health-Related Fitness Consultant; Senior Tutor, Later Life Training, Director, Equal Adventure

CONTRIBUTORS

PART 1
ESSENTIALS OF STROKE CARE

PART CONTENTS

What is a stroke?

Gillian Mead

CHAPTER CONTENTS

INTRODUCTION

The purpose of this chapter is to 'set the scene' for understanding what a stroke is, what causes a stroke, how it affects people and what its prognosis is.

DEFINITION OF A STROKE

A stroke occurs when the blood supply to part of the brain is suddenly interrupted, thus depriving the affected part of the brain of oxygen and glucose which are both vital for its normal functioning. This may cause wide-ranging neurological deficits (see also chapter 3).

Stroke is defined as 'a clinical syndrome characterised by rapidly developing clinical symptoms and/or signs of focal, and at times, global (applied to patients in deep coma and those with subarachnoid haemorrhage), loss of cerebral function with symptoms lasting more than 24 hours or leading to death, with no apparent cause other than that of vascular origin' (Hatano 1976):

- 'Focal loss of cerebral function' means that a specific area of the brain has been affected. 'Global' applies to patients in deep coma and those with subarachnoid haemorrhage.
- 'With no apparent cause other than that of vascular origin' means that other conditions mimicking stroke have been excluded or are not thought to be likely.

This definition includes stroke due to cerebral infarction (also known as 'ischaemic stroke'), intracerebral haemorrhage and most cases of subarachnoid haemorrhage (please see below for causes of stroke). This definition has stood the test of time and is still used in clinical practice today.

TYPES OF STROKE

ISCHAEMIC STROKE

Ischaemic strokes account for about 80% of strokes and are due to a blockage or reduction in the blood supply to part of the brain. (See Figure 1.1 for detailed diagrams showing the blood supply to the brain). There are several mechanisms:

- Thrombosis formation on larger intracranial vessels, e.g. middle cerebral artery.
- Embolism of a blood clot in the heart, aortic arch and carotid, i.e. a blood clot 'travels' to the brain and blocks an artery in the brain.

ESSENTIALS OF STROKE CARE

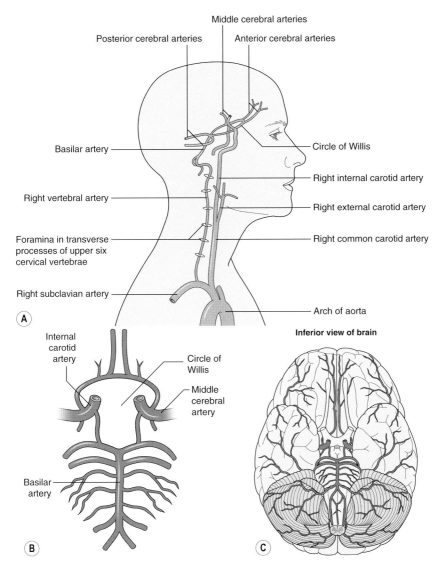

FIG 1.1   (A) Lateral view of the blood supply to the brain (for clarity, the left vertebral artery and left internal carotid artery are not shown for their entire length). (B) The basilar artery is formed when the two vertebral arteries join; the circle of Willis which lies at the base of the brain links the basilar artery with the blood supply from the internal carotid arteries. (C) View of the undersurface of the brain, including the cerebellum (in dark blue), showing how the arteries to the brain branch extensively to supply the entire brain.

- Intrinsic small vessel disease (which usually affects the small deep arteries in the brain).
- Haemodynamic causes, e.g. hypotension may cause cerebral hypoperfusion (decreased blood flow to the brain) and this may lead to so-called 'watershed infarcts'.
- Other less common causes, e.g. vasculitis (inflammation of blood vessels), intravenous drug abuse, carotid artery or vertebral artery dissection (a tear in the artery which allows blood to enter the wall of the artery and

5

split its layers), coagulopathy (any defect in the blood's clotting process), venous infarction (caused by blockage of a vein in the brain), migraine.

It is possible to identify the likely mechanism of stroke in individual patients by clues from the history or examination, e.g. a recent heart attack would suggest a cardioembolic source, though often one cannot pinpoint for certain what has caused a stroke.

HAEMORRHAGIC STROKE

Haemorrhagic strokes account for about 15% of strokes and are due to bleeding in the brain. Sometimes the bleeding is from an anatomically abnormal blood vessel in the brain, e.g. arteriovenous malformation, intracranial aneurysm, or from a tumour. Sometimes the cause of bleeding is uncertain and the bleeding is attributed to presumed abnormalities in smaller blood vessels, e.g. hypertensive vessel disease, amyloid angiopathy (where amyloid, a sort of protein, forms in a blood vessel wall in the brain). Patients with abnormal blood clotting, including those taking anticoagulants such as warfarin, are also more likely to suffer haemorrhagic strokes. Determining the underlying cause of haemorrhage in individual patients can be difficult, and is a subject of ongoing research. An example of an intracerebral bleed is shown in Figure 1.2.

Subarachnoid haemorrhage

Subarachnoid haemorrhage is usually due to rupture of an intracranial aneurysm (a weak or thin spot on a blood vessel in the brain that balloons out and fills with blood), and typically presents with 'thunderclap headache' with or without neurological signs or reduced consciousness. Subarachnoid haemorrhages are usually managed by neurosurgeons or neuroradiologists. Treatment includes inserting a coil or clipping the aneurysm to prevent further bleeding.

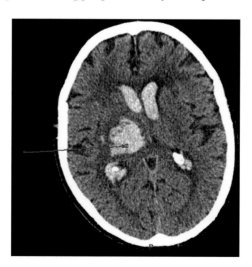

FIG 1.2 This image shows an intracerebral and intraventricular haemorrhage of a 75-year-old man. He presented with sudden onset right-sided weakness and reduced conscious level. The initial source of haemorrhage is from a bleed in the left basal ganglia (marked); blood then spread into the ventricles. Note that the blood on this image appears as white 'blobs'. *With permission from NHS Lothian.*

Patients with subarachnoid haemorrhages are generally not admitted to stroke units but they may be referred for exercise after discharge from hospital.

DIFFERENTIATING BETWEEN ISCHAEMIC AND HAEMORRHAGIC STROKE

It is essential to differentiate ischaemic from haemorrhagic stroke as this dictates treatment. For example, in the acute phase, thrombolysis ('clot busting') and aspirin can be administered to patients with ischaemic (but not haemorrhagic) strokes. The only reliable method to differentiate between the two main types of stroke is to perform brain imaging. On brain computed tomography (CT), acute haemorrhages always show up as a white area (Fig. 1.2), though over the subsequent few days the haemorrhage gradually darkens and may become indistinguishable from a cerebral infarct (Wardlaw et al. 2003). Signs of ischaemic stroke on CT include brain swelling, hypodensity (darker area) and occasionally a blood clot in one of the cerebral arteries. Some patients with ischaemic stroke have a normal CT scan, particularly if they are scanned very early after onset of symptoms.

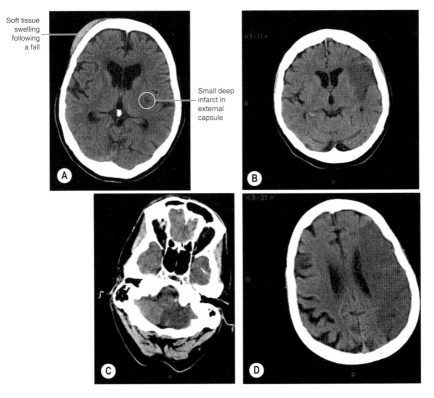

FIG 1.3 Series of CT scans of ischaemic strokes. The infarcts are blacker than surrounding brain. (A) Small deep infarct in the left external capsule of the brain; note also soft tissue swelling on right side of scalp. (B) Cortical infarct on Left in the territory of the middle cerebral artery. (C) Left cerebellar infarct (an example of a posterior circulation infarct). (D) Large infarct on left side of brain with swelling and midline shift. *With permission of NHS Lothian.*

The scans shown in Figure 1.3 are typical from patients with ischaemic stroke. When interpreting a scan, one has to imagine looking up from the feet, so the left side of the brain is on the right hand side of the image. The front part of the brain is at the top of the image, and the back of the brain is at the bottom of the image. The scanner moves from the top of the head down to the cervical spine, and creates a series of 'slices' of brain images.

TRANSIENT ISCHAEMIC ATTACKS

Transient ischaemic attacks (TIAs) are defined as 'sudden onset of focal neurological disturbance, assumed to be vascular in origin' lasting for less than 24 hours (Hatano 1976). In practice, most TIAs last for less than an hour. They are almost always due to short-lived episodes of cerebral ischaemia which resolve spontaneously. The risk factors for TIAs are very similar to the risk factors for ischaemic strokes. A TIA is a 'warning' sign that the person is at high risk from a stroke, and needs to be referred for urgent medical assessment.

IMPACT OF STROKE

Stroke is the third most common cause of death and the commonest cause of disability. In the UK, there are 150 000 new strokes per year (Office of National Statistics 2001).

INCIDENCE

'Incidence' is a measure of the risk of developing some new condition within a specified period of time. Stroke incidence has been falling in recent years, at least in the developed world. In Oxfordshire in the early 1980s, the incidence of stroke was around 2 in 1000 people per year (Bamford et al. 1988). Twenty years later, the incidence of stroke had fallen by 29% (Rothwell et al. 2004). This was attributed to better prevention of a first-ever stroke, e.g. by the more widespread use of blood pressure lowering medication (for high blood pressure) and statins (to reduce cholesterol) and is in spite of an increase in the number of older people in the population.

Stroke is a global problem. Estimates of the incidence of stroke in different parts of the world vary depending on how 'cases' of stroke are identified (Feigin 2007). It is clear, though, that stroke incidence increases with age; in a review of 15 stroke incidence studies in the developed world, the rate of stroke in those aged <45 years ranged from 0.1 to 0.3 per 1000 person-years, whilst for those aged 75–84 years, the range was 12 to 20 per 1000 person-years. In terms of premature deaths and years of life lost, stroke is a greater problem in low-income and middle-income countries (Strong et al. 2007).

PREVALENCE

Prevalence is a measure of the total number of cases of disease in a population. The prevalence of stroke increases with age. For people over the age of 65, the number with a stroke ranges from 46 to 73 per 1000 population; in other words, around 1 in 20 people over the age of 65 may be living with the effects of stroke (Feigin et al. 2003). This represents the number of people who could potentially benefit from the provision of Exercise after Stroke services.

COST OF STROKE TO THE NATION

A recent UK study estimated that the cost of treatment and loss of productivity arising from stroke amounted to a total societal cost of £8.9 billion a year, with treatment costs accounting for approximately 5% of total UK National Health Service costs (Saka et al. 2009). The financial cost of stroke includes many different components; the main ones in the first year of stroke are the costs of acute hospitalisation, inpatient rehabilitation and nursing home care (Dewey et al. 2001). Indirect costs, which were defined as the time lost from productive activity, made up 6% of the costs. Other costs include the cost of re-hospitalisation for recurrent stroke, medication, community rehabilitation, respite care and investigations.

DIAGNOSING STROKE

The diagnosis of a stroke is based on clinical symptoms and signs (p. 4). Other medical conditions can 'mimic' stroke. Around one-fifth of patients presenting to hospital with stroke-like symptoms turn out not to have had a stroke (Hand et al. 2006), but another diagnosis such as seizures, sepsis, toxic or metabolic causes (e.g. hypoglycaemia) or a space occupying lesion (e.g. a tumour or brain abscess) (Hand et al. 2006). Migraine can also mimic stroke or TIA.

Making an accurate clinical diagnosis of stroke or 'mimic' is important because this will dictate subsequent medical management, including emergency treatments. Hence, an accurate clinical history and examination is essential. If a patient is confused or has difficulty speaking, it is essential to obtain a history from a witness (if available).

Sometimes it is difficult to distinguish for certain between a stroke and a 'mimic' on clinical criteria alone. Brain imaging can help diagnose some 'stroke mimics' such as space occupying lesions.

NEUROLOGICAL EFFECTS OF A STROKE

The neurological effects of a stroke depend on which blood vessel has become blocked or has burst (see Fig. 1.1, which shows the blood supply to the brain).

In order to understand the neurological effects of stroke, it is first necessary to understand the function of different parts of the brain and how they work together. The following section provides a 'bird's eye view of the brain', which inevitably provides a very simplified picture of this most complex organ. Further details of the short-term and longer-terms effects of stroke are provided in chapter 3.

THE RELATIONSHIP BETWEEN THE BRAIN AND BEHAVIOUR: A BIRD'S EYE VIEW

The brain consists of two hemispheres (left and right) which are connected through the corpus callosum, which contains around 200 million fibres. Each hemisphere comprises four lobes. Figure 1.4A is a lateral view of the brain (i.e. looking from the side), showing its gross anatomy.

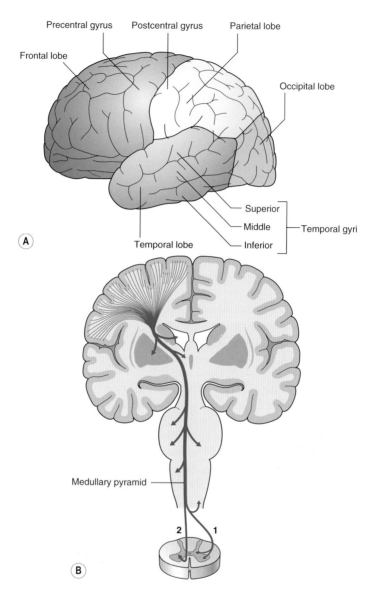

Precentral gyrus   Postcentral gyrus   Parietal lobe

Frontal lobe

Occipital lobe

Superior

Middle — Temporal gyri

(A)   Temporal lobe   Inferior

Medullary pyramid

2   1

(B)

FIG 1.4 (A) Lateral view of the brain (i.e. looking from the side), showing its gross anatomy. (B) Diagrammatic representation of the pyramidal tract and its major connections through collateral branches: 1, crossed corticospinal; 2, uncrossed corticospinal. Note that the pyramidal tract crosses over, so that the left cortex supplies the right side of the body, and vice versa.

The neurological effects of stroke largely depend on the part of the brain that has been affected. As most of the neural pathways from the brain cross over on their way to the rest of the body, a stroke in the left hemisphere will manifest itself primarily in the right side of the body and vice versa (Fig. 1.4B).

Tucked underneath is the cerebellum (or 'little brain'), which plays an important role in movement and coordination (Fig. 1.1C).

Occipital lobe

The main function of this lobe at the back of the brain is processing visual information. When looking straight ahead, one can discern a left visual field (extending from one's midline towards the left), and a right visual field (extending from midline to the right) (Fig. 1.5). Information from the left visual field is gathered in the occipital lobe of the right hemisphere and vice versa. All visual information is collated in the back of the occipital lobe, from where different aspects of visual information (e.g. colour, motion and form) are relayed in the first instance to other occipital areas for further processing.

Parietal lobe

The parietal lobe integrates visual information and information from sensors in the skin, muscle and other soft tissues. Together this information tells us about the position and movement of our body in space and allows

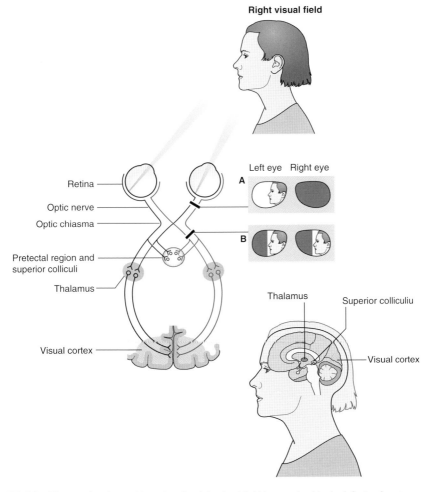

FIG 1.5 The visual pathway. Note that the right visual field is perceived in the left visual cortex. A and B indicate the impact of lesions to the visual system. A lesion at B results in homonymous hemianopia.

us to distinguish left from right, up from down, and back from front. The right parietal lobe plays an important role in focusing attention, and guiding action, e.g. stepping around an obstacle. Someone with a stroke affecting the parietal lobe may have difficulty feeling the affected side of their body, demonstrate confusion with their body schema (e.g. mixing up left with right), or have difficulty reaching for objects. Some people demonstrate neglect, i.e. they 'ignore' the affected side of their body, or apraxia, i.e. difficulty undertaking a goal-orientated activity such as dressing even when they have normal strength, sensation and comprehension.

Temporal lobe

This lobe integrates sensory information, including vision, hearing, taste and smell, to enable us to recognise objects. The temporal lobe is also involved in the comprehension of speech as well as memory and emotion. Problems with speech comprehension usually occur if the left rather than the right temporal lobe is affected. The right temporal lobe is involved with music recognition, including the musical element of speech.

Frontal lobe

The frontal lobe governs action, from the initial intention (e.g. I would like to get a glass of water) through to the actual action. The very front of this lobe governs behaviour, e.g. making plans and setting goals, checking whether these are achieved, solving problems along the way and ensuring that behaviour is appropriate. Information from this part of the brain is relayed to other areas that are involved in planning action, including motor programming, and, finally, to the end station in the motor cortex from where motor commands are relayed down to the spinal cord. A stroke affecting the motor cortex in the frontal lobe will directly affect movement. Problems with motor programming may also be observed. Speech expression may be although comprehension may be more or less intact.

The brain as an integrated system

Although different parts of the brain have different functions the brain operates as an integrated system. For example, the function of reaching for a ball requires the brain to process visual information about the object and its location, recall the type of object, integrate visual with somatosensory information, generate an appropriate motor programme, and execute this – while maintaining balance.

CONSEQUENCES OF STROKE

The consequences of stroke can be divided into those that occur at the time of the stroke as a direct result of the stroke, and those consequences which develop later, e.g. infections, spasticity, pain, depression. This chapter will provide a succinct overview of the immediate neurological effects of stroke. These may improve over time, but many stroke survivors will be left with residual neurological deficits that need to be taken into account by exercise professionals delivering exercise after stroke. Chapter 3 will cover the complications from stroke and long-term post-stroke problems in more detail.

Although every stroke is different, there are recognisable patterns of neurological deficits that occur together. For example, a patient with an occlusion of the main stem of the left middle cerebral artery will generally present with sudden onset of right-sided weakness, right-sided sensory loss, language disturbance and a visual problem known as right homonymous hemianopia and other neurological problems such as right-sided inattention and dyspraxia.

MOTOR SYMPTOMS

These include:

- Weakness on one side of the body (usually on the opposite side of the body from the brain lesion), sometimes called 'hemiparesis or hemiplegia'.
- Poor balance (patients may have a 'staggering' gait, which is sometimes known as 'ataxia') and/or incoordination of a limb. This typically occurs when the stroke affects the cerebellum, which is responsible for control of movement and balance, but can also be a problem with hemiparesis.

The specific effects of a stroke depend on which area of the brain has been affected. The 'motor homunculus' in the frontal lobe represents the projection of the human body on the 'motor strip' of the motor cortex, as illustrated in Figure 1.6. Large areas of the motor strip are dedicated to the face and hands, which require sophisticated motor control. Areas which do not require such sophistication have a smaller representation, e.g. the back.

DYSARTHRIA

Dysarthria is a motor speech difficulty, typically producing slurred speech. Persisting dysarthria after stroke is more often associated with a sub-cortical, posterior circulation or brainstem stroke where the nerves controlling

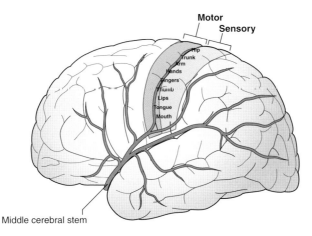

FIG 1.6 A lateral view of the brain showing the location of the motor and sensory cortex. Note that a large proportion of the motor and sensory cortex presents the mouth, tongue, face, lips, thumb, fingers and hands, compared with the hip and trunk.

the muscles of the face, mouth and throat have been affected resulting in difficulties producing clear, intelligible speech. Patients may also 'drool' or 'dribble'.

SWALLOWING PROBLEMS

Over 50% of those who have a stroke may experience difficulties eating or drinking. This problem is known as 'dysphagia', and is caused by loss of strength or control over the muscles involved in the actions of chewing and swallowing. The signs of dysphagia include coughing and choking when trying to swallow food or fluids, food sticking in the mouth, dribbling or drooling, and the voice sounding wet after eating or drinking. Dysphagia often improves over time, but some patients are left with such severe dysphagia that they require food and fluids to be delivered through feeding tubes.

LANGUAGE PROBLEMS

Communication requires language processing. In most people, it is mainly the left hemisphere that is responsible for language processing, and so the more severe difficulties in both understanding and expressing verbally are commonly experienced after a stroke in the left hemisphere. Many areas of the brain also have a role in communication, e.g. the occipital lobe is involved in visual perception and processing which is required in reading and writing. Signals are then relayed to the parietal lobe which is involved in interpreting auditory and visual signals, the temporal lobe is involved in the comprehension of speech and the frontal lobe is involved in the production of a verbal response.

The right hemisphere is also involved in language production. Strokes in the right hemisphere may cause more subtle problems in communication, e.g. difficulty interpreting and using facial expressions, a change in tone of speech, often sounding monotonous, and a breakdown in normal conversational skills, such as turn taking.

SENSORY SYMPTOMS

The human sensory systems include vision, hearing, taste, touch (temperature, light, crude, and vibration), smell, proprioception (joint/limb position and movement), orientation in space and perception of time. Basic sensory information is relayed to higher centres of the nervous system where the information is integrated to allow us to make sense of the information.

Sensory symptoms in stroke include loss of sensation, sometimes described by patients as 'numbness' or abnormal sensation (e.g. 'pins and needles'). Sensation is commonly impaired after stroke with some 50–60% of patients having a sensation-related impairment (Sullivan and Hedman 2008). Unimpaired sensory function is necessary for normal interaction with the environment and plays an important role in the control of movement.

PERCEPTUAL PROBLEMS

To 'attend to' something means to be 'perceptually selective', as not all sensory stimuli that we are exposed to become part of our conscious experience, e.g. we do not normally feel our clothing against our skin after getting dressed. Attentional problems may be present with or without sensory impairment. A stroke survivor may be unaware of auditory, visual or tactile stimuli on the contralateral side to the stroke lesion (i.e. the affected side of the body). A stroke survivor may not recognise the presence of a sensory stimulus such as a cup (object agnosia). Some stroke survivors do not recognise familiar faces (face agnosia), while some do not even seem to recognise that they have had a stroke (anosognosia). Agnosia is more common after right hemisphere strokes than after left hemisphere strokes.

VISUAL PROBLEMS

Visual problems can be a direct neurological consequence of a stroke, and may have an important impact on everyday activities. The type of defect depends on the part of the visual pathway affected by the stroke (Fig. 1.5). Common types of visual problems after stroke include:

- Field defects, including homonymous hemianopia, quadrantanopia, scotomas, wedge-shaped defects and cortical blindness
- Double vision
- Gaze palsies
- Visual inattention.

These impairments will be explained in more detail in chapter 3.

DYSPRAXIA

This refers to a range of complex disorders involving motor function, where a patient with apparently preserved motor and sensory function who is able to understand instructions is unable to carry out voluntary movements (Wade et al. 1985). Dyspraxia may have a profound impact on everyday activities, e.g. a patient may not be able to light a match or make a cup of tea, even though he has no motor or sensory deficit.

MEMORY AND THINKING PROBLEMS

These can occur as a direct consequence of the stroke, or as a result of a complication such as an infection. Memory and thinking problems may improve over time, or may remain a long-term problem.

EMOTIONAL CHANGES

These may include labile mood (characterised by extreme uncontrolled crying), laughing, mood swings and irritability.

INCONTINENCE OF URINE AND FAECES

Bladder and bowel problems can occur as a direct consequence of a stroke. For example, in patients with severe cortical strokes, urinary and faecal incontinence is common. Urinary retention, i.e. inability to empty the bladder, may also occur.

CLASSIFYING STROKE

The clinical presentation of stroke is highly variable, causes are diverse and prognosis is also variable. Hence, it is useful to classify patients who have had a stroke. The Oxfordshire Community Stroke Project (OCSP) classification is a widely used and well-known clinical classification (Bamford et al. 1991). This classification uses clinical symptoms and signs to categorise patients into one of four subtypes. Patients referred for exercise may have been assigned an OCSP classification at the time of stroke onset, and so exercise professionals and health professionals delivering exercise need a working knowledge of the classification.

OXFORDSHIRE COMMUNITY STROKE PROJECT CLASSIFICATION

- Total anterior circulation syndrome (TACS): triad of hemiparesis (or hemisensory loss), dysphasia (or other new higher cortical dysfunction) and homonymous hemianopia.
- Partial anterior circulation syndrome (PACS): only two of the features of TACS including isolated higher cortical dysfunction or isolated motor or sensory deficits which are anatomically less extensive than lacunar syndrome.
- Lacunar syndrome (LACS): pure motor stroke, pure sensory stroke, sensorimotor stroke and ataxic hemiparesis.
- Posterior circulation syndrome (POCS): homonymous hemianopia, brain stem or cerebellar signs.

The OCSP classification helps to determine the likely cause, site of the brain lesion and prognosis. For example, in patients with ischaemic stroke, ipsilateral (i.e. on the same side of the body as the brain lesion) carotid disease is more common in PACS and TACS than in the other subtypes. The site and extent of the brain lesion is correctly predicted in around 80% of patients (Mead et al. 2000), with TACS typically having large cortical infarcts (Fig. 1.3D), PACS having smaller cortical infarcts (Fig. 1.3B), LACS having small deep infarcts (Fig. 1.3A) and POCS having posterior circulation infarcts (Fig. 1.3C).

The OCSP classification also helps determine likely prognosis. For example, only 4% of TACS will be independent in the longer term, and PACS tend to have the highest rate of early stroke recurrence (Bamford et al. 1991). TACS are least likely to walk again, and take the longest when they do achieve it (Smith and Baer 1999).

RISK FACTORS FOR STROKE

Risk factors can be divided into non-modifiable or modifiable. Non-modifiable risk factors for stroke include age, gender, low birth weight, race, ethnicity and genetic factors. Well-documented and modifiable risk factors include hypertension, cigarette smoke, diabetes, atrial fibrillation (the most common sort of irregular heart rhythm) and other cardiac conditions, high lipid and cholesterol levels, carotid artery stenosis (narrowing of the carotid artery), sickle cell disease, postmenopausal hormone therapy, poor diet, physical inactivity, obesity and body fat distribution.

The most commonly seen risk factors for ischaemic stroke and TIAs include:

- High blood pressure (hypertension)
- Smoking
- High cholesterol
- Diabetes
- Atrial fibrillation
- Ischaemic heart disease.

Other factors also increase the risk of stroke. These include:

OBESITY

As body mass index increases in men, so does the risk of stroke. This seems to be independent of the effects of hypertension, diabetes and cholesterol (Kurth et al. 2002). An increased waist-hip ratio is a stronger stroke risk factor than body mass index alone in men (Suk et al. 2003).

REDUCED PHYSICAL ACTIVITY

Moderate physical activity reduces the risk of both ischaemic and haemorrhagic stroke in men (Lee and Paffenbarger 1998, Lee et al. 2003) and women (Hu et al. 2000), independently of other stroke risk factors. Higher levels of physical activity have a better protective effect than moderate levels of activity.

High blood pressure is the most important risk factor for haemorrhagic strokes. Bleeding disorders are also a risk factor for haemorrhagic strokes.

PREVENTION OF STROKE

Strokes can be prevented by targeting the modifiable risk factors, by addressing lifestyle (e.g. stopping smoking, increasing physical activity) or by treating with drugs (e.g. warfarin for people with atrial fibrillation). This risk reduction strategy applies to prevention of a first ever in a lifetime stroke (sometimes known as primary prevention) or the prevention of a recurrent stroke (secondary prevention). Secondary prevention is an integral aspect of stroke management and will be discussed in more detail in chapter 2.

PROGNOSIS AFTER STROKE

The outcome after stroke is highly variable; some patients make a complete recovery, whilst some are left dependent and some die. After stroke, there are several important questions that patients and families ask: (a) Will I die? (b) Will I become independent? (c) Will this happen again?

WILL I DIE? CASE FATALITY AFTER STROKE

The 30-day case fatality in the Oxford Vascular study (OXVASC) (Rothwell et al. 2004) was 17.2%, i.e. similar to the previous population based study (OCSP) in the same geographical area (Bamford et al. 1991), and to the Borders Stroke study (case fatality was 15.9%) (Syme et al. 2005). Case fatality rates are much higher for inpatients than for outpatients (Syme et al. 2005), and for patients with more severe strokes (e.g. TACS) than for mild strokes (Bamford et al. 1991).

WILL I BECOME INDEPENDENT AFTER STROKE? PREDICTING RECOVERY

In the OCSP, which was a population based study, 50% of stroke patients were independent at 30 days, 52% at 6 months and 49% at 1 year (Bamford et al. 1991).

In a recent study of 5048 patients recruited to 21 acute stroke trials, 39% had recovered (Barthel Index ≥95) and the others had either not made a functional recovery or had died (König et al. 2008).

There are multiple publications describing recovery of specific neurological impairments, e.g. motor recovery (Langhorne et al. 2009) and language recovery (Plowman et al. 2011), to which the reader is referred for a more detailed discussion.

WILL I HAVE ANOTHER STROKE?

Estimates of rates of stroke recurrence vary, depending on type of patients included (e.g. minor strokes only or all strokes), definition of stroke recurrence and population studied. In a population based study in South London, the risk of a recurrent stroke was 7% at 1 year, 16% at 5 years and 25% at 10 years (Mohan et al. 2009). OXVASC found a rate of recurrent events in those presenting with minor stroke or TIA of 12% at 7 days and 18% at 3 months (Coull et al. 2004). The OXVASC data emphasise the importance of rapid assessment of patients with TIA and minor stroke, and the South London stroke study provides support for ongoing monitoring and management of vascular risk factors in people with previous strokes.

PREDICTING OUTCOME FOR INDIVIDUAL PATIENTS

Various prognostic models have been developed, but none is sufficiently precise to predict final outcome for individual patients (Reid et al. 2010). Generally speaking, the more severe the initial stroke, the less likelihood there is of a functional recovery. Increasing age and prior dependence are also negative prognostic factors.

In practice, stroke physicians are often guarded about prognosis in the early days after stroke. Later in the stroke journey, as the rate of neurological recovery begins to plateau, it becomes easier to predict likely outcome. Ongoing research is trying to find out why patterns of recovery are quite so variable.

SUMMARY POINTS

- Stroke is the third most common cause of death and the commonest cause of adult disability.
- Causes of stroke include non-modifiable and modifiable risk factors. Lack of physical activity is a modifiable risk factor for stroke.
- The majority of strokes are ischaemic, i.e. due to a blocked blood vessel.
- Brain scanning is essential to distinguish between ischaemic and haemorrhagic stroke.
- The pattern of neurological deficits depends on the part of brain affected.
- When assessing someone with a stroke, the stroke team will try to identify stroke risk factors, and then modify these if possible to reduce the risk of further strokes.
- Prognosis of stroke is variable, and depends on many factors, including stroke severity, age and prior level of independence.

REFERENCES

Bamford, J., Sandercock, P., Dennis, M., et al., 1991. Classification and natural history of clinically identifiable subtypes of cerebral infarction. Lancet 337, 1521–1526.

Bamford, J., Sandercock, P., Dennis, M., et al., 1988. A prospective study of acute cerebrovascular disease in the community: the Oxfordshire Community Stroke Project 1981-1986. Methodology, demography and incident cases of first-ever stroke. J. Neurol. Neurosurg. Psychiatry 51, 1373–1380.

Coull, A.J., Lovett, J.K., Rothwell, P.M., et al., 2004. Population based study of early risk of stroke after transient ischaemic attack or minor stroke: implications for public education and organisation of services. BMJ. doi:10.1136/bmj.37991.635266.44 (published 26 January 2004).

Dewey, H.M., Thrift, A.G., Mihalopoulos, C., et al., 2001. Cost of stroke in Australia from a societal perspective. Results from the North East Melbourne Stroke Incidence Study (NEMESIS). Stroke 32, 2409.

Feigin, V.L., Lawes, C.M.M., Bennett, D.A., et al., 2003. Stroke epidemiology: a review of population based studies of incidence, prevalence, and case-fatality in the late 20th century. Lancet Neurol. 2, 43–53.

Feigin, V.L., 2007. Stroke in developing countries: can the epidemic be stopped and outcomes improved? Lancet Neurol. 6, 94–97.

Hand, P.J., Kwan, J., Lindley, R.I., et al., 2006. Distinguishing between stroke and mimic at the bedside: the Brain Attack Study. Stroke 37, 769–775.

Hatano, S., 1976. Experience from a multicentre stroke register: a preliminary report. Bull. WHO 54, 541.

Hu, F.B., Stampfer, M.J., Colditz, G.A., et al., 2000. Physical activity and risk of stroke in women. JAMA 283, 2961–2967.

König, I.R., Ziegler, A., Bluhmki, E., et al., 2008. Predicting long-term outcome after acute ischemic stroke: a simple index works in patients from controlled clinical trials. Stroke 39, 1821–1826.

Kurth, T., Gaziano, J.M., Berger, K., et al., 2002. Body mass index and risk of stroke. Arch. Intern. Med. 162, 2557–2562.

Langhorne, P., Coupar, A., Pollock, A., 2009. Motor recovery after stroke: a systematic review. Lancet Neurol. 8, 741–754.

Lee, I.M., Paffenbarger, R.S., 1998. Physical activity and stroke incidence. The Harvard Alumni Health Study. Stroke 29, 2049–2054.

Lee, C.D., Folsom, A.R., Blair, S.N., 2003. Physical activity and stroke risk. A meta-analysis. Stroke 34, 2475–2481.

What is a stroke?

Mead, G.E., Lewis, S.C., Dennis, M.S., et al., 2000. How well does the Oxfordshire Community Stroke Project Classification predict the site and size of infarct on brain imaging? J. Neurol. Neurosurg. Psychiatry 68, 558–562.

Mohan, K.M., Crichton, S.L., Grieve, A.P., et al., 2009. Frequency and predictors for the risk of stroke recurrence up to 10 years after stroke: the South London Stroke Register. J. Neurol. Neurosurg. Psychiatry 80, 1012–1018. doi:10.1136/jnnp. 2008.170456.

Office of National Statistics, 2001. Stroke incidence and risk factors in a population based cohort study. Health Statistics Quarterly 12.

Plowman, E., Hentz, B., Ellis, C., 2011. Post-stroke aphasia prognosis: a review of patient-related and stroke-related factors. J. Eval. Clin. Pract. 17. doi:10.1111/j.1365-2753.2011.01650.x.

Reid, J.M., Gubitz, G.J., Dai, D., et al., 2010. Predicting functional outcome after stroke by modelling baseline clinical and CT variables. Age Ageing 39, 360–366.

Rothwell, P.M., Coull, A.J., Giles, M.F., et al., 2004. Change in stroke incidence, mortality, case fatality, severity and risk factors in Oxfordshire, UK from 1981 to 2004 (Oxford Vascular Study). Lancet 363, 1925–1933.

Saka, O., McGuire, A., Wolfe, C., 2009. Cost of stroke in the United Kingdom. Age Ageing 38, 27–32.

Smith, M.T., Baer, G.D., 1999. Achievement of simple mobility milestones after stroke. Arch. Phys. Med. Rehabil. 80, 442–447.

Strong, K., Mathers, C., Bonita, R., 2007. Preventing stroke: saving lives around the world. Lancet Neurol. 6, 182–187.

Suk, S.H., Boden-Albala, B., Pittman, J.G., et al., 2003. Northern Manhattan Stroke Study. Abdominal obesity and risk of ischaemic stroke: the Northern Manhattan Stroke Study. Stroke 34, 1586–1592.

Sullivan, J.E., Hedman, L.D., 2008. Sensory dysfunction following stroke: incidence, significance, examination, and intervention. Top. Stroke Rehabil. 15, 200–217.

Syme, P.D., Byrne, A.W., Chen, R., et al., 2005. Community-based stroke incidence in a Scottish population. The Scottish Borders Stroke Study. Stroke 36, 1837–1843.

Wade, D.T., Langton Hewer, R., Skilbeck, C.E., et al., 1985. Stroke: A critical approach to diagnosis, treatment and management. Chapman and Hall Medical, Boca Raton.

Wardlaw, J.M., Keir, S.L., Dennis, M.S., 2003. The impact of delays in computed tomography of the brain on the accuracy of diagnosis and subsequent management in patients with minor stroke. J. Neurol. Neurosurg. Psychiatry 74, 77–81.

The management of stroke

Gillian Mead • John M.A. Dennis

2

CHAPTER CONTENTS

21

INTRODUCTION

The management of stroke is a complex area, which is rapidly evolving. This chapter will focus on the key aspects of stroke management. The term 'patient' is used in the context of hospital-based care, whilst the term 'stroke survivor' is used after discharge from hospital. It is important that exercise professionals understand what tests may have been performed, how the patient would have been treated in the earlier part of their stroke journey, and what drugs they may be taking to prevent further strokes.

The term 'health-care professional' is used to describe those clinicians involved in the clinical care of patients during their hospital admission and rehabilitation. The term 'exercise professional' is used to describe the person who designs and delivers the exercise programme. Exercise professionals may have come from different backgrounds, including exercise science and other exercise-related professions, and physiotherapists who have had the required training (chapter 10).

INVESTIGATIONS FOR STROKE

Patients with acute stroke will undergo a brain scan, blood tests, a chest X-ray and an electrocardiogram to determine the type of stroke and its possible causes, and to identify co-morbid diseases.

BRAIN SCAN

Most patients undergo a computed tomography (CT) scan and a few will undergo magnetic resonance imaging (MRI). The most important reason for performing a brain scan is to distinguish between an ischaemic stroke and a haemorrhagic stroke (chapter 1) because there are fundamental differences in their management.

BLOOD TESTS

Blood tests do not make a diagnosis of stroke, but may identify potential causes of the stroke and evidence of co-morbid diseases, e.g. kidney disease. The common blood tests that are performed after stroke are shown in Box 2.1.

OTHER TESTS

Other tests that are commonly performed in stroke are shown in Box 2.2.

STROKE MANAGEMENT

AN OVERVIEW

Stroke management can be broadly divided into:

- Acute treatments: these include medical treatments provided very early in the stroke journey.
- Rehabilitation: this is provided by a multidisciplinary team and aims to minimise long-term disability after stroke.
- Secondary prevention: to prevent further stroke. This includes lifestyle advice, drugs and sometimes surgical interventions.

BOX 2.1 Commonly performed blood tests for stroke

- Cholesterol (to detect high levels)
- Blood glucose (this will detect diabetes)
- Haemoglobin. Low levels may indicate anaemia. If anaemia is found, then drugs that increase the risk of bleeding, such as aspirin, should be started only cautiously, if at all; and the cause of the anaemia should be investigated. High levels of haemoglobin (polycythaemia) may make the blood more liable to clot and is thus a risk factor for stroke.
- Electrolytes, i.e. sodium and potassium. Drugs used for secondary stroke prevention may alter electrolyte levels so it is important to have baseline values. For example, bendrofluazide is a common cause of a low sodium level.
- Urea and creatinine. These assess kidney function. Some drugs for secondary stroke prevention can affect kidney function and may need to be avoided in patients with abnormal kidney function.
- Erythrocyte sedimentation rate. This will detect inflammation, which may be associated with stroke.

BOX 2.2 Tests commonly performed in stroke

- An electrocardiogram (ECG):
  - This will determine heart rhythm and will identify other evidence of heart disease, e.g. recent acute coronary event (e.g. heart attack).
- Imaging the carotid arteries:
  - Patients with minor non-disabling ischaemic strokes, in the anterior circulation, typically partial anterior circulation syndrome or lacunar syndrome, will undergo carotid Doppler imaging, to identify those with a narrowing in the carotid artery, who may be suitable for carotid endarterectomy (surgical removal of a 'narrowing' in the carotid artery).
  - Other modalities of carotid imaging including magnetic resonance angiography.
- Echocardiography:
  - Some patients with ischaemic strokes and transient ischaemic attacks (TIAs) may also undergo ultrasound examination of the heart, to identify blood clots in the heart (i.e. source of embolus), to look for a patent foramen ovale (sometimes called a 'hole in the heart') and to visualise other aspects of heart structure.

These three components of stroke management all start at the time of stroke onset, but as time goes on the focus of stroke management moves from acute treatment towards rehabilitation. Most patients with stroke (but usually not TIAs) will require admission to hospital for treatment. Those with minor strokes who recover quickly may not need hospital admission, but appropriate investigations must be performed and secondary prevention initiated as soon as possible.

In the following section, we will describe in more detail acute stroke treatments, secondary prevention and rehabilitation.

ACUTE TREATMENTS

Acute treatments can be divided into those which are specific to stroke, and those which are 'general supportive treatments'.

Stroke-specific treatments

In this section, we describe stroke-specific treatments. Generally speaking, the specific treatments that are effective for patients with ischaemic stroke tend to increase bleeding risk, and are therefore not given to patients with haemorrhagic strokes.

Aspirin

This has a small beneficial effect if administered within 48 hours of onset of ischaemic stroke (Sandercock et al. 2003). It is an antiplatelet drug which reduces the 'stickiness' of the blood. It is given to the vast majority of people who have had an ischaemic stroke.

Thrombolysis

Recombinant tissue plasminogen activator (rt-PA) (a 'clot-busting' drug) is licenced for intravenous administration to patients with acute ischaemic stroke within 3 hours of onset of symptoms. It is given via a small drip placed into a vein, usually in the arm. On the basis of a recent trial, some physicians will now administer it up to 4.5 hours after onset of symptoms (Hacke et al. 2008). It significantly reduces the risk of death and disability (Wardlaw et al. 2010) by dissolving the blood clot in the artery which has caused the stroke. It is therefore not surprising that the main side effect of thrombolysis is bleeding into the brain, which occurs in about 1 in 30 patients. Overall, the net benefit of rt-PA is one more independent survivor for every 10 patients treated. Around 10–15% of all stroke patients are suitable for thrombolysis. The remaining patients will not receive thrombolysis for various reasons, e.g. time of stroke onset unknown (and so doctors cannot be sure that treatment can be administered within the narrow time window), stroke symptoms improving rapidly at the time of admission to hospital, very mild neurological symptoms, high risk of bleeding, anaemia or receiving anticoagulation with warfarin.

The sooner thrombolysis is given, the better the outcome. This is why there have been major public health campaigns to raise awareness of stroke, so that people with suspected stroke symptoms seek urgent medical attention.

Hemicraniectomy for 'malignant middle cerebral artery territory infarction' for ischaemic stroke

Younger patients (<65 years) with large middle cerebral artery territory infarcts are at high risk of fatal brain swelling. Surgical treatment to 'lift' part of the skull to provide space for brain swelling reduces mortality (Vahedi et al. 2007). Currently, very few patients require this treatment in clinical practice.

Mechanical retrieval of blood clot/intra-arterial thrombolysis for ischaemic stroke

Very small tubes, called catheters, can be inserted via an artery in the groin into the arteries in the brain, to extract blood clot. This procedure is performed under X-ray guidance by a specialist doctor called an interventional neuroradiologist. This procedure is considered if there are medical reasons why intravenous thrombolysis cannot be given, e.g. recent bleeding, recent stroke. Thrombolysis can also be administered directly into the blood clot through these intra-arterial catheters.

Specific management of haemorrhagic strokes

After haemorrhagic strokes, drugs which increase the risk of bleeding (e.g. aspirin and warfarin) will usually be discontinued for at least 1–2 weeks (Sacco et al. 2006). The effect of an anticoagulant is sometimes reversed (e.g. with vitamin K). If oral anticoagulants are considered to be essential for the long-term management of another condition (e.g. in patients with prosthetic heart valves), they may be restarted at some stage after the stroke.

Neurosurgery is very occasionally performed for haemorrhagic strokes to remove the bleeding, particularly if it has occurred in the cerebellum. Patients with aneurysmal subarachnoid haemorrhage require specialist neurological care and almost always undergo either clipping or coiling of the aneurysm to prevent further bleeding.

Stroke units for the management of both ischaemic and haemorrhagic stroke

Stroke patients who require hospital admission should be managed on a stroke unit. Organised inpatient (stroke unit) care is a term used to describe the focusing of care for stroke patients in hospital under a multidisciplinary team who specialise in stroke management (Stroke Unit Trialists Collaboration 2007). Further details of the multidisciplinary team are discussed later in this chapter.

A stroke unit may be based on a dedicated ward, with a mobile stroke team or within a generic disability service (Stroke Unit Trialists Collaboration 2007). Patients who receive organised inpatient care in a stroke unit are more likely to be alive, independent and living at home 1 year after the stroke. This applies to both ischaemic and haemorrhagic stroke, to mild strokes and more severe strokes, and to stroke patients of all ages.

Stroke unit care is complex, dynamic and comprises a number of components (e.g. intensive interdisciplinary teamwork, responsiveness and specialist interventions), which can be difficult to pin down. This type of care is sometimes referred to as a 'black box'.

Exactly which components of the 'black box' of stroke unit care are effective are not certain. Possible reasons for better outcomes in stroke units include early prescription of aspirin (Indredavik et al. 1999), better diagnostic procedures (e.g. carotid imaging and hence more rapid carotid endarterectomy), better or more focused nursing care, early mobilisation of patients, prevention of medical complications, more effective rehabilitation procedures (Langhorne and Dennis 1998), specially trained staff, team work and enhanced involvement of relatives (Indredavik et al. 1999).

General supportive care

General supportive care is important for patients with both haemorrhagic and ischaemic stroke. The following interventions may be needed.

Intravenous fluids

These may be required for patients who have dysphagia and who cannot swallow safely. Some patients may be dehydrated on admission, or may become dehydrated during their admission.

Feeding

Patients with acute stroke may be too drowsy to eat or drink safely, or may have dysphagia (Barer 1989). They are at risk of aspiration, i.e. breathing in foreign materials into the lungs, which can lead to inflammation and infection in the lungs. A modified texture diet (e.g. puréed food) and thickened fluids can be provided to reduce the risk of aspiration. Those at high risk of aspiration may require feeding via a nasogastric tube (a tube inserted into the stomach via the nose). Early feeding with a nasogastric tube leads to a small non-significant reduction in case fatality, though this is offset by a slight increase in the proportion of patients surviving with dependence (The FOOD Trial Collaboration 2005). If dysphagia improves over time, the nasogastric tube can be removed. If dysphagia persists, a more permanent method of artificial feeding may be required. The most common technique used is a percutaneous endoscopic gastroenterostomy (PEG) tube, inserted through the abdominal wall into the stomach.

It is unlikely that patients with PEG tubes will attend exercise programmes because these tubes are generally needed for patients with more severe strokes. Patients with modified consistency diets and/or thickened fluids may well attend exercise programmes; the exercise professional must be aware of this, so that normal consistency food or unthickened fluids are not given inappropriately during or after an exercise session.

Urinary catheter

Urinary catheters are required for retention of urine (i.e. bladder does not empty). Sometimes catheters are inserted for incontinence of urine, particularly if the incontinence is likely to contribute to the development of pressure sores. However, the routine insertion of catheters for incontinence is generally avoided as they predispose to urinary tract infections. Some stroke patients require catheterisation in the short term, whilst a few may need long-term catheterisation.

Oxygen

This may be required for patients with low oxygen levels in the blood (hypoxia). Common reasons for hypoxia include aspiration of food or fluids into the lungs, pneumonia or co-existing lung disease. It is unlikely that stroke patients attending exercise programmes will be using long-term oxygen, unless they have co-existing chronic lung disease.

REHABILITATION AND THE ROLE OF THE MULTIDISCIPLINARY TEAM OF HEALTH-CARE PROFESSIONALS

An overview of the role of the multidisciplinary team

Characteristics of a multidisciplinary team

Patients with residual neurological deficits usually undergo rehabilitation on a specialist stroke unit if requiring inpatient care, or as part of a community rehabilitation service or early supported discharge service. The aim of rehabilitation is to minimise the functional impact of the stroke and maximise independence. Rehabilitation generally starts as soon as possible and when the patient is sufficiently medically stable. Patients are typically treated by a multidisciplinary team of health-care professionals. The 'core' members of a team generally include doctors, nurses, physiotherapists, occupational therapists, dieticians, speech and language therapists, and social workers. Some teams also include psychologists and pharmacists. Teams may work in different ways in different parts of the world. In the UK, multidisciplinary teams who care for patients on stroke units provide specialist treatments. Teams typically meet once a week to discuss patients' progress in key areas (e.g. continence, mobility, activities of daily living, mood), agree goals, solve problems and plan discharge and future care, in collaboration with the patients and their families. The team may ask for advice from other specialists, including psychologists, orthotists, orthoptists, pharmacists, radiologists, vascular surgeons and psychiatrists. Other medical specialists may also contribute to the provision of care, e.g. gastrointestinal specialists are responsible for PEG tube insertion.

Although each professional has had specific training in different areas and has specific roles in stroke management, the success of rehabilitation depends on close team-working and some degree of role blurring to ensure a patient-centred approach. If rehabilitation continues after discharge from hospital, a new multidisciplinary team will take over the care of the patient in the community.

Working with families and carers

The multidisciplinary team works very closely with relatives and carers, providing information about the aims of and progress with rehabilitation. Later in the patient journey, relatives play a key role in helping to plan discharge, particularly when they are likely to be involved in providing hands-on care for the stroke survivor after discharge from hospital. The needs of carers must be considered when planning discharge, and the multidisciplinary team needs to ensure that carers are given as much support as possible, particularly if they are taking on a new caring role.

Key members of the multidisciplinary team

A description of core members of the multidisciplinary team is provided on page 28; for more detailed information about the roles of the team members and the interventions they provide, please see Scottish Intercollegiate Guideline Network Stroke Rehabilitation Guideline Number 118 (SIGN 2010). Table 2.1 summarises the key aims of therapy, describes commonly used interventions and the usual professional lead.

Table 2.1	Key aims of therapy, typical intervention and the usual professional lead(s)	
Key aim: optimisation of:	**Typical intervention(s)**	**Professional lead(s)**
Medical management of acute stroke	Acute treatment, e.g. thrombolysis	Physician and nurse
	Management of medical complications	Physician and nurse
	Secondary prevention	Physician and pharmacist
Daily care	24 hour assisted care input	Nurse
Administration of medications	Assistance to administer if required	Nurse
Nutrition	Assessment of swallowing to determine the safety of oral feeding	Speech and language therapist
	Swallow retraining	Speech and language therapist
	Diet texture modification	Dietician
	Nutritional supplements	Dietician
	Assistance with oral feeding	Nurse
	Tube (nasogastric or percutaneous enterogastrostomy tube)	Nurse, physician, speech and language therapist, dietician, gastrointestinal physician for PEG tube insertion
Respiratory function	Ensuring clear airways and appropriate functional breathing	Physiotherapist and physician
Physiological functioning	Physiological monitoring (pulse, blood pressure and blood oxygen levels)	Nurse
Pressure area care	Correct positioning, regular turning and pressure relieving mattresses to avoid skin breakdown over pressure areas, e.g. sacrum, heels	Nurse and physiotherapist
Continence	Assessment of continence	Nurse and physician
	Regular toileting	Nurse
	Drugs for urinary incontinence	Physician
	Avoiding constipation	Nurse and physician
	Bowel regime for faecal incontinence	Nurse
Communication	Language retraining	Speech and language therapist
	Word-finding skills	
	Speech production	
	Listening and interpreting skills	
	Communication aids	
Mood	Screen for depression	Nurse
	Treat depression (antidepressants, clinical psychologist advice, non-pharmacological treatment, e.g. cognitive behavioural therapy)	Stroke physician, clinical psychologist
	Identify and treat anxiety	Stroke physician and nurse
Independent mobility	Gait re-education	Physiotherapy
	Negotiating stairs, stepping	
	Provision of walking aids	
	Balance re-education	
	Ocular-vestibular re-education	
	Transfers (e.g. sit-to-stand)	

Key aim: optimisation of:	Typical intervention(s)	Professional lead(s)
Functional upper limb movement	Facilitation of components of upper limb movement and support function Reach and grasp retraining Functional strengthening	Physiotherapist and occupational therapist
Task development involving upper limb	Functional retraining of real-life scenarios Activities of daily living, e.g. washing dressing and food preparation Eating and drinking skills Compensatory strategies	Occupational therapist
Cognitive and executive function	Re-education of task sequencing Cognitive retraining Compensatory strategies	Occupational therapist
Vision	Re-education of visuospatial awareness Scanning techniques	Occupational therapist and physiotherapist Orthoptist
Fitness and endurance rehabilitation	Early strengthening of muscles for active movements Functional endurance in activities of daily living	Physiotherapist
Neuro-biomechanics	Appropriate lower limb and hand/wrist biomechanics Splinting or other orthoses	Orthotist
Transition to self-management of stroke as a chronic disease – when appropriate	Knowledge of lifestyle factors that may help reduce the risk of recurrent stroke	All
Providing for long-term care needs	Training relatives to provide hands-on care Arranging care in the community Advising on financial benefits available to stroke survivors and their carers	Nurse, physiotherapist, occupational therapist Social worker Social worker

Table 2.1 *Key aims of therapy, typical intervention and the usual professional lead(s)—cont'd*

The links between the multidisciplinary team and the exercise professional

The information in Table 2.1 may help the exercise professional understand which health professional might be best placed to deal with new complications that might arise during an exercise programme. The table lists the key roles of each health-care professional (please note that the information provided is not exhaustive). Referral mechanisms back to the health-care professionals may vary according to the type of stroke service and its geographical location. Chapters 9 and 13 discuss referral routes related to community-based Exercise after Stroke services in further detail.

Stroke physician

Stroke physicians play a critical role in the diagnosis of stroke, identifying the cause of stroke, providing medical treatment in the acute phase and optimising secondary prevention. They also identify and treat complications from stroke. Traditionally, it has been the stroke physician who oversees the rehabilitation, leads the multidisciplinary team meeting and guides discharge planning. Some patients die, predictably over the first few weeks – particularly those with severe strokes – and this may cause a range of distressing symptoms that need to be managed, even if death is inevitable (Royal College of Physicians Stroke Intercollegiate Working Party 2008). Stroke physicians guide the management of patients who are dying, seeking advice from specialist palliative care teams if needed.

Nurse

Nurses have a diverse role in the management of stroke. Nurses care for people during inpatient stay, and may also provide long-term care and support. They wash and dress patients, administer medication and provide palliative care. They lead the management of continence, assist patients with feeding, insert nasogastric tubes, monitor patients' physiological status and position the patient (which helps prevent the development of pressure sores). They also play a central role in talking to families, giving updates on progress and directing families to other members of the multidisciplinary team for specific information.

Physiotherapist

The Chartered Society of Physiotherapy (CSP) in the UK defines the essence of physiotherapy as '...*a health care profession concerned with human function and movement and maximising potential*' (CSP Curriculum Framework 2002).

Physiotherapy generally starts as soon as possible after admission to hospital. The initial assessment will include: level of consciousness, ability to follow commands, airway patency and the function of the respiratory system. The physiotherapist will also assess sensation, joint and muscle movement and limb positions; resting muscle tone, static and dynamic postural alignment and symmetry; balance in sitting, standing and movement; strength and coordination of movement and how easily the patient can change position and move around. Physiotherapists use physical interventions to reduce impairments, including exercises aimed at improving upper limb function, balance, gait and transfers, and other interventions such as functional electrical stimulation of weak muscles.

Some of the interventions provided by physiotherapists may include elements of physical fitness training. For example, strength training of muscle groups where weakness is present can lead to significant improvements in function, but this has to be balanced with the risk of affecting postural tone problems and joint injury where movement control is poor.

Some physiotherapists may introduce aerobic exercise training towards the end of rehabilitation, or use other training modalities, e.g. treadmill training, to help improve mobility. If this exercise is provided as part of inpatient rehabilitation, the exercise professional should be provided with information about the duration, frequency and intensity of any exercise training already provided, in order to help plan future exercise training.

Occupational therapist

Occupational therapists help people engage as independently as possible in the activities (occupations) which enhance their health and wellbeing (College of Occupational Therapists 2011). The occupational therapist works in partnership with the patient, carer and other health-care and voluntary personnel at all stages of the patient's journey from inpatient acute care and rehabilitation through to outpatient and community care.

The occupational therapist will identify the individual aspects which make up a person's ability to carry out selected activities (i.e. physical, cognitive, perceptual, psychological, social, environmental and spiritual) and will set jointly agreed goals. They will use purposeful activity to promote the restoration of function and to maximise participation in meaningful activities, i.e. occupations of self-care, as well as domestic, social, leisure and work roles.

Speech and language therapist

Speech and language therapists manage disorders of speech, language, communication and swallowing. They work closely with parents, carers and other professionals (Royal College of Speech and Language Therapists 2011). The speech and language therapist is responsible for assessing, diagnosing and treating communication and swallowing difficulties (Table 2.1 and chapter 7).

For patients who cannot eat or drink anything safely, the speech and language therapist may recommend tube feeding. Other patients may manage to take food and fluid safely if their diet is changed, e.g. puréed food and thickened liquids. Sometimes different positions can make swallowing easier.

The speech and language therapist may recommend exercises aimed to facilitate facial muscles, develop lip closure and tongue placement, which will help improve swallowing. Treatment strategies are also offered for aphasia (chapter 7).

Dietician

Registered dieticians assess, diagnose and treat diet and nutrition problems at an individual and wider public health level (The British Dietetic Association 2011).

The dietician will advise on the most appropriate foods, nutritional components and supplements for stroke survivors, and plays a central role in prescribing nutritional support for patients with dysphagia who are being tube-fed. For patients able to swallow who may be underweight, they may advise on diet and supplementary feeds, and in people who are overweight they may advise on weight loss.

Social worker

Social workers protect vulnerable people, enhance relationships and help families to stay together, where possible, and enable people to live fulfilled lives as independently as they can (The College of Social Work 2011).

Social workers generally become involved later in the stroke journey, when the long-term care needs become clearer. A social worker will assess care needs, help organise financial support and organise home care, e.g. carers visiting at home to help with washing, dressing and bathing. If a person cannot be supported at home, the social worker will advise on alternative placements, e.g. nursing homes.

Orthotist

Orthotists are responsible for the assessment, diagnosis, measurement, prescription, supply and review of orthoses. These devices use biomechanical principles to apply forces to one or more body segments to effect change in movement pattern, prevent deformity and/or relieve pain. This includes ankle-foot orthoses (AFO) which are made from stiff plastic and worn on the lower part of the leg and foot to control the motion and prevent deformities of the ankle and foot (Fig. 2.1). Ankle-foot orthoses facilitate function of the affected leg during gait and standing, aligning the lower leg correctly during the stance phase of gait. Orthotists may also provide hand and wrists splints to help prevent the development of contractures.

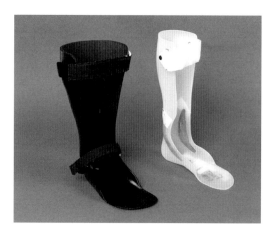

FIG 2.1 Orthotists may provide ankle-foot orthoses as shown above.

Clinical psychologist

Clinical psychologists aim to reduce psychological distress and enhance and promote psychological wellbeing. Although many people make a good recovery following stroke, some stroke survivors need additional help to enable them to cope with the cognitive, emotional and physical effects of stroke and its impact on their lives. Sometimes, the carer needs help. A referral to clinical psychology is made if psychological factors related to a patient's stroke are causing significant emotional distress or reducing their potential for independence.

Orthoptist

Orthoptists are concerned with the diagnosis and treatment of ocular motility (eye movements) and problems relating to vision (British and Irish Orthoptic Society 2011). An orthoptist can assess and diagnose visual problems, provide treatments (e.g. prisms for double vision) and advise on ways to cope with visual problems.

Pharmacist

Pharmacists are experts in medicines and how they work (Royal Pharmaceutical Society 2011). They provide advice on medication-related issues, e.g. which drugs can be provided by tube feeding, drug interactions, secondary prevention and monitoring of warfarin.

SECONDARY PREVENTION

After an ischaemic stroke or TIA the risk of a recurrent event is about 10% in the first week (Coull et al. 2004), so early secondary prevention is critical to prevent further vascular events. There are different service models that can help achieve early secondary prevention; in one area in Scotland, for example, a telephone 'hotline' has been established whereby any primary care physician can call a stroke physician for urgent advice on management (Kerr et al. 2010).

The key approaches to secondary prevention are detailed in the following section; lifestyle advice is provided to all patients with stroke, and blood pressure lowering should be considered irrespective of pathological stroke type.

Lifestyle advice

Patients are given general advice about stopping smoking, losing weight (if overweight), avoiding heavy alcohol consumption and reducing salt intake (Sacco et al. 2006). Patients are also advised to increase levels of physical activity, though the best type, frequency and intensity of physical activity is uncertain (chapters 4 and 10). Such advice is given to patients with both haemorrhagic and ischaemic stroke.

Blood pressure lowering

Blood pressure lowering should be considered after ischaemic stroke, haemorrhagic stroke and TIA. This is usually achieved by drug treatment (PROGRESS Collaborative Group 2001). Most stroke physicians would aim for a target blood pressure of less than 130/170 mmHg using various drugs such as thiazide diuretics, angiotensin converting enzyme inhibitors, calcium antagonists, beta blockers or alpha blockers. If blood pressure is persistently elevated above this level when patients attend for exercise sessions, it is important to report back to the patient's general practitioner. However, provided that resting levels do not exceed 200 mmHg systolic or 110 mmHg diastolic (chapter 9), there is no absolute need to discontinue exercise sessions.

Drugs for secondary prevention after ischaemic stroke and transient ischaemic attack

Several different drugs may be prescribed to reduce the risk of recurrent stroke, which are described below. Exercise professionals need to understand the effects of common drugs in the context of exercise, but they would not advise on medication.

Antiplatelet drugs

These drugs reduce stroke risk by at least one-quarter (Antithrombotic Trialists Collaboration 2002). Aspirin is the most commonly used antiplatelet drug. It is often prescribed in combination with another antiplatelet drug called dipyridamole slow release (side effects include headaches, dizziness and nausea). Increasingly, clopidogrel, which is also an antiplatelet drug, is being given instead of the combination of aspirin and dipyridamole. Antiplatelet drugs increase the risk of bruising and bleeding.

Statins

There are several different types of statins; the commonly used ones include simvastatin, atorvastatin and pravastatin. Statins reduce cholesterol levels and so reduce the risk of recurrent vascular events (Heart Protection Study Collaborative Group 2002). Side effects of statins include abnormal liver function tests, sometimes even jaundice, and muscle aching. It may be difficult to distinguish between the muscle aches caused by a statin and muscle aches caused as a result of starting exercise classes. Any concerns about muscle pains in patients attending exercise sessions who are taking statins should be raised with the patient's general practitioner.

Blood pressure reduction

There are a number of different drugs that can be used for blood pressure reduction after stroke. Side effects of all these drugs include dizziness and postural hypotension, i.e. a fall in blood pressure on standing up. This might be relevant to the delivery of specific exercises, e.g. sit to stand.

There are other side effects of specific types of drugs. For example, diuretics can cause abnormalities of salt levels (e.g. low sodium), angiotensin converting enzyme inhibitors (examples include enalapril, lisinopril and ramipril) can cause renal failure, and calcium antagonists can cause swollen ankles. Beta blockers are often used for blood pressure control; these slow the heart rate and so there may not be the usual heart rate response to exercise.

Anticoagulation

Atrial fibrillation (an irregular heart rate which occurs as a result of disorganised and irregular contraction of the atria) is an important risk factor for stroke. Anticoagulation with warfarin reduces the risk of a further stroke by about two-thirds. The most common, and important, side effects of warfarin are bleeding and easy bruising. Thus, it is particularly important that the exercise professional ensures that the stroke survivor does not bump into equipment or fall during an exercise sessions. Stroke survivors who take warfarin need to have blood tests performed regularly to monitor levels of anticoagulation.

Carotid endarterectomy

Patients with ischaemic stroke or TIA who have a narrowing in the internal carotid artery, which supplies blood to the side of the brain affected by the stroke, are usually offered carotid endarterectomy. This is a surgical procedure to remove the 'narrowing', performed under local or general anaesthetic. There is a 3–5% risk of stroke as a result of the surgery, but overall there is a substantial reduction in the long-term risk of stroke.

Drugs for secondary prevention after haemorrhagic stroke

Anticoagulants (e.g. warfarin) and antiplatelet drugs (e.g. aspirin) are usually *discontinued* in the short term, but may be restarted in the longer term, depending on the original reason for their prescription. For example, if a patient has severe angina and requires an antiplatelet drug, the stroke physician and cardiologist together may agree that the long-term risk of further bleeding into the brain is less than the risk of an acute coronary event. Blood pressure reduction is important in haemorrhagic strokes as well as in ischaemic stroke and TIA.

EARLY SUPPORTED DISCHARGE AND COMMUNITY REHABILITATION

There is persuasive evidence to support other interventions later in the stroke pathway; these include early supported discharge from hospital (Early Supported Discharge Trialists 2005) and community rehabilitation by multidisciplinary teams (Outpatient Service Trialists 2003). When targeted community-based rehabilitation is given, seven patients are spared a poor long-term outcome for every 100 stroke patients treated (Outpatient Service Trialists 2003)

   Services have been developed that offer patients an early discharge from hospital with more rehabilitation at home (early supported discharge) (Langhorne et al. 2007). A systematic review of 12 trials (1659 patients) of early supported discharge found that it reduced the risk of death or dependency, equivalent of five fewer adverse outcomes for every 100 patients receiving the early supported discharge. Early supported discharge services are now being set up; as these services become more widespread, it is likely that referral to Exercise after Stroke services will occur after the patient has been discharged from an early supported discharge service.

STROKE AS A LONG-TERM CONDITION

There is an increasing awareness that the effects of stroke can last a lifetime, and stroke is now being viewed as a long-term condition (Brainin et al. 2011). The area of 'Life after Stroke' is becoming an important focus for further research and service development. Chapter 3 describes some of the long-term effects of stroke, all of which are relevant to the delivery of exercise after stroke.

In order to address the long-term needs of stroke survivors, they need to be reviewed after discharge from hospital. The National Stroke Strategy for England and Wales states that stroke survivors and their carers should be offered a review from primary care services of their health and social care status and secondary prevention needs, typically within 6 weeks of discharge home or to a care home, and again by 6 months of leaving hospital. This should be followed by annual health and social care check, which facilitates a clear pathway back to further specialist review, advice, information, support and rehabilitation, where required (Department of Health 2007). These primary care reviews should check that the stroke survivor has been prescribed appropriate drugs for secondary prevention, that stroke risk factors are being managed appropriately (e.g. smoking, obesity), that long-term post-stroke problems have been addressed (e.g. spasticity, incontinence, mood disorders). The reviews should also support return to work if appropriate, and ensure that carers' needs have been identified and met. These reviews provide an excellent opportunity to refer the stroke survivor to an Exercise after Stroke service, if this has not already been done.

SUMMARY POINTS

- Patients with stroke will undergo investigations to determine the type of stroke, to seek causes of the stroke and to identify co-morbidities.
- Stroke treatment can be broadly divided into acute treatment, rehabilitation and secondary prevention.
- There is increasing recognition that stroke is a long-term condition and that stroke survivors need to be under regular review. Such reviews provide an excellent opportunity to refer to Exercise after Stroke services if this has not already been done.

REFERENCES

Antithrombotic Trialists Collaboration, 2002. Collaborative overview of randomized trials of antiplatelet therapy a: prevention of death, myocardial infarction and stroke by prolonged antiplatelet therapy in various categories of patients. BMJ 308, 81–106.

Barer, D.H., 1989. The natural history and functional consequences of dysphagia after hemispheric stroke. J. Neurol. Neurosurg. Psychiatry 52, 236–241.

Brainin, M., Norrving, B., Sunnerhagen, K.S., et al., 2011. Poststroke chronic disease management: towards improved identification and interventions for poststroke spasticity-related complications. Int. J. Stroke 6, 42–46.

British and Irish Orthoptic Society. Available online at http://www. orthoptics.org.uk/patients/orthoptics (accessed 11.04.2011).

College of Occupational Therapists. Available online at http://www.cot. co.uk/Homepage/About_Occupational_Therapy/ (accessed 11.04.2011).

Coull, A.J., Lovett, J.K., Rothwell, P.M., et al., 2004. Population based study of early risk of stroke after transient ischaemic attack or minor stroke: implications for public education and organization of services. BMJ 328, 326. doi:10.1136/bmj.37991.635266.44.

Department of Health, 2007. National stroke strategy. Department of Health, London.

Early Supported Discharged Trialists, 2005. Services for reducing duration of hospital care for acute stroke patients. Cochrane Database Syst. Rev. 2, CD000443. doi:10.1002/14651858.

Hacke, W., Kaste, M., Bluhmki, E., et al., 2008. Thrombolysis with alteplase 3 to 4.5 hours after acute ischemic stroke. N. Engl. J. Med. 359, 1317–1329.

Heart Protection Study Collaborative Group, 2002. MRC/BHF Heart Protection Study of cholesterol lowering with simvastatin in 20,536 high-risk individuals: a randomised placebo-controlled trial. Lancet 360, 7–22.

Indredavik, B., Bakke, F., Slordahl, S.A., et al., 1999. Treatment in a combined acute and rehabilitation stroke unit: which aspects are most important. Stroke 30, 917–923.

Kerr, E., Arulraj, N., Scott, M., et al., 2010. A telephone hotline for transient ischaemic attack and stroke: prospective audit of a model to improve rapid access to specialist stroke care. BMJ 341, c3265.

Langhorne, P., Dennis, M.S., on behalf of the Stroke Unit Trialists' Collaboration, 1998. Stroke units: an evidence based approach. BMJ Books, London.

Langhorne, P., Holmqvist, P., Widen, L., Early Supported Discharge Trialists, 2007. Early supported discharge after stroke. Int. J. Rehabil. 39, 103–108.

Outpatient Service Trialists, 2003. Therapy-based rehabilitation services for stroke patients at home. Cochrane Database Syst. Rev. 1, CD002925. doi:10.1002/14651858.

PROGRESS Collaborative Group, 2001. Randomised trial of a perindopril-based blood pressure lowering regimen among 6105 individuals with previous stroke or transient ischaemic attack. Lancet 358, 1033–1041.

Royal College of Speech and Language Therapists. Available online at. http://www.rcslt.org (accessed 11.04.2011).

Royal College of Physicians Intercollegiate Stroke Working Party, 2008. National clinical guidelines for stroke, third ed. Royal College of Physicians, London.

Royal Pharmaceutical Society. Available online at http://www.rpharms.com/about-pharmacy/what-do-pharmacists-do-.asp (accessed 11.04.2011).

Sacco, R.L., Adams, R., Albers, G., 2006. Guidelines for prevention of stroke in patients with ischaemic stroke or transient ischaemic attack: a statement for healthcare professionals from the American Heart Association/American Stroke Association Council on Stroke. Stroke 37, 577–617.

Sandercock, P., Gubitz, G., Foley, P., et al., 2003. Antiplatelet therapy for acute ischaemic stroke. Cochrane Database Syst. Rev. 2, CD000029. doi:10.1002/14651858.

Scottish Intercollegiate Guidelines Network, 2010. Guideline 118: Management of patients with stroke: rehabilitation, prevention and management of complications, and discharge planning. A national clinical guideline. Scottish Intercollegiate Guidelines Network (SIGN), Edinburgh. Available online at http://www.sign.ac.uk/guidelines/fulltext/118/index.html (accessed 12.11.2010).

Stroke Unit Trialists Collaboration, 2007. Organised inpatient (stroke unit) care for stroke. Cochrane Database Syst. Rev. 4, CD000197. doi:10.1002/14651858.

The British Dietetic Association. Available online at www.bda.uk.com (accessed 11.04.2011).

The Chartered Society of Physiotherapy, 2002. Curriculum framework for qualifying programmes in physiotherapy. The Chartered Society of Physiotherapy, London.

The College of Social Work. Available online at http://www.basw.co.uk/ (accessed 11.04.2011).

The FOOD Trial Collaboration, 2005. Effect of timing and method of enteral tube feeding for dysphagic stroke patients (FOOD): a multicentre randomised controlled trial. Lancet 365, 764–772.

Vahedi, K., Hofmeijer, J., Juettler, E., et al., 2007. Early decompressive surgery in malignant infarction of the middle cerebral artery: a pooled analysis of three randomized controlled trials. Lancet 6, 215–222.

Wardlaw, J.M., Murray, V., Berge, E., del Zoppo, G.J., 2010. Thrombolysis for acute ischemic stroke. Stroke 41, e445–e446.

Post-stroke problems

Frederike van Wijck • Mark Smith •
Pauline Halliday • Gillian Mead

3

CHAPTER CONTENTS

INTRODUCTION

Approximately 50% of people who survive a stroke are left with long-term disabilities (Mackay and Mensah 2004) and stroke is the major cause of adult disability. Post-stroke problems may be the direct result of the stroke, indirectly related to the neurological event (e.g. due to reduced activity following stroke), or associated with the longer-term effects of disuse, inactivity and changes in lifestyle after stroke.

In addition, stroke survivors may have co-morbidities, such as diabetes or heart disease, that exist alongside the stroke and which may have a further impact on their ability to undertake exercise.

The purpose of this chapter is to raise awareness of the most common post-stroke problems and explore how they may affect a stroke survivor's ability to engage in physical activity. It builds on the descriptions of post-stroke neurological deficits introduced in chapter 1, but goes into more detail, introduces the important longer-term post-stroke problems as well as co-morbidities, and considers their broad implications for exercise. The latter will be discussed in more detail in chapter 10, which focuses on the design of exercise programmes after stroke.

This chapter will cover problems with movement and functional activity, sensation and perception, pain, cognitive problems, emotional difficulties, psychosocial issues and other post-stroke problems such as fatigue. We will explain why a comprehensive, bio-psychosocial approach is necessary to fully understand these problems and their impact on the lives of stroke survivors and their families.

PROBLEMS WITH MOVEMENT AND FUNCTIONAL ACTIVITY AFTER STROKE

MOTOR IMPAIRMENTS

As described in chapter 2, motor symptoms following stroke may include weakness, spasticity and contractures, which indirectly may lead to loss of range of movement.

Weakness

Weakness, also known as hemiparesis or hemiplegia, primarily affects the side of the body opposite to the side of the brain lesion. However, as will be detailed in chapter 4, it is important to note that the so-called 'unaffected side' is often also weaker than normal (Andrews and Bohannon 2000).

In the hemiparetic lower limb, weakness of the extensor muscles is common, which may cause difficulties with rising from a chair, walking and stair climbing (Saunders et al. 2008). Weakness of the muscles that extend the ankle and lift the forefoot (i.e. the ankle dorsiflexors) is common and can impair heel strike during gait, a problem known as a 'drop-foot'. This is an important problem, as lack of foot clearance increases the risk of falls. As a compensatory measure, people with a drop-foot may be fitted with a splint or orthosis (e.g. an ankle-foot orthosis or AFO), while others may use an electrical stimulation device that controls ankle movement during walking (Burridge et al. 1998, Taylor et al. 1999).

Weakness of trunk musculature may affect postural stability and balance; importantly it may also affect the use of the upper limb because the necessary base of support (i.e. stability of the shoulder girdle in relation to the trunk) is lacking.

In the upper limb, weakness may affect all muscle groups, including shoulder flexors and abductors, and elbow flexors and extensors, often making it difficult to reach and grasp objects. Weakness affecting muscles of the wrist and hand may impair hand function, including grip strength and dexterity (Boissy et al. 1999). Some people with stroke may be able to grasp an object, but uncontrolled activity of the finger flexors together with weakness of the extensors may make it difficult to release the object.

Implications for exercise. Exercise professionals need to carefully monitor stroke survivors who have a drop-foot. It is essential that those who have been fitted with an orthosis or electrical stimulation device wear this when they exercise. If a stroke survivor chooses not to wear their device because of a poor fit, they should be referred back to their orthotist or other appropriate health professional for an assessment.

Weakness in other muscle groups may constitute a hazard (e.g. insufficient grip force to hold on to the handle bar of a static bicycle) and must be carefully monitored.

Spasticity

Spasticity[1] is a complex topic. It is a motor disorder, characterised by abnormal muscle activation, which can be felt by both the stroke survivor and the therapist as increased resistance to movement when a muscle is passively stretched. In this book, we will use the definition from a European Union Consortium, which described spasticity as: *'Disordered sensori-motor control, resulting from an upper motor neurone lesion, presenting as intermittent or sustained involuntary activation of muscles'* (Pandyan et al. 2005, p. 5).

Spasticity is common after stroke; around 38% of stroke survivors are estimated to develop spasticity over the first year (Watkins et al. 2002). In the acute stage after stroke, the brain is in a state of 'shock' and muscle activation may be temporarily absent, resulting in abnormally low tone or flaccidity. When the brain begins to recover, hyperactive reflexes and abnormal muscle activity emerge, often together with paresis. This combination makes it difficult for the stroke survivor to move and maintain an optimum posture. This can lead to further problems, as abnormally high tone together with weakness reduces range of movement. If this situation persists, connective tissue within and around the muscle will begin to shorten and form adhesions, thereby increasing the biomechanical stiffness of the muscle even further. Thus, disordered muscle activation is a direct result of the stroke, whereas changes in connective tissue are an indirect problem.

Entire patterns of muscle hyperactivity may be seen, known as 'associated reactions'. For example, when a person with stroke tries to walk, the sheer effort may spark off hyperactivity in the upper limb, resulting in a flexor pattern involving the shoulder, elbow, wrist and hand (Fig. 3.1). When the level of effort reduces, the associated reaction also usually diminishes.

There are other factors that may trigger spasticity in people with a neurological condition, e.g. pain, an ingrown toenail, pressure sores or a urinary tract infection (Barnes 2001).

The term 'spasticity' is often used interchangeably with 'high tone' or 'hypertonia' (Edwards 2002). However, it is important to differentiate between these concepts, which are related but not the same. Loosely described, 'tone' reflects the tightness of a muscle or muscle group. Normally, muscle tone increases when we prepare for action, while it reduces when we relax. It is important to understand that muscle tone is a combination of neurogenic (i.e. muscle activation) and biomechanical factors. In fact, in fully relaxed muscles of healthy people, muscle activation may be entirely absent, and muscle tone is purely caused by biomechanical factors (Walsh 1992). These include the length and tension of connective tissue within and around the muscle. At a microscopic level, this includes cross-bridges between actin and myosin filaments within muscle fibres, which may be resolved through gentle, repetitive movement, which in turn reduces soft tissue stiffness (Walsh 1992). This phenomenon is known as 'thixotropy'[2] (Walsh 1992), a familiar analogy of which is stirring a pot of paint before using it to decorate a wall: the stirring action breaks the connections

---

[1]Spasticity: from the Greek σπαστικοσ, meaning 'to tug or draw' (Sheean 1998, p. 7).
[2]Thixotropy: from the Greek θιξις (touch) and τροπη (turning) (Walsh 1992, p. 84).

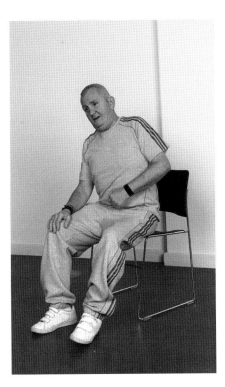

FIG 3.1   Example of an associated reaction. Note in particular the elbow flexion - an involuntary reaction during a strenuous task.

between the molecules and makes the paint more 'runny'. Thixotropy is dependent on temperature and thus the soft tissue stiffness experienced by stroke survivors may be partially attributable to thixotropy caused by lack of movement and further compounded by decreased temperature caused by reduced circulation of the affected limb.

Traditionally, physiotherapists have been cautious about using exercise (particularly strength training) with stroke survivors, for fear that this might increase spasticity and affect motor recovery (Bobath 1990). However, a recent systematic review indicates that spasticity is not increased by exercise (Borges et al. 2009). Although the precise impact of exercise on spasticity is not fully understood, it is important that exercise professionals have a good understanding of this phenomenon in order to enable stroke survivors who have spasticity to engage with exercise safely and effectively.

Spasms are short-lived involuntary contractions that often produce a pain that is similar to athletic cramping. They should not necessarily prevent the continuation of a resistive exercise, unless they present on a frequent basis. Long periods of forceful contractions in major muscle groups can cause painful muscle spasms. They can often be reduced or stopped altogether by gently and slowly stretching the muscle group affected (often self-managed by the individual) while weight bearing can also reduce them.

Clonus is an involuntary, rhythmic contraction of a muscle that often sustains itself, having been provoked by a fast stretch (Sheean 2001).

Treatment

Treatment for spasticity is usually required when it interferes with function and hygiene, or causes pain, or when long-term complications are expected (Barnes 2001, Thompson 1998). Given that other factors (e.g. pain) can contribute to spasticity, these problems need to be carefully examined and treated where possible. Drug treatment may be either systemic (i.e. the drug affects the entire central nervous system, such as oral baclofen) or local (i.e. the drug affects a specific location only, such as phenol or botulinum toxin) (Ward and Ko Ko 2001). Systemic, oral anti-spastic medication may have unwanted side effects such as drowsiness (Ward and Ko Ko 2001), which could affect a person's ability to exercise safely. Therefore, if spasticity is a local problem (e.g. mainly affecting wrist and finger flexors, or hip adductors), focal pharmacological agents tend to be preferred. Botulinum toxin type A is used increasingly, as there are usually few side effects, while its administration (i.e. by injection) is relatively straightforward (Davis and Barnes 2001). Other focal techniques include nerve blocks, which are undertaken by injecting alcohol into the nerve, or surgery by cutting through a specific nerve known to be the cause of the spasticity; however, these treatments are not routine and require further evaluation (Scottish Intercollegiate Guidelines Network 2010).

A number of different physiotherapy techniques are used to reduce hypertonia, although it is often not clear whether the intervention targets neurogenic, biomechanical, or both factors. Examples are electrical stimulation, stretching, splinting, positioning, or serial casting, whereby the position of a joint (e.g. the ankle) is increased in a step-wise manner to gradually stretch soft tissue around it (e.g. the plantar flexors of the ankle). However, there is no evidence that electrical stimulation (Pomeroy et al. 2006), stretching (Katalinic et al. 2010) or splinting (Lannin et al. 2007, Lannin and Herbert 2003) have any effect on spasticity, while there is insufficient evidence to support serial casting (Mortenson and Eng 2003).

Implications for exercise. For exercise professionals it is important to carefully monitor stroke survivors with spasticity. It may be possible to tailor an exercise for a stroke survivor with spasticity, ensuring that they can still undertake the exercise safely and effectively. Where this is not possible, an alternative may need to be found, or advice should be sought from the participant's physiotherapist. Relaxation and/or muscle stretching following exercise may be beneficial to reduce any remaining spasticity.

Contractures

A contracture is a fixed deformity of a joint with a permanent loss of joint range of movement. This usually happens when joint movement has been reduced for some time. Contractures of the wrist flexors have been reported within 6–8 weeks of stroke (Pandyan et al. 2003). Contractures tend to be due to persistently increased muscle tone, permanent biomechanical changes in soft tissue around a joint, muscle weakness and inactivity. Contractures may cause pain and, in more extreme cases, secondary complications such as pressure sores at points of contact, e.g. the inner aspect of the knees in a stroke survivor with contractures of the adductors of the hip (Edwards 2002).

To prevent or treat contractures, therapists may use splinting and careful positioning, as well as assisted movement immediately after stroke, to ensure that joints and muscles are taken through their full range of pain-free movement. Strategies aimed at treating contractures overlap with some that are used to reduce hypertonia, discussed above.

Implications for exercise. Exercise professionals need to know if a stroke survivor has a contracture, as this is a fixed deformity around which any exercise needs to be tailored. If the stroke survivor has been given a splint, this needs to be worn during exercise. Whether or not a stroke survivor wears a splint, careful positioning of the affected limb is essential to avoid any damage to soft tissue. Exercise professionals should liaise with the stroke survivor's therapist or orthotist if they are unsure about the safety of a particular exercise.

PROBLEMS WITH BALANCE, SIT TO STAND, WALKING, REACHING AND GRASPING, AND SWALLOWING

Reduced motor control, including abnormalities in the production of force, timing and sequencing of movement, may affect a wide range of functional activity such as reaching and grasping, balance and walking, and transfers such as rising to stand.

Balance

Stroke survivors may have difficulty maintaining their balance during sitting, standing and/or walking (Bonan et al. 2004) and as a result may be at risk of falling. Impaired balance may occur as a direct result of a stroke without limb weakness, or the paresis and/or sensory symptoms may cause people to be unsteady.

Implications for exercise. Stroke survivors with impaired balance who participate in exercise classes will attempt to steady themselves, often using their unaffected hand, by holding on to equipment in the gym and care must be taken to maintain their safety. Exercise stations need to be set up in such a way that support (e.g. a chair, or a wall) is available in case a person becomes unsteady.

Sit to stand

Weakness and sensory loss in the trunk and affected leg may cause stroke survivors to stand up asymmetrically, usually bearing more weight on the stronger leg. This may then make it difficult for them to begin walking safely.

Implications for exercise. Stroke survivors may need to be reminded to try and stand up symmetrically when rising from sitting, which in turn will help to activate weak leg muscles through visual, vestibular, proprioceptive and tactile feedback (Shumway-Cook and Woollacott 2007). The choice of chair height could also be considered as it will be easier to stand up symmetrically from a higher seat.

Walking (gait)

Around three-quarters of stroke survivors will walk independently, but on average at a much lower speed than normal (Ada et al. 2003). The symptoms of stroke can cause a variety of walking problems that may arise as a result of weakness, loss of sensation, abnormal muscle tone, lack of visuospatial awareness, impaired balance and coordination problems (Michael et al. 2005). Stroke gait is usually characterised by a short stance phase on the affected leg (i.e. the amount of time the foot is placed on the ground), coupled with a quick step with the stronger leg. People often fail to 'step through' with the stronger leg as it can then be difficult to relax the affected leg muscles sufficiently to take the next step (Woolley 2001). There may also be a degree of asymmetry of the trunk, usually side-flexed towards the stronger side.

Some stroke survivors may have a 'staggering' or 'uncoordinated' gait, which is known as 'ataxia'. This is a specific feature of a stroke in the cerebellum (which is responsible for control of movement and balance), but may also result from hemiparesis, where there is insufficient muscle force to control the movement.

Implications for exercise. It is common for stroke survivors to use walking aids which may involve both hands, such as a mobilator, a stick or a tripod in the unaffected hand (Laufer 2004). Care must be taken in the gym environment to ensure that those who use walking aids can move around safely.

Reaching and grasping

Earlier, we mentioned how weakness of the muscles around the shoulder, elbow, wrist and finger joints could affect the ability to reach, grasp and release objects. This may be compounded if there are soft tissue adhesions that limit range of movement, and/or spasticity affecting the ease and accuracy with which movement can be completed. In addition, there may be coordination difficulties that affect function of the arm and hand. Reaching in stroke survivors is slower, less smooth and more variable (van Vliet and Sheridan 2007), suggesting that more time is needed to take in the necessary visual and proprioceptive information and plan the activity step-by-step.

Implications for exercise. There are some typical compensatory movements that can be observed in stroke survivors, which include bending the trunk, often combined with elevating the shoulder girdle (Archambault et al. 1999). To maximise the training effect of arm exercises (Michaelsen et al. 2006), exercise professionals should emphasise an upright, symmetrical posture during reaching exercises and help stroke survivors avoid such compensatory movements. Exercise professionals should be aware that stroke survivors may not have sufficient grip force to hold objects in their hand and care must be taken, e.g. when working with a pole or weight.

Swallowing

As mentioned in chapter 1, more than half of stroke survivors may experience difficulties with swallowing (dysphagia) (Gordon et al. 1987), which is caused by reduced strength and/or coordination of muscles involved in chewing and swallowing, as well as potentially altered sensation in the pharynx. Dysphagia is a risk factor as people may choke when trying to swallow food or liquids. Some stroke survivors whose swallow has been affected can be given texture-modified diets (e.g. puréed food) and their fluids can be thickened to reduce the risk of aspiration (i.e. when secretions or foreign material enter the airways).

Implications for exercise. Exercise professionals need to be aware when an individual has dysphagia, and check whether they are taking – if allowed – the right type of fluid during exercise.

COMMON INTERVENTIONS TO IMPROVE MOTOR FUNCTION AFTER STROKE

As described in chapter 2, treatment to improve motor function after stroke is based on a detailed, ongoing assessment of the individual and may involve input from the multidisciplinary team. Commonly used therapeutic strategies include specialist facilitation techniques to elicit muscle activity and improve strength and coordination (Baer and Durward 2004, Carr and Shepherd 2003, Jackson 2004, Raine 2009). In hydrotherapy, buoyancy of the water can be instrumental in facilitating movement in cases where muscle force is insufficient to act against gravity on land. Electrical stimulation or functional electrical stimulation (FES) may be used to induce or augment muscle contraction, e.g. to improve grasping (Popovic et al. 2005) or heel strike during walking (Burridge and McLellan 2000). Current practice involves intensive, functional, task-specific practice where possible (French et al. 2007, Langhorne et al. 2009, Steultjens et al. 2003, van Peppen et al. 2004). The rationale for this type of practice is based on the idea that each functional activity is subserved by dedicated neural networks. When practising often enough, these networks will become more efficient, finally leading to long-term neuroplastic changes (Carey et al. 2005, Nudo et al. 2000). Although evidence is still lacking in some areas of physical rehabilitation after stroke, examples of intensive, task-specific practice that are currently recommended (Scottish Intercollegiate Guidelines Network 2010) are constraint-induced movement therapy (Wolf et al. 2008), where the affected arm is forced to participate in functional activity as the other arm is prevented from being used for a considerable period each day (e.g. as the hand is placed in a mitt) and robotic devices that enable repetitive practice in purpose-designed activities (Mehrholz et al. 2008). Another example is gait training (either over ground or on a treadmill), which is recommended to improve walking (Scottish Intercollegiate Guidelines Network 2010).

BLADDER AND BOWEL PROBLEMS AFTER STROKE

Motor control problems after stroke may also affect bladder and bowel function and incontinence is common after stroke, particularly in people who have survived a more severe stroke. This includes faecal and urinary incontinence, constipation and urinary retention. Not all of these problems are directly related to the stroke, however; constipation may be related to dehydration, drugs (e.g. painkillers), reduced mobility and low-fibre diet, while urinary incontinence may be caused by urine infection and diuretics. Urinary retention is another problem that may occur soon after stroke, and may be exacerbated by constipation, drugs and immobility.

It is estimated that around 40–60% of patients with acute stroke have urinary incontinence and that this problem persists in 15% of stroke survivors at 1 year after stroke (Thomas et al. 2008). The first stage of managing incontinence is to identify and treat reversible causes, which may be unrelated to stroke. Sometimes a so-called 'unstable bladder' may contribute to the problems, and this may respond to drugs such as tolterodine. Regular toileting may also help and some stroke survivors who are unaware of the status of their bladder may have been advised to go to the toilet at specific times (a strategy known as 'timed voiding'). Stroke survivors who still have urinary incontinence after careful assessment and specific treatment may require 'pad and pants' to contain the urine. Sometimes sheaths are used for men. As a last resort, a catheter may be inserted, but catheters carry a risk of infection and are generally avoided as a way to manage incontinence.

Implications for exercise. It is unlikely that those with faecal incontinence would be referred for exercise, but people with less severe bladder and bowel problems may be referred. Stroke survivors may also have pre-existing stress incontinence (i.e. leakage of urine during coughing or sneezing) and may experience leakage of urine during exercise. It is important for the exercise professional to be aware of these problems, and check that the necessary toilet facilities are available and accessible. Stroke survivors may also wish to empty their bladders before they begin exercising.

PROBLEMS WITH SENSATION AND PERCEPTION AFTER STROKE

As mentioned in chapter 1, 50–60% of stroke survivors have some form of sensory impairment, though the reported prevalence varies widely (Carey 1995). We will now provide more details on the most common sensory impairments after stroke and explore their potential impact on the ability to engage in exercise.

Perceptual problems following stroke can affect visual, tactile, proprioceptive and auditory modalities and include more complex perceptual disorders such as inattention (neglect) and agnosia (i.e. failure of recognition in the presence of adequate sensory input).

VISUAL PROBLEMS

Following stroke, a large proportion of stroke survivors may have visual problems (Rowe et al. 2009). These may be a direct effect of the stroke itself, as will be explained below, or caused by premorbid factors. Many stroke survivors will have had significant visual problems prior to their stroke, including cataracts, age-related macular degeneration, glaucoma or diabetic retinopathy. Visual impairment may affect the ability to perform activities of daily living such as reading and driving, while they reduce quality of life and may increase the risk of falls, particularly in unfamiliar environments such as gym settings.

The type of visual impairment depends on the part of the visual pathway affected by the stroke (Fig. 3.2), and on pre-existing visual problems. Common visual impairments after stroke include double vision (diplopia), gaze palsy (difficulty controlling eye movements, due to paresis of extraocular muscles), visual inattention (also known as unilateral neglect, see below) and visual

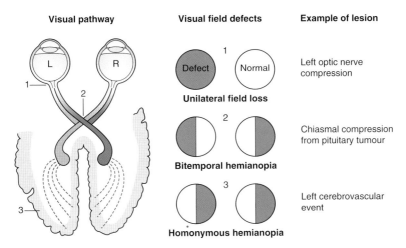

Visual pathway **Visual field defects** **Example of lesion**

1

Defect Normal

Left optic nerve
compression

Unilateral field loss

2

Chiasmal compression
from pituitary tumour

Bitemporal hemianopia

3

Left cerebrovascular
event

Homonymous hemianopia

FIG 3.2 Three common visual field defects, including homonymous hemianopia due to a stroke.
Image from http://www.dwp.gov.uk/img/visual-stroke.jpg reused with permission and courtesy of Frank Munro.

field defects, including homonymous hemianopia. Homonymous hemianopia is a condition whereby the same field (homonymous) of view is
obscured (anopia or anopsia) in both eyes (Fig. 3.2). From chapter 1, we
know that the left occipital lobe receives information from the right visual
field and the other way round. Hence, if a stroke affects the left occipital
lobe, the person is likely to have difficulty perceiving their right visual field
in both eyes.

The management of vision after stroke requires a multidisciplinary
approach (Scottish Intercollegiate Guidelines Network 2010). For example,
the physiotherapist and occupational therapist can provide exercises and
advice on ways to manage visual impairments during activities of daily
living, while ophthalmologists, orthoptists and opticians also play an important role in examining and prescribing treatments for visual impairment after
stroke.

Implications for exercise. Exercise professionals need to know if a stroke
survivor has visual problems, as this has implications for the stroke survivor's own safety and that of others. Wherever possible, the exercise professional should position themselves in the stroke survivor's preserved field of
view, and ensure they can see objects and people around them. Chapter 9 will
detail the risk assessments that the exercise professional needs to undertake
prior to exercise, which involves removing clutter and ensuring adequate
lighting to prevent falls.

AUDITORY PROBLEMS

Hearing loss towards the affected side is not uncommon after stroke and,
given that stroke affects older people who may already have developed a
hearing impairment, many stroke survivors who are referred for exercise
are likely to have hearing difficulties. These may be further compounded if
background music is used.

Implications for exercise. It is important to ensure that the environment is as noise-free as possible, that hearing aids are worn and working and that instructions are delivered in the clearest way possible, positioning stroke survivors in such a way that they can use the side where hearing is best.

PROBLEMS WITH TACTILE AND PROPRIOCEPTIVE SENSATION

Sensory function

Sensory modalities may be affected by stroke, causing sensory information to be absent, diminished, distorted or amplified. For the stroke survivor, sensory impairment can be disturbing. For example, some may experience a burning sensation in their hand when gripping an object. Sensory impairment may also be detrimental to motor recovery, for example upper limb function is hampered by severe sensory impairment despite the presence of active movement (Carey 1995, De Souza 1983). This is because sensory information is required to coordinate fine, skilled movement such as writing or doing buttons.

Implications for exercise. During exercise, it is important to ensure that head, trunk and limbs are in good alignment for function so that the sensory feedback to the central nervous system is as 'normal' as possible to optimise movement. Orthotic devices may have been provided to maintain optimum alignment of, as well as to protect, joints and soft tissue, particularly at the ankle, shoulder, hand and wrist. In the presence of sensory loss, people with stroke may have to compensate by looking at their limbs as they move them, in order to perform accurate and coordinated actions. This may be particularly important when using equipment such as static bicycles, treadmills and weight-training machines. Great care must be taken to ensure that the skin is protected by avoiding damage through knocks from parts of gym equipment.

Stereognosis

Occasionally, stroke survivors with right hemisphere damage can present with a sensory problem known as astereognosis. People with asterognosis may be unable to recognise objects through touch alone (i.e. with vision occluded) (Turvey et al. 1998) and may have difficulty with using equipment and dressing. Treatment for this problem includes allowing the individual to examine objects thoroughly through touch and using this sensory information to provide clues to the objects used (e.g. examining a cup with a handle would allow the individual to identify a key characteristic about the object, indicating how this would be used).

Implications for exercise. Exercise professionals should be aware that some stroke survivors may have difficulty using objects because of astereognosis. Where this is the case, stroke survivors should be encouraged to look at objects before using them in an exercise.

Proprioception

Normally, people have an awareness of where their limbs are in space, without having to look at them. This is called proprioception and is achieved through specific receptors within muscles, tendons and joint capsules, signalling information about posture and movement directly to the central nervous system. In normal circumstances, individuals have no conscious awareness of this process. Stroke survivors can often have difficulty monitoring where their limbs are in relation to their body because this signalling can be interrupted, corrupted or absent altogether. As a result they can misplace their limbs or not position limbs appropriately for activities, e.g. they may be found with their affected arm hanging over the side of the wheelchair, their fingers at risk of being caught in the spokes.

Implications for exercise. Diminished proprioception can make activities in the gym setting difficult or even hazardous. However, as indicated earlier, stroke survivors can be taught to compensate for this by using visual feedback (i.e. to look at the affected limb and use visual feedback to provide sensory information on the limb's positioning). Exercise professionals can use verbal prompts to remind stroke survivors to look at their affected limbs if required.

DISORDERS OF THERMAL SENSATION

Stroke survivors with any type of stroke can experience disordered perception of warm/cool and/or hot/cold sensation in comparison with healthy people (Choi-Kwon et al. 2006). This may not be immediately apparent as people may not be aware of it themselves. Disorders of thermal sensation may also be associated with the development of central post-stroke pain (Bowsher 2001). Some stroke survivors with disturbed thermal sensation can experience pain when touching normally non-painful stimuli, such as cold metal; this is known as allodynia.

Implications for exercise. Care must be taken to ensure that participants involved in exercise programmes are not at risk of touching potentially damaging hot or cold sources such as water taps, radiators or liquids.

DISORDERS OF TASTE

About 30% of stroke survivors have reduced taste after a stroke (Heckmann et al. 2005). This may affect appetite which partially explains poor nutritional status following stroke (Poels et al. 2006). Whether improvements in taste occur in the longer term is uncertain.

UNILATERAL NEGLECT

Also known as unilateral neglect, contralateral neglect, visuospatial neglect or hemi-inattention, unilateral neglect is a phenomenon whereby a person fails to attend to, perceive stimuli in, or move towards their affected side (Manly and Robertson 2003). Following a stroke, a person may be unaware of auditory, visual or tactile stimuli on the side opposite to the lesion (i.e. the affected side). They may fail to notice objects or people on their affected side and walk into them. They may also fail to notice that their affected side (e.g. their arm) is in an unsafe position and at risk of being harmed. There are a number of possible causes for this complex problem, including disorders with attention (see below), reduced sensation or perception of the affected side, or a combination of these factors. Neglect is particularly commonly found in people with a large stroke affecting the right hemisphere.

COMMON INTERVENTIONS FOR SENSORY/PERCEPTUAL PROBLEMS AFTER STROKE

As with other impairments after stroke, altered sensation and perception tend to improve over time. Reported interventions to treat loss of sensation include the application of heat and cold packs (Chen et al. 2002); sensory retraining (Byl et al. 2003, Smania et al. 2003, Yekutiel and Guttman 1993); weight bearing through the hemiplegic upper limb while wearing an inflatable splint (Feys et al. 1998) and intermittent compression of the arm (Cambier et al. 2003). While there have been encouraging results from these studies, small participant numbers and methodological weaknesses mean that it is not possible at this stage to recommend specific treatments to improve sensory recovery after stroke.

Implications for exercise. It is important that exercise professionals closely monitor participants with stroke with regard to the safe use of equipment, as impairments of attention and/or sensation may put them and others at risk of accident or injury. As described for stroke survivors with diminished proprioception, exercise professionals can use verbal prompts to remind stroke survivors to pay attention to the affected side of their body and/or space, as required (Bowen et al. 2003).

PAIN AFTER STROKE

Pain is a considerable problem after stroke with up to 42% of stroke survivors reporting it (Jönsson et al. 2006, Kong et al. 2004). The most common types of pain experienced by people after stroke are musculoskeletal pain (Chakour et al. 1996), hemiplegic shoulder pain (Ratnasabapathy et al. 2003) and pain of central origin as a direct consequence of the stroke (Bowsher 2005). Whilst stroke survivors may find it hard to explain the nature of their pain, it is important to take a careful history, as this is likely to provide important clues to the cause of their pain.

CENTRAL POST-STROKE PAIN

Central post-stroke pain used to be known as 'thalamic pain' as this part of the brain was thought to be implicated in all cases. However, central post-stroke pain is a direct result of damage to the spinothalamocortical system and may typically be described as 'burning', 'shooting' or pricking', or may be felt as a cold, dead, throbbing feeling. It may be triggered and worsened by touch or cold, and is often highly reactive to movement (or lack thereof).

HEMIPLEGIC SHOULDER PAIN

The glenohumeral joint (the joint between the arm and the scapula) is biomechanically unstable because the socket formed by the scapula is too shallow to stabilise the ball-shaped upper part of the humerus. Thus, the shoulder complex is largely controlled by muscles. This design allows for maximum mobility in order to be able to position the hand anywhere within a wide envelope, but at the expense of stability. Paresis and loss of proprioception after stroke may thus render the shoulder complex unstable and prone to damage (Bender and McKenna 2001). Hemiplegic shoulder pain (HSP) is common after stroke, affecting around 25% of stroke survivors (Lindgren et al. 2007, Ratnasabapathy et al. 2003). HSP generally persists (Ratnasabapathy et al. 2003) and, when present, is usually moderate to severe (Lindgren et al. 2007). HSP is more common in people with impaired motor function following a severe stroke, where the glenohumeral joint may be partially dislocated (known as a subluxation). The causes of HSP are poorly understood but are probably multifactorial and may include damage to the capsule surrounding the joint, bursitis, subluxation, rotator-cuff tears (Gardner et al. 2002) and so-called 'shoulder-hand syndrome' (Lo et al. 2003), in which the affected limb is painful, swollen and changed in colour. In many cases, HSP may result from accidental damage caused by incorrect moving and handling, e.g. 'underarm' assistance with transfers or pulling on the affected arm (Pong et al. 2009). It may interfere with rehabilitation, especially with attempting repeated exercises, and can affect sleeping and mood (Kucukdeveci et al. 1996).

Implications for exercise. When delivering exercise classes to stroke survivors with shoulder pain, it is important to seek advice from the person's physiotherapist about the types of movements that may exacerbate the condition. Under no circumstances should the exercise professional pull people with stroke by the arm – whether they have shoulder pain or not – as this is likely to either cause or exacerbate shoulder problems.

OTHER CAUSES OF PAIN

Complex regional pain syndrome is a condition commonly seen in relation to paresis, which may occur in around 10% of people with stroke. The symptoms include pain and inflammation resulting in swelling, redness, heat and stiffness in the affected part. In extreme cases it can result in further paresis, tremors and muscle spasms (Veldman et al. 1993).

Arthritis is an example of a non-stroke-related condition that may cause pain in stroke survivors (Chakour et al. 1996). Arthritic pain symptoms can be exacerbated when combined with the abnormal biomechanics of movement through motor weakness after a stroke. Commonly affected areas include the low back, hip and knee.

Implications for exercise. Adequate analgesia and the performance of exercises in such a way as to minimise painful movements is likely to make exercising more enjoyable for people with stroke, and increase their capacity to improve physical fitness. Exercise professionals should liaise with the stroke survivor's health professional to determine the optimum type and intensity of exercise for people with arthritis.

COMMONLY USED PAIN MANAGEMENT STRATEGIES IN STROKE

Musculoskeletal pain after stroke may be prevented or reduced through correct positioning and alignment during rest and movement (NHS QIS 2011). Simple analgesics such as aspirin or paracetamol may help; sometimes stronger opiate-based medication is required. Whilst anti-inflammatory drugs such as ibuprofen may reduce the symptoms, they are generally avoided because of their multiple side effects, including bleeding from the gastrointestinal tract. Stroke survivors should seek medical advice before taking non-prescribed analgesic drugs.

The optimum treatment for HSP is uncertain. Shoulder strapping may delay onset of pain, but does not decrease it or increase function (Ada et al. 2009). There is insufficient evidence regarding the effectiveness of shoulder slings (Ada et al. 2009), therapeutic exercise, shoulder supports, drugs, local treatments (e.g. steroid injections), other physical treatments (e.g. acupuncture or transcutaneous electrical nerve stimulation) or surgery. Functional electrical stimulation (FES) of muscles around the shoulder can reduce the loss of passive lateral rotation in the shoulder, often associated with HSP, but it has not been shown to prevent or successfully treat this condition (Price and Pandyan 2008).

Central post-stroke pain is often difficult to treat but may respond to antidepressants, anticonvulsants and anti-arryhthmic drugs (Royal College of Physicians 2008a, Scottish Intercollegiate Guidelines Network 2010). First-line treatment is usually a small dose of amitryptiline or gabapentin.

In summary, people with stroke may experience pain to high levels with up to 33% developing HSP, around 25% having symptoms of complex regional pain syndrome, up to 8% having central post-stroke pain and about 50% having generalized musculoskeletal pain.

Implications for exercise. Exercise professionals should be cognisant of the fact that participants with stroke may experience some form of pain, either as a direct consequence of the stroke, or as a secondary problem. Careful assessment and monitoring are therefore required to ensure that exercises are tailored appropriately. If pain worsens, further consultation from the stroke survivor's health-care professional may be necessary.

COGNITIVE PROBLEMS AFTER STROKE

People with stroke may have had cognitive impairment (i.e. problems with mental processes such as thinking, remembering and problem solving) prior to their stroke, which may be worsened as a result of their stroke, while others without prior cognitive impairment may develop it following their stroke. Estimates of the prevalence of cognitive impairment after stroke vary. One study found that 26% had cognitive impairment 1 month post stroke and 21% at 6 and 12 months post stroke (House et al. 1990), while another study of stroke survivors admitted to hospital found a frequency of confusion of 36% (Langhorne et al. 2000). Cognitive impairment may affect a person's ability to participate safely in exercise classes, as will be explained below.

IMPAIRED ATTENTION

In normal circumstances, we can effortlessly select, focus and concentrate on information – or choose to ignore it! Following a stroke, however, the attentional system may be affected, resulting in a reduced ability to take in and process information and remain focused. People with attentional problems may appear drowsy, easily distracted, have difficulty maintaining attention or doing more than one thing at once. People with attentional problems may find it difficult to learn a new task that has several components. They will require guidance and practice within a new environment to master skills and only when they have been given opportunities to practise will they be able to carry out tasks more automatically, with little or no supervision.

Implications for exercise. When exercising in a gym, sensory inputs are likely to be received from multiple sources at any one time (e.g. visual information about other people moving around, verbal instructions from the exercise professional, proprioceptive and tactile information from their own movement). In healthy people, such situations involve competition between signals coming into the attentional system and not all information can be attended to. In stroke survivors in whom attentional capacity is compromised already, multiple sensory inputs may lead to information overload. Individuals with attentional difficulties work better in quieter surroundings with fewer distractions when learning a new skill. It is therefore important to create an environment where undesirable sensory stimuli (such as noise or pain) are kept to a minimum – at least in the early stages of learning new activities. 'Noise' can be introduced when the participant is safe and becoming more skilled. An example is walking and talking at the same time, which requires the person to process information about two tasks simultaneously (known as 'dual tasking').

IMPAIRED MEMORY

Given the high prevalence of attentional difficulties after stroke, it is perhaps not surprising that memory problems may also occur. Memory problems can be manifest in the short term and improve over time, or may remain a long-term problem.

Implications for exercise. Exercise professionals should not assume that stroke survivors will remember instructions, advice or exercises in the same way as their age-matched healthy counterparts, and extra reminders may be required for some individuals. Memory impairments can not only affect the way stroke survivors remember instructions given in the past, but also cause problems when using forward planning – known as prospective memory (e.g. remembering when to come to the next class). There are many ways in which a stroke survivor can be helped with memory difficulties, such as using a diary, visual information (e.g. watching someone carry out a technique) or written instructions, while the occupational therapist may be able to provide tips on how to help such stroke survivors.

EXECUTIVE DYSFUNCTION

Executive dysfunction (also known as dysexecutive function or dysexecutive syndrome) is often seen in people with lesions affecting the frontal lobe, although other brain areas (including the cerebellum) may also be involved. Executive dysfunction indicates a constellation of problems associated with organising and supervising one's behaviour, and has been described *as '... the abilities that enable a person to establish new behaviour patterns and ways of thinking and to introspect upon them'* (Burgess 2003, p. 302).

People with executive dysfunction may have problems with organising and prioritising tasks, starting an activity and distinguishing between relevant and non-relevant information. They may have difficulty planning for future events and estimating the time needed to complete tasks. They may be easily distracted and miss important information, have difficulty shifting attention and can get stuck on a thought. They may become drowsy or unable to sustain alertness unless actively engaged, may process information very slowly or may have trouble slowing down enough to process information effectively. They can often have low tolerance for frustration and be extremely sensitive to criticism. Difficult emotions can quickly become overwhelming and emotional reactions may be intense. Short-term and working memory may be impaired and they may have difficulty regulating their behaviour, including inhibiting unwanted behaviour. With a diminished 'supervisory' function, they can also react impulsively and have difficulty using feedback from others.

Crucially, people affected by executive dysfunction are often unaware of their problems, which may cause upset amongst people around them.

Implications for exercise. Box 3.1 provides some pointers for both exercise professionals and stroke survivors regarding the management of executive dysfunction in an exercise setting.

BOX 3.1 Managing executive dysfunction after stroke in an exercise setting: pointers for exercise professionals and stroke survivors	
Tips for the exercise professional	**Tips for the stroke survivor**
• Goal setting: provide the individual with specific goals to help focus attention • Attention: if a stroke survivor has problems with attention and is easily distracted, choose a quieter time to attend the gym • Reduce noise and other forms of distraction as much as possible • Comprehension check: provide instructions clearly and at a steady pace. Ask the individual to repeat the instructions/information to check their understanding • Feedback: this should be honest and constructive. End sessions on positive aspects of the individual's achievements	• Take a step back – don't rush in. Think about things for a few moments (think about the instructions you have been given for equipment, repetitions, etc.) • Think about what you want to achieve, set yourself a goal • If you have a problem getting started, think again about what you are trying to achieve • Make a list of steps needed to achieve the task • Simplify the task – break it down into small steps, and write them down • Use checklists and always check your work: follow the steps in the correct order, ticking off each one as you have achieved it • Remove distractions if possible • 'Talk' to yourself: at first, whisper, and then talk silently to yourself to remind yourself to stay focused • Use external cues (cue cards, bleeping watches) • Work at your best time of day – not when you are tired • Take breaks • In the middle of tasks, check everything is going according to plan • Check that you have achieved what you want to accomplish • Reward yourself for achieving specific tasks.
Adapted from Powell and Malia (2006) with kind permission of Speechmark Publishing Ltd and Trevor Powell.	

DYSPRAXIA

Dyspraxia is a term used to describe a variety of disorders of movement that are neurologically induced, acquired or developmental in origin (Rothi and Heilman 1997). Damage to the cerebellum, basal ganglia, motor or sensory cortex can all cause problems with movement such as abnormal muscle tone, loss of strength and coordination. Dyspraxia, which is a more complex problem, involves the parietal lobes, corpus callosum and frontal lobes and causes problems with skilled action, i.e. sequenced movements that require practice (Grieve 1999). A stroke survivor with dyspraxia can have problems with everyday tasks such as dressing, putting on glasses and operating equipment – despite having preserved movement and sensation in their limbs. Common problems for stroke survivors with dyspraxia include:

- Perseveration: where the stroke survivor has difficulty moving from one part of an activity to the next (e.g. continually washing face instead of completing the task by drying their face).
- Fragmented responses: where the stroke survivor tends to stop/start continually as the motor planning is disrupted.
- Inappropriate use of objects: using an object for the wrong purpose, e.g. using a toothbrush as a shaver.
- Vocal overflow: where the stroke survivor continually provides a running commentary on what they are doing.
- Right/left confusion: where the stroke survivor has difficulty telling right from left. Stroke survivors with this problem may have difficulty using mirror images of themselves.

So although dyspraxia manifests itself through disordered action, the problem is not one of movement per se. Rather, dyspraxia is a cognitive problem, which may arise in different stages of planning and executing an action, e.g. in integrating sensory information about objects to be used, sequencing the different stages of an activity and knowing when to stop.

Although there is a need for more research into the treatment of dyspraxia, there is evidence that people perform better in a familiar setting with feedback being given to the individual (tactile and proprioceptive) before and during the activity (Bonfils 1996).

Implications for exercise. Dyspraxia may affect a person's ability to imitate movement, and stroke survivors with dyspraxia may have difficulty imitating a demonstration of an exercise. Using equipment for exercises (e.g. Theraband) may be problematic and the exercise professional needs to carefully monitor that stroke survivors with dyspraxia are able to undertake such exercises safely. It may also be beneficial for the exercise professional to spend time with the stroke survivor in the exercise setting to allow familiarisation with equipment, the routine and the exercise plan. A stroke survivor with dyspraxia will often improve with regular practice; however, feedback, activities and routine need to remain similar in order that the activity can become more automatic.

The Psychology Concise Guidelines for Stroke (Royal College of Physicians 2008b) recommend that all stroke survivors with dyspraxia be provided with appropriate interventions to treat or help compensate for specific deficits.

Thus, the exercise professional should liaise with the stroke survivor's occupational therapist to discuss how exercises could be structured to enable better participation in an exercise class.

EMOTIONAL PROBLEMS AFTER STROKE

In a recent survey of stroke survivors in the UK, emotional problems were identified by 39% of respondents as an unmet need after stroke (McKevitt et al. 2010). Emotional problems after stroke include emotional lability (i.e. uncontrolled crying or laughing), mood swings, reduced patience and increased frustration, reduced confidence, more dissatisfaction and a less agreeable nature, depression and anxiety (Stone et al. 2004). Some of these changes may occur as a direct effect of the stroke, others may be a result of the psychosocial impact of the stroke on the life of the survivor and their family. Regardless of the cause, for the exercise professional it is important to have an understanding of and empathy for an individual's emotional difficulties.

The most common types of mood disorders following a stroke are depression, anxiety and emotionalism, which will be described in more detail below.

DEPRESSION

People with depression typically experience low mood, negative thoughts, fatigue, sleep disturbance, changes in appetite and social withdrawal. The prevalence of depression after stroke is around 33% (Hackett et al. 2005), although estimates vary. Depression after stroke may impede recovery and also contributes to carer stress (Berg et al. 2005). Sometimes it can be difficult to diagnose depression after stroke because communication problems such as aphasia make it difficult for stroke survivors to clearly express their feelings.

Depression is not always treated adequately because of uncertainty about whether low mood is really depression, or an 'understandable' reaction to the experience of stroke. If one considers the potential impact of stroke, not just on physical function, but also on autonomy, work, leisure and relationships, it is perhaps not surprising that some stroke survivors develop depression. Additionally, it can be difficult to diagnose depression in stroke survivors with aphasia.

The Cochrane systematic review of interventions for the treatment of depression after stroke demonstrated that antidepressant drugs improve mood, but may cause adverse effects such as confusion and constipation or diarrhoea (Hackett et al. 2008). This review also found that there was little information on the effects of the antidepressants on seizures, falls or delirium – adverse events that are common in older people, or those using a combination of medication for co-morbidities. Compared to standard care, there was no evidence of benefit from any type of psychotherapy (which in this review included cognitive-behavioural therapy and motivational interviewing). This review concluded that there is currently a lack of evidence regarding the best type of routine treatment for depression after stroke. However, in clinical practice, antidepressants are widely used because they are both clinically and cost-effective, while not all stroke services may have access to psychotherapy or counselling services.

ANXIETY

Anxiety is characterised by fear and apprehension, and although it is normal for anyone to experience anxiety from time to time about specific situations, people with an anxiety disorder experience disproportionate apprehension and distress (e.g. palpitations, excessive perspiration or dizziness) during daily events. Stroke survivors suffering from anxiety may report being fearful of having another stroke, having a fall or causing embarrassment in social situations, which in turn may lead to social withdrawal and depression.

Following discharge from hospital after stroke, anxiety symptoms often persist and may actually increase over time (Langhorne et al. 2000). A cross-sectional study found a frequency of anxiety of 21% at 3 months (Barker-Collo 2007) and between 3% and 49% up to 5 years after stroke (Burvill et al. 1995, Langhorne et al. 2000).

There are currently no systematic reviews of the effects of interventions for anxiety after stroke, although a protocol for a Cochrane systematic review to evaluate the effects of pharmacological and psychological treatments has been published (Campbell et al. 2010).

Implications for exercise. For exercise professionals it is important to understand that stroke survivors may be anxious about the risk of another stroke as a result of exercise, or of experiencing a fall. It is important to address such fears and carefully explain the actual risks and benefits to stroke survivors to avoid unnecessary drop-out and withdrawal.

EMOTIONALISM

Emotionalism (also known as emotional lability) is a condition where a person has difficulty moderating their emotional expressions. The emotionally labile stroke survivor may suddenly start to laugh or cry. The trigger to these outbursts may not always be clear, and the emotional response is often out of proportion and sometimes inappropriate given the context in which the outburst takes place. In the eyes of the stroke survivor and their family, these outbursts are often felt to be 'out of character', which can cause further distress. Emotionalism affects about 20–25% of survivors in the first 6 months after stroke, although even at 1 year between 10% and 15% of stroke survivors still experience some emotionalism (Hackett et al. 2010).

A systematic review of all available evidence on treatment for emotionalism after stroke only found trials using antidepressant drugs. These appeared to be effective in reducing symptoms of emotionalism (Hackett et al. 2010), but there was little information on adverse effects. There did not appear to be any randomised controlled trials on psychological interventions for emotionalism after stroke, and further research is required to make recommendations on how best to treat emotionalism after stroke.

Implications for exercise. Exercise professionals should be aware of stroke survivors who have emotionalism, and be sensitive to their needs. Stroke survivors may feel embarrassed when they experience an outburst, and may wish to stop exercising until they are ready to resume. Exercise professionals could ask, in a private moment with an individual stroke survivor, what they would like the exercise professional to do in case they experience an outburst.

OTHER POST-STROKE PROBLEMS

PROBLEMS WITH SPEECH AND LANGUAGE

Communication requires language processing and this can be variably affected after a stroke, depending on the location and severity of the stroke. Many areas of the brain are involved when we are communicating with each other; however, in the majority of individuals it is the left hemisphere that is primarily involved in language processing.

The more severe difficulties in both understanding and expressing ourselves verbally are experienced after a stroke in the left hemisphere.

Language processing involves:

- Understanding what is being said
- Communicating fluently, finding the right words
- Understanding when reading
- Being able to write meaningful messages.

To succeed in all the above tasks, different areas of the brain are activated. For example, the occipital lobe is involved in visual perception and processing as is required in reading and writing, signals are then relayed to the parietal lobe which is involved in interpreting auditory and visual signals; the temporal lobe is involved in the comprehension of speech and the frontal lobe is involved in the planning and production of a verbal response. All these areas have to be working well together to avoid any disruption in the process of communication. A language problem acquired after stroke is known as aphasia (sometimes referred to as dysphasia) and can present in many different ways depending on the nature and severity of the stroke.

In addition to language difficulties, people can present with a motor speech difficulty, which is known as dysarthria. Persisting dysarthria after stroke is more often associated with a sub-cortical, posterior circulation or brainstem stroke where the nerves controlling the muscles of the face, mouth and throat have been affected, resulting in difficulties producing clear, intelligible speech.

Either type of communication disability can be intensely frustrating for the person with stroke. It is important to note the differences between a language disorder (aphasia) and a speech disorder (dysarthria) in order to select the more appropriate strategies to minimise the barriers to communication.

Implications for exercise. Good communication is essential for a successful collaboration between the stroke survivor and the exercise professional. Chapter 7, which is dedicated to the topic of communication, discusses the intricacies of successful communication in more depth and explores the implications of communication impairment for stroke survivors engaging in exercise.

FATIGUE

Fatigue is common after stroke: depending on the population studied and the definition of fatigue used, the prevalence of fatigue after stroke ranges from 16% to 70% (Lynch et al. 2007). In community-dwelling stroke survivors, fatigue is defined as a situation where 'over the past month, there has been at least a two week period when the stroke survivor has experienced fatigue, a lack of energy or an increased need to rest every day or nearly every day'. This fatigue makes taking part in everyday activities difficult (Lynch et al. 2007). In a recent needs survey amongst stroke survivors in the UK, 43% of respondents identified fatigue as one of their 'unmet needs' (McKevitt et al. 2010).

The literature on fatigue in neurological conditions sometimes differentiates between central fatigue (implying a problem with the brain) and peripheral fatigue (implying a problem with the muscles). It is unclear whether this conceptual framework for fatigue after stroke is appropriate. Some stroke survivors say that their fatigue is more 'mental' than 'physical' whilst some say it is a combination of mental and physical fatigue, and others do not differentiate between mental and physical fatigue.

Fatigue after stroke seems to be more common in stroke survivors who had fatigue before their stroke (Choi-Kwon et al. 2005) and it has been found to be associated with depression (de Groot et al. 2003) – though whether fatigue causes depression or whether depression causes fatigue is uncertain. One large study of stroke survivors found associations between fatigue and lower mood, being older and being female, but together these factors explained only about 30% of the variation in fatigue. This suggests that other factors, as yet not identified, may also contribute to fatigue after stroke (Mead et al. 2011). Fatigue is found even in those who are highly motivated to exercise. Further research is required to investigate factors associated with fatigue and how best to treat it.

One interesting theory is that fatigue may be related to physical deconditioning which is common after stroke (see chapter 4). It is also possible that fatigue is related to a reduction in information processing capacity. We have already seen that a stroke may impair attention and memory. In addition, it is worth remembering that, after a stroke, many activities that were previously automatic (e.g. getting dressed, walking or talking) need to be relearned. This process places an additional burden on the already diminished resources for attention and memory, rendering previously automatic tasks effortful. In summary, 'fatigue' is a complex phenomenon, comprising both physical and psychological dimensions.

Currently there is no known treatment for fatigue. Generally, physicians identify any reversible medical cause (e.g. anaemia, hypothyroidism), determine whether or not the stroke survivor has depression, and review whether any specific medication may be causing fatigue. They may also suggest a gradual increase in physical activity as a treatment for fatigue, although whether this is effective is not yet known.

Implications for exercise. The presence of fatigue may influence the stroke survivor's ability to participate in exercise. Exercise professionals should, therefore, bear in mind that the starting level and the rate of progression need to be adapted to stroke survivors, taking into account the high level of fatigue in this group.

SEIZURES

A hospital-based study found that 8.9% of stroke survivors with stroke had seizures within 9 months and that haemorrhagic stroke and cortical location were risk factors for seizures (Bladin et al. 2000). In the Oxfordshire

Community Stroke Project (Bamford et al. 1991), the risk of a first seizure, excluding those occurring at the time of stroke onset, was 5% in the first year after stroke and 1–2% thereafter. Around half of stroke survivors who have a seizure after stroke will go on to have a recurrent one.

Generally most doctors start anticonvulsants only after a second seizure, because of the side effects of these drugs.

Implications for exercise. It is important for exercise professionals to check whether a participant has had seizures, or is taking anticonvulsant drugs, and know what to do in case someone experiences a seizure.

FALLS, OSTEOPOROSIS AND FRACTURES

Falls

Falls are common after discharge from hospital, with estimates of the proportion of stroke survivors having a fall ranging from half (Mackintosh et al. 2005) to three-quarters (Forster and Young 1995) in the first 6 months after discharge. There are multiple reasons why stroke survivors fall, including stroke-related factors (e.g. muscle weakness, reduced reaction time, lack of balance and coordination, and loss of awareness of body schema), environmental factors (e.g. ill-fitting or inappropriate footwear, slippery floors, inadequate supervision) and drugs (e.g. sedatives and anti-hypertensives). Less than 5% of falls result in serious injury, but fear of falls and loss of confidence is common (Nyberg and Gustafson 1995).

Although further research is required in this area, there are some interesting preliminary data suggesting that group exercise programmes that include agility exercises may reduce the risk of falls (Marigold et al. 2005). One small study found that low-dose vitamin D reduces falls risk and also hip fractures in women after stroke (Sato et al. 2005a), possibly by increasing muscle strength. English and Hillier (2010) undertook a review of circuit class therapy to improve mobility after stroke, and found that there were more falls in the intervention group than in the control group during the delivery of the circuit class therapy. This was attributed to the fact that the circuit class challenged balance function. However, none of the falls were serious, but this review demonstrates that the risk of falls from participation in exercise should be carefully evaluated.

Osteoporosis and fractures

Osteoporosis, particularly on the hemiparetic side, may occur in stroke survivors with reduced mobility due to reduced weight bearing, leading to a reduction of the bone mineral demand from the bone. Within 2 years following stroke, the risk of fracture is 4% and the risk of hip fracture is 1.1% (Dennis et al. 2002). This is 1.4 times the rate of hip fracture in the general population. Fracture risk is increased after stroke because stroke survivors are at risk of both falls and of developing osteoporosis.

Bisphosphonates may reduce fracture risk, either when given as a single dose intravenously (Poole et al. 2007) or as daily dose post stroke (Sato et al. 2005b). Further trials of bisphosphonates after stroke are being planned to try to confirm these findings in a larger group of stroke survivors.

Implications for exercise. Exercise professionals should put design measures in place (e.g. adaptations to pace, transitions between exercises and direction changes, etc.) to minimise the risk of falls for stroke survivors. These, together with other measures (e.g. removing clutter, using adequate lighting) will be further discussed in chapter 9.

CO-MORBIDITIES

INTRODUCTION

Co-morbidities can be defined as one or more diagnosable medical conditions which exist in addition to the most significant condition. Stroke survivors may well have one or more co-morbidities which must be taken into consideration when delivering exercise.

An extensive review of all possible co-morbidities is beyond the scope of this chapter. We shall concentrate on the most common and important co-morbidities that are likely to be experienced by a stroke survivor attending exercise classes, based on the co-morbidities that we reported in the STARTER trial (Mead et al. 2007). We will discuss their management, their relevance to the safe delivery of exercise, and we will give *general* advice about how they should be managed in an exercise setting. Please note the important recommendation in Box 3.2.

BOX 3.2 Recommendation regarding the management of co-morbidities in the context of exercise after stroke

We strongly recommend that, should an exercise professional have any uncertainties about the influence of any co-morbidity on the delivery of exercise to individual stroke survivors, they *must* consult with the referring health-care professional before prescribing exercise.

HYPERTENSION

Blood pressure is determined by how much blood the heart pumps and how much resistance there is to blood flow. Hypertension (high blood pressure) is defined as a systolic blood pressure of more than 140 mmHg and a diastolic blood pressure of more than 80 mmHg. Most people with high blood pressure have no symptoms whatsoever, and in more than 90% of people no cause can be found.

There are several different types of medication that can be used to reduce high blood pressure. The common ones include thiazide diuretics, angiotensin converting enzyme (ACE) inhibitors, calcium antagonists, beta-blockers and centrally acting drugs such as alpha blockers.

During an exercise class, it is highly unlikely that hypertension per se will cause any symptoms. It is more likely that that the drugs used to treat hypertension may cause problems. For example, many of the antihypertensive drugs have the potential to cause postural hypotension and dizziness, which can be risks especially when changing position (e.g. rising to stand). Patients taking beta-blockers will not experience the usual increase in heart rate with exercise, which means that pulse rate cannot be used to monitor the intensity of exercise.

ISCHAEMIC HEART DISEASE

This is characterised by reduced blood supply to the heart, usually due to narrowing of the arteries that supply the heart muscle. The most important clinical manifestations of ischaemic heart disease are:

- Angina
- Acute coronary events (including heart attacks)
- Cardiac failure
- Cardiac arrthymias (the most common of which is atrial fibrillation)

It has been estimated that up to 75% of people after stroke will have co-existing cardiac disease (Gordon et al. 2004), some of which may be 'silent', i.e. cause no symptoms. Whilst exercise is of benefit to patients with ischaemic heart disease (as it is after stroke), exercise may carry risks, particularly if it is vigorous. Stroke survivors should seek advice from their general practitioner before attending classes, and undergo a thorough assessment as detailed in chapter 9.

ANGINA

The most common symptom of angina is central chest pain (or ache) on exertion which is relieved by rest, though the pain may only affect the arm or jaw, and occasionally the only symptom may be breathlessness on exertion.

The management of angina includes drugs, usually aspirin and glyceryl trinitrate (GTN) spray. Some people may also require cholesterol lowering drugs, isosorbide mononitrate, nitrate patches, beta-blockers, calcium antagonists and potassium channel activators (e.g. nicorandil). Some patients may also undergo angioplasty (whereby a 'balloon' is inserted into the narrowed artery and then inflated), stenting (a metal 'cylinder' which is placed inside the artery to stop it from closing) or a coronary artery bypass.

Generally speaking, stroke survivors should exercise within the limitations of their angina. Some patients may be advised to take their GTN spray before exercise. Should a stroke survivor develop angina during an exercise class, the exercise professional should stop the exercise, ask the stroke survivor to sit down, and suggests he/she take a GTN spray (if used). The spray should be used at 5 minute intervals up to three times, but, if there is no relief, the exercise professional should call for an emergency ambulance.

ACUTE CORONARY EVENTS

Acute coronary events, including heart attacks, are characterised by severe central chest pain, unrelieved by rest, and which are often associated with nausea and sweating, and are usually caused by formation of a blood clot on a narrowed artery supplying the heart muscle. Clearly, if the stroke survivor develops symptoms of an acute coronary event during an exercise class, the exercise professional should call for an emergency ambulance.

CARDIAC FAILURE

Cardiac failure is characterised by breathlessness (on exertion and/or lying down), and ankle swelling. Fatigue is also a common symptom of cardiac failure. Treatment includes diuretics, ACE inhibitors, spironolactone, beta-blockers, and, for patients in atrial fibrillation, digoxin. The breathlessness and fatigue are likely to limit exercise tolerance and therefore the exercise programme should be tailored accordingly. The drugs used for treatment of cardiac failure may induce postural hypotension, which may cause dizziness during exercise classes.

ARRHYTHMIAS (OR ABNORMAL HEART RHYTHM)

The most common arrhythmia is atrial fibrillation. Symptoms include palpitations, breathlessness and fatigue, although atrial fibrillation often causes no symptoms at all. Medical management includes aspirin or warfarin (to reduce the risk of stroke) and digoxin (to prevent the heart rate from rising too high). Other arrhythmias include heart block (which may require treatment with a pacemaker). Providing the pacemaker is working normally, there should be no particular problems for stroke survivors attending exercise classes. Less common arrhythmias include ventricular tachycardia (fast and regular rhythm originating from the ventricle). This is a serious rhythm which may cause chest pain, breathlessness and palpitations, and may lead to ventricular fibrillation which can be fatal. Patients who have had previous episodes of ventricular tachycardia would almost certainly be taking medication to prevent further episodes.

DIABETES MELLITUS

Diabetes mellitus is defined as a metabolic disorder of multiple aetiology characterised by chronic hyperglycaemia with disturbances of carbohydrate, protein and fat metabolism resulting from defects in insulin secretion, insulin action, or both. The clinical diagnosis of diabetes is often indicated by the presence of symptoms such as polyuria (passing large volumes of urine, in the adult >2.5 litres per day), polydipsia (drinking large volumes of liquid) and unexplained weight loss, and is confirmed by measurement of abnormally high blood glucose (hyperglycaemia). Diabetes increases the risk of vascular disease including stroke and ischaemic heart disease. Exercise may help normalise blood sugar levels and reduce the risk of vascular complications.

Drugs given to patients with diabetes include insulin and/or oral medication to reduce blood sugar. The main side effect of treatment is hypoglycaemia, i.e. low blood sugar. This may be characterised by dizziness, faintness or sweating, and, if left untreated, may progress to coma and death.

Exercising muscles require additional glucose, which means that exercise may precipitate hypoglycaemia ('hypo'). Stroke survivors with diabetes should seek medical advice before taking up exercise classes. Various strategies can be used to reduce the risk of hypoglycaemia during a class, including reducing the usual insulin dose prior to exercise, taking additional carbohydrate before exercise and avoiding injecting insulin into exercising muscles, as this increases the absorption of insulin and so the risk of hypogly-caemia. Although advice on the management of individual stroke survivors will vary, one reasonable approach is to check the blood sugar twice before exercise (30 minutes apart); if less than 5.5 mmol/l the stroke survivor should ingest carbohydrate, check blood sugar immediately afterwards and again 30 minutes later. If the stroke survivor is new to exercise or increasing the exer-cise duration, blood sugar should be checked every 30 minutes.

Hypoglycaemia in patients with diabetes can present with shaking, confusion and aggressive behaviour. Should a stroke survivor develop symp-toms of a 'hypo' during an exercise class, they should stop the exercise and take oral carbohydrate. If the stroke survivor becomes unconscious, this is a medical emergency and he/she requires intravenous glucose or intramus-cular glucagon, which stimulates the liver to release glucose. The exercise professional should call for an emergency ambulance and inform emergency services that the stroke survivor is diabetic.

Should stroke survivors have 'hypos' during classes, they should discuss with their doctor whether further changes are required to their insulin or oral hypoglycaemic drugs. It is important to remember that beta-blocker drugs may attenuate symptoms of hypoglycaemia. This means that if a diabetic per-son is taking a beta-blocker, they may become hypoglycaemic without the usual 'warning' signs such as sweating and dizziness.

Exercise may also precipitate hyperglycaemia. If pre-exercise blood glucose levels are >13 mmol/l, one should not exercise; if pre-exercise blood glucose levels are 10–13 mmol/l, levels should be checked again 10 minutes after starting exercise and people should only continue if the level has fallen.

ARTHRITIS

Osteoarthritis is the most common form of arthritis, which becomes more common as people get older. It can affect the hands, feet, spine, hips, knees and feet. Its exact cause is uncertain. The main symptoms are pain and stiff-ness. Treatment includes simple analgesics such as paracetamol, non-steroidal anti-inflammatory drugs, local steroid injections, braces and joint replace-ment. Aerobic and strengthening exercises seem to improve pain and func-tion to a similar extent to non-steroidal anti-inflammatory drugs (Bischoff and Roos 2003), without the side effects. Hence, if stroke survivors also have arthritis, they can be reassured that exercise may well improve their arthritic pain. This needs to be carefully monitored in class, however, and if symptoms exacerbate, the stroke survivor should be advised to consult their referring health-care professional.

ASTHMA

Asthma is a clinical diagnosis. Central to all definitions is the presence of symptoms (more than one of wheeze, breathlessness, chest tightness, cough) and of variable airflow obstruction. Treatment includes inhaled bronchodi-lators, inhaled steroids and oral steroids. Some patients seem to experience worsening of their asthma during exercise – the term exercise-induced asthma is used to describe these patients, but frequently it is expression of poorly controlled asthma and, therefore, regular treatment including inhaled steroids should be reviewed.

The exercise professional should seek advice from the general practitioner about how to manage a stroke survivor's asthma in the context of exercise. Generally speaking, the stroke survivor should not exercise if their asthma is poorly controlled. If the asthma is well controlled, one reasonable approach is to take bronchodilator medication about 10 minutes prior to exercise. If the stroke survivor develops asthma during an exercise class, he/she should stop the exercise, take his/her bronchodilator medication, and only start exercise again if symptoms resolve. If the symptoms return, the stroke survivor should stop exercise again and seek medical advice before exercising again.

CHRONIC OBSTRUCTIVE PULMONARY DISEASE

Chronic obstructive pulmonary disease (COPD) is a term used for a number of conditions, including chronic bronchitis and emphysema. COPD leads to damaged airways in the lungs, causing them to become narrower and making it harder for air to get in and out of the lungs. The word 'chronic' means that the problem is long term. Exercise may improve symptoms of COPD – and, indeed, pulmonary rehabilitation services are being set up that are based on exercise. A typical pulmonary rehabilitation course includes a physical exercise programme, carefully designed for each individual, giving advice on lung health and coping with breathlessness, and a friendly, supportive atmosphere (British Lung Foundation 2011).

If a stroke survivor has COPD, they are likely to become more breathless during exercise than a stroke survivor without COPD, so this needs to be taken into account when tailoring the exercise programme. There may be benefit in the stroke survivor taking inhaled bronchodilators 30 minutes before exercise, as for asthma.

PSYCHOSOCIAL ISSUES AFTER STROKE

To many stroke survivors, a stroke means a crisis. In chapter 8, John Brown poignantly and eloquently describes how a stroke affected his life – and how rebuilding it, with the support of loved ones and professionals, took years of determination, patience and sheer hard work. Others who have experienced a stroke have also indicated that life needs to be 'reconstructed' after stroke (Reed et al. 2010). Psychosocial issues, including socio-economic difficulties, are amongst the most enduring factors affecting life after stroke. A survey of stroke survivor needs, undertaken by The Stroke Association in the UK (McKevitt et al. 2010), provides a stark overview of unmet needs. The most commonly reported were: memory problems, fatigue, concentration problems, emotional difficulties and reading difficulties.

As we have seen above, some post-stroke problems are caused by the direct impact of the stroke; however, for many stroke survivors, a complex interaction between biological, psychological, social and economic factors is at play. For example, a person who has physically recovered well enough to return to work may find that their executive dysfunction (a direct effect of the stroke) renders a job that requires initiative and planning unsustainable. Feeling dejected and hopeless, the person spirals into depression and becomes withdrawn and inactive. This inactivity starts to affect their physical function and confidence, making it even harder for them to engage in activity, while a lack of income reduces their financial resources required to attend leisure facilities.

The overview of post-stroke problems in this chapter is intended to make exercise professionals more aware of the complexities of life after stroke and more sensitive towards the needs of stroke survivors. The experiences of stroke survivors participating in exercise programmes designed for people with stroke indicate that these were instrumental in helping them rebuild their confidence and self-esteem, creating a safe and enjoyable environment where they felt supported to work on their own recovery (Carin-Levy et al. 2009, Reed et al. 2010, Sharma et al. 2011). Through the provision of such opportunities, exercise professionals can make an important contribution to the lives of stroke survivors.

SUMMARY POINTS

- A stroke may impact on a myriad of functions, either directly, as a result of the brain lesion, or indirectly, e.g. as a result of reduced mobility.
- With stroke affecting the brain as an information processing system, the exercise professional should not only consider the demands that physical activity places on the cardiorespiratory and musculoskeletal systems, but also on perceptual and cognitive systems.
- Some impairments (e.g. reduced movement) are directly visible, but others (e.g. impaired attention, memory or understanding) may be more 'hidden'. To ensure that stroke survivors are able to engage safely in physical activity, exercise professionals need to anticipate and carefully monitor any potential difficulties, and tailor activities as appropriate. The following questions may serve to prompt the exercise professional to look out for any – visible or invisible – impairments, e.g.:
  - Is the stroke survivor able to hear and understand the instructions, or could this be impaired by hearing impairment, aphasia or cognitive impairment?
  - Can they fully see the professional and the equipment – or is there a visual impairment, or hemispatial neglect?
  - When using equipment, is the stroke survivor put at risk by any perceptual impairment, or by dyspraxia?
  - Does the stroke survivor have spasticity that affects their safety (e.g. their ability to keep their foot on the bicycle pedal, or their hand on the handlebar)?
  - If the stroke survivor experiences any shoulder pain, is the exercise safe? If so, how does their pain respond to exercise?
  - Is the stroke survivor keeping to their number of repetitions, or does their executive dysfunction interfere?
- Psychosocial issues, including socio-economic difficulties, are amongst the most enduring factors affecting health and wellbeing after stroke, through a complex bio-psychosocial and economic interplay of factors. It is important for exercise professionals to be aware of such issues, in

order to develop a deeper understanding of the needs of their participants and their families.

- Stroke survivors may have co-existing health conditions (co-morbidities) such as heart disease or diabetes, which may also impact on their ability to engage in physical activity. Advice from referring health-care professionals is required for exercise professionals to safely tailor exercises to suit individuals with stroke and co-morbidities.
- We have discussed the management of co-morbidities and their relevance to the safe delivery of exercise. We have given *general* advice about how they should be managed in an exercise setting. We strongly recommend that, should an exercise professional have any uncertainties about the influence of these co-morbidities on the delivery of exercise to individual stroke survivors, they must consult with the referring clinical team before prescribing exercise.

Chapters 9 and 10 will present further detail on how to prepare, design and implement an exercise programme for people with stroke.

REFERENCES

Ada, L., Foongchomcheay, A., Canning, C.G., 2009. Supportive devices for preventing and treating subluxation of the shoulder after stroke. Cochrane Database Syst. Rev. 1, CD003863. doi:10.1002/14651858.

Ada, L., Dean, C.M., Hall, J.M., et al., 2003. A treadmill and overground walking program improves walking in persons residing in the community after stroke: a placebo-controlled, randomized trial. Arch. Phys. Med. Rehabil. 84, 1486–1491.

Andrews, A., Bohannon, R., 2000. Distribution of muscle strength impairments following stroke. Clin. Rehabil. 14, 79–87.

Archambault, P., Pigeon, P., Feldman, A.G., et al., 1999. Recruitment and sequencing of different degrees of freedom during pointing movements involving the trunk in healthy and hemiparetic subjects. Exp. Brain Res. 126, 55.

Baer, G., Durward, D., 2004. Stroke. In: Stokes, M. (Ed.), Physical management in neurological rehabilitation, second ed. Elsevier Mosby, London, pp. 75–102.

Bamford, J., Sandercock, P., Dennis, M., et al., 1991. Classification and natural history of clinically identifiable subtypes of cerebral infarction. Lancet 337, 1521–1526.

Barker-Collo, S.L., 2007. Depression and anxiety 3 month post-stroke: prevalence and correlates. Arch. Clin. Neuropsychol. 22, 519–531.

Barnes, M.P., 2001. An overview of the clinical management of spasticity. In: Barnes, M.P., Johnson, G.R. (Eds.), Upper motor neuron syndrome and spasticity. Clinical management and neurophysiology. Cambridge University Press, Cambridge, pp. 1–11.

Bender, L., McKenna, K., 2001. Hemiplegic shoulder pain: defining the problem and its management. Disabil. Rehabil. 23, 698–705.

Berg, A., Palomäki, H., Lönnqvist, J., et al., 2005. Depression among caregivers of stroke survivors. Stroke 36, 639–643.

Bischoff, H.A., Roos, E.M., 2003. Effectiveness and safety of strengthening, aerobic and co-ordination exercises for patients with osteoarthritis. Curr. Opin. Rheumatol. 15, 141–144.

Bladin, C.F., Alexandrov, A.V., Bellavance, A., et al., 2000. Seizures after stroke, a prospective multicenter study. Arch. Neurol. 57, 1617–1622.

Bobath, B., 1990. Adult hemiplegia: evaluation and treatment. Butterworth-Heinemann, Oxford.

Boissy, P., Bourbonnais, D., Carlotti, M.M., et al., 1999. Maximal grip force in chronic stroke subjects and its relationship to global upper extremity function. Clin. Rehabil. 13, 354–362.

Bonan, I.V., Yelnik, A.P., Colle, F.M., et al., 2004. Reliance on visual information after stroke. Part II: Effectiveness of a balance rehabilitation program with visual cue deprivation after stroke: a randomised controlled trial. Arch. Phys. Med. Rehabil. 85, 274–278.

Bonfils, K.B., 1996. The Affolter approach to treatment: a perceptual-cognitive perspective of function. In: Pedretti, L.W. (Ed.), Occupational therapy: practice skills for physical dysfunction. Mosby, St Louis.

Borges, C.A.S., Castao, K.C., Souto, P.A., et al., 2009. Effect of resisted exercise on muscular strength, spasticity and functionality in chronic hemiparetic subjects: a systematic review. J. Appl. Res. 9, 147–158.

Bowen, A., Lincoln, N.B., Dewey, M., 2003. Cognitive rehabilitation for spatial neglect following stroke (Cochrane Review). The Cochrane Library, Issue 1, 2003. Oxford. Update Software.

Bowsher, D., 2001. Stroke and central post-stroke pain in an elderly population. J. Pain 5, 258–261.

Bowsher, D., 2005. Allodynia in relation to lesion site in central post-stroke pain. J. Pain 6, 736–740.

British Lung Foundation 2011. Available online at http://www.lunguk.org/you-and-your-lungs/diagnosis-and-treatment/pulmonary-rehabilitation (accessed 09.09.2011).

Burgess, P.W., 2003. Assessment of executive function. In: Halligan, P.W., Kischka, U., Marshall, J.C. (Eds.), Handbook of clinical neuropsychology. Oxford University Press, Oxford, pp. 302–321.

Burridge, J.H., Taylor, P.N., Swain, I.D., 1998. A review of the literature published for the correction of peroneal nerve stimulation for the correction of dropped foot. Rev. Clin. Gerontol. 8, 155–161.

Burridge, J.H., McLellan, D.L., 2000. Relation between abnormal patterns of muscle activation and response to common peroneal nerve stimulation in paraplegia. J. Neurol. Neurosurg. Psychiatry 69, 353–361.

Burvill, P.W., Johnson, G.A., Jamrozik, K.D., et al., 1995. Anxiety disorders after stroke: results from the Perth Community Stroke Study. Br. J. Psychiatry 166, 328–332.

Byl, N., Roderick, J., Mohamed, O., et al., 2003. Effectiveness of sensory and motor rehabilitation of the upper limb following the principles of neuroplasticity: patients stable poststroke. Neurorehabil. Neural Repair 17, 176–191.

Cambier, D.C., de Corte, E., Danneels, L.A., et al., 2003. Treating sensory impairments in the post-stroke upper limb with intermittent pneumatic compression. Results of a preliminary trial. Clin. Rehabil. 17, 14–20.

Campbell Burton, C.A., Knapp, P., Holmes, J., et al., 2010. Interventions for treating anxiety after stroke. Cochrane Database Syst. Rev. 12, CD008860. doi:10.1002/14651858.

Carey, L.M., 1995. Somatosensory loss after stroke. Crit. Rev. Phys. Rehabil. Med. 7, 51–91.

Carey, L.M., Abbott, D.F., Egan, G.F., et al., 2005. Motor impairment and recovery in the upper limb after stroke: behavioral and neuroanatomical correlates. Stroke 36, 625–629.

Carin-Levy, G., Kendall, M., Young, A., et al., 2009. The psychosocial effects of exercise and relaxation classes for persons surviving a stroke. Can. J. Occup. Ther. 76, 73–80.

Carr, J., Shepherd, R., 2003. Stroke rehabilitation. Guidelines for exercise and training to optimise motor skill. Elsevier Butterworth Heinemann, Oxford.

Chakour, M.C., Gibson, S.J., Bradbeer, M., et al., 1996. The effect of age on Aδ- and C-fibre thermal pain perception. Pain 64, 143–152.

Chen, J.I., Ha, B., Bushnell, M.C., et al., 2002. Differentiating noxious- and innocuous-related activation of human somatosensory cortices using temporal analysis of fMRI. J. Neurophysiol. 88, 464–474.

Choi-Kwon, S., Han, S.W., Kwon, S.U., et al., 2005. Post-stroke fatigue: characteristics and related factors. Cerebrovasc. Dis. 19, 84–90.

Choi-Kwon, S., Choi, J.M., Kwon, S.U., et al., 2006. Factors that affect the quality of life at 3 years post-stroke. J. Clin. Neurol. 2, 34–41.

Davis, E.C., Barnes, M.P., 2001. The use of botulinum toxin in spasticity. In: Barnes, M.P., Johnson, G.R. (Eds.), Upper motor neuron syndrome and spasticity. Clinical management and neurophysiology. Cambridge University Press, Cambridge, pp. 206–222.

de Groot, M.H., Phillips, S.J., Eskes, G.A., 2003. Fatigue associated with stroke and other neurologic conditions: implications for stroke rehabilitation. Arch. Phys. Med. Rehabil. 84, 1714–1720.

Dennis, M.S., Lo, K.M., McDowall, M., et al., 2002. Fractures after stroke. Frequency, type and associations. Stroke 33, 728.

De Souza, L.H., 1983. The effects of sensation and motivation on regaining movement control following stroke. Physiotherapy 69, 238–240.

Edwards, S., 2002. Abnormal tone and movement as a result of neurological impairment: considerations for treatment. In: Edwards, S. (Ed.), Neurological physiotherapy. A problem-solving approach. Churchill Livingstone, Edinburgh.

English, C., Hillier, S.L., 2010. Circuit class therapy for improving mobility after stroke. Cochrane Database Syst. Rev. 7, CD007513. doi:10.1002/14651858.

French, B., Thomas, L.H., Leathley, M.J., et al., 2007. Repetitive task training for improving functional ability after stroke. Cochrane Database Syst. Rev. 4, CD006073. doi:10.1002/14651858.

Feys, H.M., De Weerdt, W.J., Selz, B.E., et al., 1998. Effect of a therapeutic intervention for hemiplegic upper limb in the acute phase after stroke: a single-blind, randomized, controlled multicenter trial. Stroke 29, 785.

Forster, A., Young, J., 1995. Incidence and consequence of falls due to stroke: a systematic review. BMJ 311, 83–86.

Gardner, M.J., Ong, B.C., Liporace, F., et al., 2002. Orthopedic issues after cerebrovascular accident. Am. J. Orthop 10, 559–568.

Grieve, J., 1999. Neuropsychology for occupational therapists, second ed. Blackwell Publishing, Oxford.

Gordon, C., Hewer, R.L., Wade, D.T., 1987. Dysphagia in acute stroke. Br. Med. J. (Clin. Res. Ed.) 295, 411–414. doi:10.1136/bmj.295.6595.411.

Gordon, N.F., Gulanick, M., Costa, F., et al., 2004. Physical activity and exercise recommendations for stroke survivors: An American Heart Association scientific statement from the Council on Clinical Cardiology, Subcommittee on Exercise, Cardiac Rehabilitation, and Prevention; the Council on Cardiovascular Nursing; the Council on Nutrition, Physical Activity, and Metabolism; and the Stroke Council. Circulation 109, 2031–2041.

Hackett, M.L., Yapa, C., Parag, V., et al., 2005. Frequency of depression after stroke: a systematic review of observational studies. Stroke 36, 1330–1340.

Hackett, M.L., Anderson, C.S., House, A., et al., 2008. Interventions for treating depression after stroke. Cochrane Database Syst. Rev. 4, CD003437. doi:10.1002/14651858.

Hackett, M.L., Yang, M., Anderson, C.S., et al., 2010. Pharmaceutical interventions for emotionalism after stroke. Cochrane Database Syst. Rev. 2, CD003690. doi:10.1002/14651858.

Heckmann, J.G., Stössel, C., Lang, C.J.G., et al., 2005. Taste disorders in acute stroke: a prospective observational study on taste disorders in 102 stroke patients. Stroke 36, 1690–1694.

House, A., Dennis, M., Warlow, C., et al., 1990. The relationship between intellectual impairment and mood disorder in the first year after stroke. Psychol. Med. 20, 805–814.

Jackson, J., 2004. Specific treatment techniques. In: Stokes, M. (Ed.), Physical management in neurological rehabilitation. Elsevier Mosby, Edinburgh, pp. 393–412.

Jönsson, A.C., Lindgren, I., Hallström, B., et al., 2006. Prevalence and intensity of pain after stroke: a population based study focusing on patients' perspectives. J. Neurol. Neurosurg. Psychiatry 77, 590–595.

Katalinic, O.M., Harvey, L.A., Herbert, R.D., et al., 2010. Stretch for the treatment and prevention of contractures. Cochrane Database Syst. Rev 9, CD007455. doi:10.1002/14651858.

Kong, K.H., Woon, V.C., Yang, S.Y., 2004. Prevalence of chronic pain and its impact on health-related quality of life in stroke survivors. Arch. Phys. Med. Rehabil. 85, 35–40.

Kucukdeveci, A.A., Tenant, P.H., Chamberlain, M.A., 1996. Sleep problems in stroke patients: relationship with shoulder pain. Clin. Rehabil. 10, 166–172.

Langhorne, P., Stott, D.J., Robertson, L., et al., 2000. Medical complications after stroke. A multicentre study. Stroke 31, 1223–1229.

Langhorne, P., Coupar, F., Pollock, A., et al., 2009. Motor recovery after stroke: a systematic review. Lancet Neurol 8, 741–754.

Lannin N.A., Cusick A., McCluskey A., et al., 2007. Effects of splinting on wrist contracture after stroke. A randomized controlled trial. Stroke 38, 111–116.

Lannin, N.A., Herbert, R.D., 2003. Is hand splinting effective for adults following stroke? A systematic review and methodological critique of published research. Clin. Rehabil. 17, 807–816.

Laufer, Y., 2004. The use of walking aids in the rehabilitation of stroke patients. Rev. Clin. Gerontol. 14, 137–144.

Lindgren, I., Jönsson, A., Norrving, B., et al., 2007. Shoulder pain after stroke a prospective population-based study. Stroke 38, 343–348.

Lo, S.F., Chen, S.Y., Lin, H.C., et al., 2003. Arthrographic and clinical findings in patients with hemiplegic shoulder pain. Arch. Phys. Med. Rehabil. 84, 1786–1791.

Lynch, J., Mead, G., Greig, C., et al., 2007. Fatigue after stroke: the development and evaluation of a case definition. J. Psychosom. Res. 63, 539–544.

Mackay, J., Mensah, G., 2004. Atlas of heart disease and stroke. World Health Organisation Press, Geneva.

Mackintosh, S.F., Hill, K., Dod, K.J., et al., 2005. Falls and injury prevention should be part of every stroke rehabilitation plan. Clin. Rehabil. 19, 441–451.

Manly, T., Robertson, I.H., 2003. The rehabilitation of attentional deficits. In: Halligan, P.W., Kischka, U., Marshall, J.C. (Eds.), Handbook of clinical neuropsychology. Oxford University Press, Oxford, pp. 89–107.

Marigold, D.S., Eng, J.J., Dawson, A.S., et al., 2005. Exercise leads to faster postural reflexes, improved balance and mobility and fewer falls in older persons with chronic stroke. J. Am. Geriatr. Soc. 53, 416–423.

Mead, G., Greig, C.A., Cunningham, I., et al., 2007. STroke: A Randomised Trial of Exercise or Relaxation (STARTER). J. Am. Geriatr. Soc. 55, 892–899.

Mead, G.E., Graham, C., Dorman, P., et al., 2011. Fatigue after stroke: baseline predictors and influence on survival. Analysis of data from UK patients recruited in the International Stroke Trial. PLoS One 6, e16988.

Mehrholz, J., Platz, T., Kugler, J., et al., 2008. Electromechanical and robot-assisted arm training for improving arm function and activities of daily living after stroke. Cochrane Database Syst. Rev. 4, CD006876. doi:10.1002/14651858.

Michael, K.M., Allen, J.K., Macko, R.F., 2005. Reduced ambulatory activity after stroke: the role of balance, gait and cardiovascular fitness. Arch. Phys. Med. Rehabil. 86, 1552–1556.

Michaelsen S.M., Dannenbaum R., Levin M.F., 2006. Task-specific training with trunk restraint on arm recovery in stroke randomized control trial. Stroke 37, 186–192.

Mortenson, P.A., Eng, J.J., 2003. The use of casts in the management of joint mobility and hypertonia following brain injury in adults: a systematic review. Phys. Ther. 83, 648–658.

NHS QIS, 2011. Pain management following acute stroke. Best practice statement 2011. NHS Quality Improvement Scotland. Available online at http://www.gla. ac.uk/media/media_193827_en.pdf (accessed 09.09.2011).

Nudo, R.J., Barbay, S., Kleim, J.A., 2000. Role of neuroplasticity in functional recovery after stroke. In: Levin, H.S., Grafman, J. (Eds.), Cerebral reorganisation of function after brain damage. Oxford University Press, New York, pp. 168–200.

Nyberg, L., Gustafson, Y., 1995. Patient falls in stroke rehabilitation, a challenge to rehabilitation strategies. Stroke 26, 838–842.

Pandyan, A.D., Cameron, M., Powell, J., 2003. Contractures in the post-stroke wrist: a pilot study of its time course of development and its association with upper limb recovery. Clin. Rehabil. 17, 88–95.

Pandyan, A.D., Gregoric, M., Barnes, M.P., et al., 2005. Spasticity: clinical perceptions, neurological realities and meaningful measurement. Disabil. Rehabil. 27, 2–6.

Pomeroy, V.M., King, L.M., Pollock, A., et al., 2006. Electrostimulation for promoting recovery of movement or functional ability after stroke. Cochrane Database Syst. Rev. 2, CD003241. doi:10.1002/14651858.

Pong, Y.P., Wang, L.Y., Wang, L. et al., 2009. Sonography of the shoulder in hemiplegic patients undergoing rehabilitation after a recent stroke. J. Clin. Ultrasound 37, 199–205.

Poole, K.E.S., Loveridge, N., Rose, C.M., et al., 2007. A single infusion of zoledronate prevents bone loss after stroke. Stroke 38, 1519–1525.

Poels, B.J., Brinkman-Zijlker, H.G., Dijkstra, P.U., et al., 2006. Malnutrition, eating difficulties and feeding dependence in a stroke rehabilitation centre. Disabil. Rehabil. 28, 637–643.

Popovic, M.R., Thrasher, T.A., Zivanovic, V., et al., 2005. Popovic neuroprosthesis for retraining reaching and grasping functions in severe hemiplegic patients. Neuromodulation: Technology at the Neural Interface 8, 58–72.

Powell, T., Malia, K., 2006. The brain injury workbook – exercises for cognitive rehabilitation. Speechmark Publishing Ltd., Milton Keynes.

Price, C.I.M., Pandyan, A.D., 2008. Electrical stimulation for preventing and treating post-stroke shoulder pain. Cochrane Database Syst. Rev. 4, CD001698. doi:10.1002/14651858.

Raine, S., 2009. The Bobath concept: developments and current theoretical underpinning. In: Raine, S., Meadows, L., Lynch-Ellerington, M. (Eds.), Bobath concept. Theory and clinical practice in neurological rehabilitation. Wiley-Blackwell, Chichester, pp. 1–22.

Ratnasabapathy, Y., Broad, J., Baskett, J., et al., 2003. Shoulder pain in people with a stroke: a population-based study. Clin. Rehabil. 17, 304–311.

Reed, M., Harrington, R., Duggan, A., et al., 2010. Meeting stroke survivors' perceived needs: a qualitative study of a community-based exercise and education scheme. Clin. Rehabil. 24, 16–25.

Rothi, L.J.G., Heilman, K.M. (Eds.), 1997. Apraxia: the neuropsychology of action. Psychology Press, Hove.

Rowe, F., Brand, D., Jackson, C., et al., 2009. Visual impairment following stroke: do stroke patients require vision assessment? Age Ageing 38, 188–193.

Royal College of Physicians, Intercollegiate Stroke Working Party, 2008a. National clinical guideline for stroke, third ed. Royal College of Physicians, London. Available online at http://www.rcplondon.ac.uk/pubs/books/stroke/stroke_guidelines_2ed.pdf.

Royal College of Physicians, 2008b. Psychology concise guidelines for stroke. Royal College of Physicians, London. Available online at http://www.rcplondon.ac.uk/clinical-standards/ceeu/Current-work/stroke/Documents/psych-concise-guide-2008.pdf (accessed 01.04.2011).

Sato, Y., Iwamoto, J., Kanoko, T., et al., 2005a. Low dose vitamin D prevents muscular atrophy and reduces falls and hip fractures in women after stroke: a randomized controlled trial. Cerebrovasc. Dis. 20, 187–192.

Sato, Y., Iwamoto, J., Kanoko, T., et al., 2005b. Risedronate sodium therapy for prevention of hip fracture in men 65 years and older after stroke. Arch. Intern. Med. 165, 1743–1748.

Saunders, D.H., Greig, C.A., Young, A., et al., 2008. Association of activity limitations and lower-limb explosive extensor power in ambulatory people with stroke. Arch. Phys. Med. Rehabil. 89, 677–683.

Scottish Intercollegiate Guidelines Network, 2010. Guideline 118: Management of patients with stroke: rehabilitation, prevention and management of complications, and discharge planning: a national clinical guideline. Scottish Intercollegiate Guidelines Network (SIGN), Edinburgh. Available online at http://www.sign.ac.uk/guidelines/fulltext/118/index.html (accessed 08.09.2011).

Sharma, H., Bulley, C., van Wijck, F., 2011. Experiences of an exercise referral scheme from the perspective of people with chronic stroke: a qualitative study. Physiotherapy doi:org/10.1016/j.physio.2011.05.004.

Sheean, G., 1998. Clinical features of spasticity and the upper motor neurone syndrome. In: Sheean G. (Ed.), Spasticity rehabilitation. Churchill Communications Europe Ltd., London, pp. 7–16.

Sheean, G., 2001. Neurophysiology of spasticity. In: Barnes, M.P., Johnson, G.R. (Eds.), Upper motor neuron syndrome and spasticity. Clinical management and neurophysiology. Cambridge University Press, Cambridge, pp. 12–18.

Shumway-Cook, A., Woollacott, M., 2007. Motor control: translating research into clinical practice. Williams and Wilkins, Baltimore.

Smania, N., Montagnana, B., Faccioli, S., et al., 2003. Rehabilitation of somatic sensation and related deficit of motor control in patients with pure sensory stroke. Arch. Phys. Med. Rehabil. 84, 1692–1702.

Steultjens, E.M., Dekker, J., Bouter, L.M., et al., 2003. Occupational therapy for stroke patients: a systematic review. Stroke 31, 676–687.

Stone, J., Townend, E., Kwan, J., et al., 2004. Personality change after stroke: some preliminary observations. J. Neurol. Neurosurg. Psychiatry 75, 1708–1713.

Taylor, P.N., Burridge, J.H., Wood, D.E., et al., 1999. Clinical use of the Odstock Drop Foot Stimulator - its effect on the speed and effort of walking. Arch. Phys. Med. Rehabil. 80, 1577–1583.

McKevitt, C., Fudge, N., Redfern, J., et al., 2010. Stroke survivor needs survey. The Stroke Association, London.

Thomas, L.H., Cross, S., Barrett, J., et al., 2008. Treatment of urinary incontinence after stroke in adults. Cochrane Database Syst. Rev. 1, CD004462.

Thompson, A.J., 1998. Spasticity rehabilitation: a rational approach to clinical management. In: Sheean, G. (Ed.), Spasticity rehabilitation. Churchill Communications Europe Ltd., London, pp. 51–56.

Turvey, M.T., Burton, G., Amazeen, E.L., et al., 1998. Perceiving the width and height of a hand-held object by dynamic touch. J. Exp. Psychol. Hum. Percept. Perform. 24, 35–48.

Van Peppen, R.P.S., Kwakkel, G., Wood-Dauphinee, S., et al., 2004. The impact of physical therapy on functional outcomes after stroke: what's the evidence? Clin. Rehabil. 18, 833–862.

van Vliet, P.M., Sheridan, M.R., 2007. Coordination between reaching and grasping in patients with hemiparesis and normal subjects. Arch. Phys. Med. Rehabil. 88, 1325–1331.

Veldman, P.H.J.M., Reyen, H.M., Evo, E.A., et al., 1993. Signs and symptoms of reflex sympathetic dystrophy: prospective study of 829 patients. Lancet 342, 1012–1016.

Walsh, E.G., 1992. Muscles, masses and motion. The physiology of normality, hypotonicity, spasticity and rigidity. MacKeith Press, London.

Ward, A.B., Ko Ko, C., 2001. Pharmacological management of spasticity. In: Barnes, M.P., Johnson, G.R. (Eds.), Upper motor neuron syndrome and spasticity. Clinical management and neurophysiology. Cambridge University Press, Cambridge, pp. 165–187.

Watkins, C., Leathley, M., Gregson, J., et al., 2002. Prevalence of spasticity post stroke. Clin. Rehabil. 16, 515.

Wolf, S.L., Winstein, C., Miller, J.P., et al., 2008. Retention of upper limb function in stroke survivors who have received constraint-induced movement therapy: the EXCITE randomised trial. Lancet Neurol. 7, 33–40.

Woolley, S.M., 2001. Characteristics of gait in hemiplegia. Top. Stroke Rehabil. 7, 1–18.

Yekutiel, M., Guttman, E., 1993. A controlled trial of the retraining of sensory function of the hand. J. Neurol. Neurosurg. Psychiatry 56, 241–244.

PART 2
FOUNDATIONS FOR EXERCISE AND FITNESS TRAINING AFTER STROKE

PART CONTENTS

Physical fitness and function after stroke

David H. Saunders • Carolyn A. Greig

CHAPTER CONTENTS

It is widely known that low levels of physical fitness can limit peoples' ability to perform physical activities. This would suggest that increasing physical fitness could be beneficial after stroke, particularly where there is loss of function and mobility. In this chapter, the components of physical fitness are outlined, alongside a description of what we know about physical fitness after stroke. Understanding these parameters of physical fitness is essential to developing exercise programmes for people following stroke.

PHYSICAL FITNESS

Physical fitness is defined by a set of physiological attributes which people have or achieve that relate to the ability to perform and tolerate physical activities. Physical activity describes all body movement produced by skeletal muscle and which substantially increases energy expenditure (USDHHS 2008). Physical activities include work performed during occupational, leisure and sporting activities but also walking, activities of daily living and maintenance of posture.

COMPONENTS OF FITNESS

The cardiorespiratory system and skeletal muscle constitute the most important physiological systems that define and influence physical fitness. The capacity of these systems is at the centre of the physical fitness concept because they interact to generate external work for all physical activities (USDHHS 2008).

This is why, in this book, we shall focus on aerobic fitness, muscle strength and muscle power:

- Cardiorespiratory fitness (sometimes termed 'aerobic fitness') is conferred by the central capacity of the circulatory and respiratory systems to supply oxygen, and the peripheral capacity of skeletal muscle to utilise oxygen. It is commonly assessed by measuring the highest rate of oxygen utilisation ($\dot{V}O_2$ peak) achievable during maximal exercise. Cardiorespiratory fitness is associated with the ability to perform and tolerate continuous physical activity, e.g. walking.
- Muscle strength is the maximum force or torque that can be generated by a specific muscle or muscle group. The measures are reported in Newtons (N) for force and Newton metres (Nm) for torque and can be normalised to body mass (e.g. $N \cdot kg^{-1}$).
- Muscle power output is defined as the greatest rate of work achieved during a single, fast, resisted contraction. Power output is the product of force and speed of movement, usually reported as a power to body mass ratio ($W \cdot kg^{-1}$). Power differs from strength in that it is a velocity-dependent characteristic. Strength and power are associated with the ability to lift objects or raise body mass, e.g. mounting a step.

The successful performance of any physical activity is not just about muscular work. Other parameters are involved which include motor control, balance, flexibility (range of motion about a joint) and body composition (e.g. lean body mass).

PLASTICITY OF FITNESS

In healthy people, physical fitness parameters show considerable variation and plasticity that is the ability to change and adapt (Fig. 4.1). Key factors in influencing fitness and plasticity are:

- *Age and gender.* In adults increasing age causes a decline in cardiorespiratory fitness of 1–2% per year, muscle strength of 1–2%, and muscle power of 3–4% per year (Young 2001). The gender difference accompanying this decline means men have the equivalent of around a 20-year fitness advantage over women. Loss of lean body mass is detectable after the age of 45 years; alongside a gender difference, this may partly explain some of the variation and plasticity (Narici and Maffulli 2010).

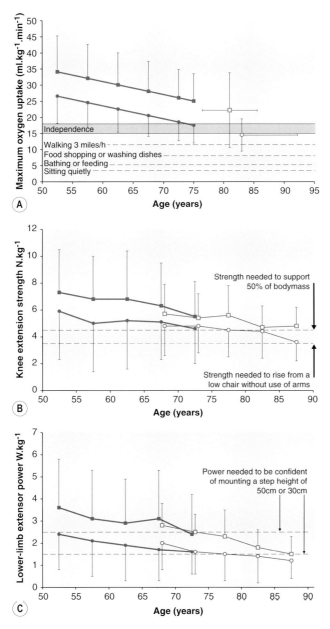

FIG 4.1 Age- and gender-related decline in cardiorespiratory fitness (♂ ■ ♀ ●; Shvartz and Reibold 1990) (♂ □ ♀ ○; Malbut et al. 2002) and musculoskeletal fitness (♂ ■ ♀ ●; Skelton et al. 1999) (♂ □ ♀ ○; Skelton et al. 1994) in healthy people aged 50 years and older. Functional thresholds (---) are marked on these data to indicate when low fitness may limit certain activities (Allied Dunbar National Fitness Survey 1992, Ainsworth et al. 2000) or threaten independence (Shephard 2009). Data points are means and error bars represent 2 standard deviations.

- *Inactivity*. Profound physical inactivity (bed rest) causes a substantial decline in cardiorespiratory fitness (12%), muscle strength (13%) and muscle power (14%) in just 10 days (Kortebein et al. 2008). Thus physical inactivity causes a deconditioning effect on fitness far faster than the effect of ageing.
- *Chronic disease*. The effects of chronic disease may reduce fitness due to inactivity and secondary consequences such as systemic inflammation (Degens and Alway 2006).
- *Activity and exercise*. All parameters of physical fitness can be improved by increased physical activity and exercise.

FUNCTIONAL IMPORTANCE OF FITNESS

Low physical fitness may be insufficient to meet the energetic demands of certain activities, thus rendering them fatiguing and uncomfortable (Fig. 4.1). For example, muscle strength and power of the lower limbs both predict the ability to perform functional activities such as stair climbing, chair rising and walking speed, but power is the strongest predictor (Cuoco et al. 2004, Puthoff and Nielsen 2007). 'Thresholds' exist for physical fitness below which independence is threatened (Fig. 4.2). For example $\dot{V}O_2$ peak values below 15–18 ml·kg^{-1}·min^{-1} (Shephard 2009; Fig. 4.1) and muscle strength of the hip flexors strength below 2.3 N·kg^{-1} (Hasegawa et al. 2008) are both associated with loss of independence. Therefore, as fitness declines (for any reason) the likelihood of activity limitations and loss of independence increases, and individuals are vulnerable to the inevitable effects of further age-related decline.

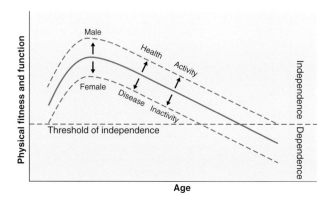

FIG 4.2 Physical fitness and function through the lifespan (——) showing the age-related decline seen during adulthood and the implications this may have for loss of independence in later life (Young 1986). The arrows indicate how factors such as gender, health status and physical activity level may influence fitness and function positively (↑) and negatively (↓) and in turn hasten or delay age-related loss of independence.

PHYSICAL FITNESS AFTER STROKE

Fitness and the ability to undertake activities of daily living have been found to be compromised following stroke with fatigue limiting walking distance.

POST-STROKE CARDIORESPIRATORY FITNESS

Measures of cardiorespiratory fitness in ambulatory stroke survivors have shown that $\dot{V}O_2$ peak is half (50% to 60%) that expected in healthy people matched for age and gender (Fig. 4.3A). The typical $\dot{V}O_2$ peak observed was ~15 ml·kg⁻¹·min⁻¹, which corresponds to that implicated in loss of independence in elderly people (15–18 ml·kg⁻¹·min⁻¹; Shephard 2009). The low values suggest some everyday activities would be difficult to perform since they recruit a high proportion of the $\dot{V}O_2$ peak, resulting in either fatigue or the need to slow down or modify the activity (Fig. 4.3B).

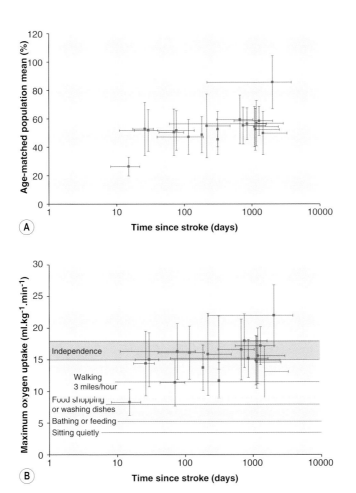

FIG 4.3 The average $\dot{V}O_2$ peak of stroke patients (19 studies; n=714, not cited) in relation to time since stroke, expressed (A) relative to a healthy, untrained age- and gender-matched population (Shvartz and Reibold 1990), and (B) corrected for body mass in relation to the energetic cost of selected physical activities (Ainsworth et al. 2000) and a proposed boundary in $\dot{V}O_2$ (around 15 to 18 ml·kg⁻¹·min⁻¹) below which a loss of independence is implicated in elderly people (Shephard 2009). Each data point is the mean $\dot{V}O_2$ value reported by each study and the error bars represent the standard deviation.

Abnormal gait and low gait speed are common post-stroke problems caused by factors such as abnormal patterns of movement, use of walking aids, hemiparesis, poor flexibility, contractures, abnormal muscle tone, antagonist coactivation and poor balance. One consequence is an increased energy expenditure which does not contribute to locomotion. Thus the $\dot{V}O_2$ cost per unit distance walked can be several times greater than in healthy people (da Cunha et al. 2002, David et al. 2006, Platts et al. 2006), even after controlling for the confounding effect of a lower gait speed. Peak $\dot{V}O_2$ is half that expected in healthy people, yet the $\dot{V}O_2$ cost of walking is typically double. This means that the high cost of even slow walking may involve drawing on a high proportion of the already diminished maximal $\dot{V}O_2$, leaving little in 'reserve'. One consequence is that walking is fatiguing and slow and there is little leeway for further deterioration in fitness before walking becomes impossible.

POST-STROKE MUSCLE STRENGTH

Observational studies comparing the isometric strength of stroke survivors with healthy adults show clear evidence of the muscle weakness, especially on the side of body affected by stroke. This is a defining feature of many types of stroke (Table 4.1).

The degree of impairment in muscle strength is highly variable and is greatest in the limbs directly affected by the stroke, e.g. strokes in the territory of the left middle cerebral artery typically cause sudden onset weakness in the right arm and leg (chapter 1). Muscle strength of the unaffected side is also lower (compared with healthy age-matched adults), although this is less pronounced in the chronic phase (>1 year; Boissy et al. 1999, Maeda et al. 2000, Ng and Hui-Chan 2005) where compensatory physical activity may contribute to a local training effect.

Trunk extension and flexion strength have also been measured in stroke survivors and shown to be lower than healthy age-matched controls in both the acute (Karatas et al. 2004) and chronic (Tanaka et al. 1998) phases of recovery. These studies suggest that strength impairment may be greater when the movement is dynamic (isokinetic) rather than static (isometric).

There are very few longitudinal studies of muscle function after stroke. These are confined exclusively to changes in strength but report conflicting results, i.e. increased strength (Newham and Hsiao 2001), unchanged (Carin-Levy et al. 2006) or decreased strength (Harris et al. 2001).

POST-STROKE MUSCLE POWER OUTPUT

Observational studies (Dawes et al. 2005, Greig et al. 2003, Saunders et al. 2008) have measured lower limb power in community-dwelling stroke patients (Table 4.2) using a Nottingham Power Rig (Bassey and Short 1990). When compared with normative data for age- and gender-matched healthy people (Skelton et al. 1999, Skelton et al. 1994), the greatest impairment in power was shown in the affected leg (<50% of healthy people). This is not surprising as chapter 1 describes that weakness of one side of the body (i.e. hemiparesis)

Table 4.1 Studies comparing bilateral measures of isometric muscle strength in stroke patients with age-matched healthy control groups

Study	Stroke patients			Strength measure	% healthy controls	
	Age Mean (SD)	n	Time since stroke Mean (SD)	Muscle group	Affected side	Unaffected side
Boissy et al. (1999)	47 (14)	15	>1 year	Handgrip	35% to 40%	107% to 115%
Brasil-Neto and de Lima (2008)	58 (11)	25	43.8 months (55.4)	Handgrip	16%	80%
Maeda et al. (2000)	69.9	40	3.5 years (~1.0)	Knee extension	63% (male) 72% (female)	103% (male) 108% (female)
Newham and Hsiao (2001)	61 (5)	12	21 days (1)	Knee flexion Knee extension	43% 56%	79% 92%
			6 months	Knee flexion Knee extension	70% 82%	90% 96%
Ng and Hui-Chan (2005)	61.7 (7.2)	11	5.6 years (3.3)	Ankle dorsiflexion Ankle plantar flexion	51% 49%	99% 95%
Horstman et al. (2008)	55.9 (10.4)	14	109 days (46)	Knee extension Knee flexion	28% 12%	68% 63%
Gerrits et al. (2009)	54 (10)	18	22 months (18)	Knee extension	42%	73%

Table 4.2 *Studies reporting explosive muscle power output (W·kg⁻¹) of the extensors of whole lower limb (knee and hip) in community-dwelling stroke survivors compared with healthy control normative data*

Study	Stroke participants		Time post stroke	% of healthy norms*	
	Age Mean (SD)	n (m/f)**	Mean	Affected side	Unaffected side
Dawes et al. (2005)	46.8 (8)	14 (8/6)	>6 months	31%[†]	57%[†]
Greig et al. (2003)	73.5 (8.7)	11 (9/2)	14 months	48%	51%
Saunders et al. (2008)	71.85 (9.9)	66 (36/30)	152 days	42%	54%

*Age- and gender-matched norms established using same equipment (Allied Dunbar National Fitness Survey 1992, Skelton et al. 1994, Skelton et al. 1999).
**m, male; f, female.
[†]Stronger side assumed to be 'unaffected'.

is common after stroke. Importantly though, power output of the 'unaffected' lower limb was also only 50% to 60% of healthy people. These data suggest a substantial impairment in power output after stroke, at least as great as for muscle strength, affecting both sides of the body (albeit more so on the hemiparetic (primarily affected) side).

WHY IS FITNESS LOW AFTER STROKE?

Since many stroke survivors are elderly (>70 years), age-related low levels of fitness and muscle mass are common. In addition, a number of factors directly and indirectly associated with stroke reduce fitness further:

- *Indirect pre-stroke factors.* Low fitness may predate stroke since cardiorespiratory fitness is a risk factor for stroke (Hooker et al. 2008) and muscle strength deteriorates faster in those developing chronic diseases (Rantanen et al. 1998). Low fitness could also be due to the effects of physical inactivity (Wendel-Vos et al. 2004), co-morbid diseases (Degens and Alway 2006) and smoking (Al Obaidi et al. 2004).
- *Direct effect of stroke.* The direct neurological effect of a stroke lesion anywhere in the motor tract (e.g. motor cortex, internal capsule) can lead to a hemiparesis due to reduced motor neuron recruitment. Any reduction in muscle mass that can be activated to perform physical activity thus imposes an immediate impairment in all aspects of physical fitness and economy of walking.
- *Indirect post-stoke factors.* Post-stroke physical inactivity has the potential to lead to further declines in physical fitness. For example, non-ambulatory patients are inactive for more of the day (98%) than those able to walk independently (40.5% of day) (Bernhardt et al. 2007). Co-morbid disease could also influence post-stroke fitness, e.g. the $\dot{V}O_2$ peak is lower in stroke patients who also have coronary artery disease compared with those who do not (Mackay-Lyons and Makrides 2002).

Low values of physical fitness are likely to limit functional abilities of people with stroke in the same way that they would for healthy elderly people (Fig. 4.1). Since fitness has been shown to be lower after stroke, the risk of crossing a 'threshold of independence' (Fig. 4.2) increases.

CARDIORESPIRATORY FITNESS AND POST-STROKE FUNCTION

Observational studies have determined the strength of simple (bivariate) associations between cardiorespiratory fitness and walking performance (Table 4.3). Although the data vary, low $\dot{V}O_2$ peak tends to give a modest prediction of reduced comfortable walking speed and a stronger prediction of walking performance during a 6-minute walking test. Continuous activities such as walking rely upon cardiorespiratory fitness. However, more complex (multivariate) analyses show that additional stroke impairments associated with other components of fitness also influence walking (Michael and Macko 2007, Pang et al. 2005, Patterson et al. 2007). These analyses identify balance, strength and tone as important determinants of walking performance, which may 'swamp' the influence of $\dot{V}O_2$ peak. $\dot{V}O_2$ peak, balance and leg strength are all independently predictive of the 6-minute walking test performance; for the slowest walkers only balance predicts walking, and for the fastest only $\dot{V}O_2$ peak (Patterson et al. 2007).

Associations between low $\dot{V}O_2$ peak and other activity limitations have been reported including maximum walking speed (r=0.68; Kelly et al. 2003) and Barthel Index score <90, which is a global index of activity limitation (Mackay-Lyons and Makrides 2002).

These data only indicate a *connection* between fitness and function. We cannot conclude that low fitness *causes* poor function since it is also plausible that poor post-stroke mobility causes fitness to deteriorate. However, these data do allow us to hypothesise that improving fitness through exercise interventions may improve function such as walking performance.

MUSCLE STRENGTH AND FUNCTION

A number of studies have examined associations between muscle strength and post-stroke function. Most of the available data are for community-dwelling stroke survivors relate to lower limb strength and function. For example, comfortable walking speed and walking endurance (6-minute walking test; Table 11.1) were predicted by the dynamic knee extension strength of affected and unaffected legs (Patterson et al. 2007). Similar data show that indices of walking speed were predicted by the dynamic strength of the affected leg, but not the unaffected leg (Flansbjer et al. 2006). Almost without exception other similar data show the strongest relationship with the affected limb. Lower limb strength, in particular of the affected side, plays an important role in other activity limitations such as chair rising and stair climbing performance (Flansbjer et al. 2006, Kim and Eng 2003, Lomaglio and Eng 2005).

Several studies have examined the association of muscle strength with activity limitation in combination with factors such as age and gender, and impairments including balance, sensation, motor function and muscle tone

Table 4.3 Studies reporting bivariate associations between $\dot{V}O_2$ peak and measures of continuous walking performance after stroke

| Study | Participants | | Time post stroke (days) Mean (SD) | Exercise mode for $\dot{V}O_2$ peak | Association between $\dot{V}O_2$ peak and walking | |
	Age Mean (SD)	n			Comfortable walking speed	6-Minute walking test
Kelly et al. (2003)	60.8 (16.4)	17	29.2 (11.0)	Cycle ergometer	r = 0.736, P < 0.001	r = 0.84, P < 0.001
Ryan et al. (2002)	65 (9)	60	1096 (1351)	Treadmill	r = 0.53, P < 0.01	–
Eng et al. (2004)	62.5 (8.6)	12	1278 (731)	Cycle ergometer	r = 0.32, NS	r = 0.37, NS
Michael and Macko (2007)	65	50	314	Treadmill	r = 0.290, NS	–
Patterson et al. (2007)	64 (10)	74	1146 (1796)	Treadmill	r = 0.54, P < 0.001	r = 0.64, P < 0.001
Courbon et al. (2006)	53.5 (7.65)	21	746 (852)	Cycle ergometer	–	r = 0.602, P < 0.0032
Pang et al. (2005)	65.3 (8.7)	63	2009 (1790)	Cycle ergometer	–	r = 0.402, P < 0.005

NS, not significant.

(Flansbjer et al. 2006, Hsu et al. 2003, Le Brasseur et al. 2006, Nadeau et al. 1999, Patterson et al. 2007, Pohl et al. 2002, Suzuki et al. 1999). These multivariate analyses indicate that all these factors independently influence indices of walking (maximum walking speed, comfortable walking speed, 6-minute walking test). However, it is muscle strength during hip flexion and knee flexion/extension of the affected leg which often emerge as key factors predicting walking performance, and, to a lesser extent, negotiating stairs (Flansbjer et al. 2006, Le Brasseur et al. 2006).

These data suggest that improving the low muscle strength of stroke patients, particularly of the affected lower limb, could improve functional activities such as walking. In addition, other post-stroke impairments are involved in walking, including balance. Balance could also be addressed during exercise training interventions.

MUSCLE POWER AND FUNCTION

Small studies exploring associations between power output and walking performance after stroke report contradictory results (Bohannon 1992, Dawes et al. 2004). The latter study showed that lower limb extensor power was not significantly associated with comfortable walking speed, but that asymmetry in power between limbs was predictive of comfortable walking speeds.

Multivariate analyses (statistical analyses that describe the relationship between several different factors) have shown that power of the knee extensors, particularly of the affected side, was the most important factor that predicted comfortable walking speed and stair climbing performance (Le Brasseur et al. 2006). Lower limb extensor power of either leg has also been shown to be the only factor that predicts comfortable walking speed, chair rising and timed up-and-go (Table 11.1) from within multivariate analyses which include age, gender, time since stroke, stature, smoking, use of walking aids (Table 11.1), incidence of key co-morbid diseases (Saunders et al. 2008).

The few data that directly compare the influence of strength and power after stroke suggest comfortable walking speed is similarly predicted by both fitness variables (Bohannon 1992, Le Brasseur et al. 2006). However, power explained more than double the variation in stair climbing time than strength (Le Brasseur et al. 2006).

These data allow us to hypothesise that interventions to increase muscle power may benefit performance in a range of physical activities commonly limited after stroke, including walking.

A MODEL OF THE ROLE OF POST-STROKE FITNESS IMPAIRMENT

In healthy elderly people physical fitness is often low and associated with activity limitation and dependence. Physical fitness after stroke is low due to the effects of age and also because of physical inactivity, co-morbid diseases and smoking both before and after stroke. The observational data presented in this chapter show associations between fitness and function. These do not imply causal effects (i.e. that low physical fitness is a direct cause of activity limitation and dependence)

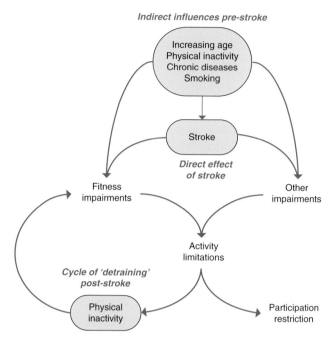

FIG 4.4 Model of the possible causes and influences of post-stroke fitness impairments. Fitness is low in people with stroke due to the combined influence of indirect factors which pre-date stroke and the direct neurological effects of stroke. Low fitness and other impairments may interact to cause or exacerbate post-stroke activity limitations and participation restrictions; these precipitate further physical inactivity leading to a 'cycle of detraining' in which fitness impairments and activity limitations continue to develop.

but they do allow one to hypothesise that low fitness, along with other impairments, may exacerbate the direct effects of stroke and drive post-stroke activity limitations. A simple model of these relationships is summarised in Figure 4.4.

Since physical fitness can be increased by exercise training, the model in Figure 4.4 suggests that fitness improvements could help counteract problems linked to low fitness and physical inactivity, and compensate for the effects of other stroke-related impairments. This causal effect will be examined in the next chapter using controlled experimental data.

SUMMARY POINTS

PHYSICAL FITNESS

- Cardiorespiratory fitness, muscle strength and muscle power largely define the capacity to perform, and comfortably tolerate, physical activities.
- Physical fitness is lower in women than in men and deteriorates in both men and women with increasing age.
- Physical fitness is impaired by physical inactivity, chronic diseases and smoking.
- Low physical fitness is linked to activity limitations.
- Physical fitness can be improved with physical activity or exercise.

FITNESS AFTER STROKE

- Cardiorespiratory fitness:
  - $\dot{V}O_2$ peak is 50–60% of that expected in healthy people.
  - Economy of walking is often lower than in healthy people.
  - Cardiorespiratory fitness 'reserve' is low.
- Muscle strength:
  - Impaired after stroke; degree of impairment is highly variable.
  - Impairment is bilateral but greater on the affected side.
- Muscle power:
  - Leg power is 40–60% of that expected in healthy people.
  - Impairment is bilateral but greater on the affected side.
  - Degree of impairment is at least as great as muscle strength.
- Fitness impairments may arise from direct neurological effects of stroke, plus physical inactivity, co-morbid disease and smoking.
- Fitness impairments persist into the chronic stage of recovery.

FUNCTIONAL CONSEQUENCES OF IMPAIRMENT

- Low fitness is associated with some common post-stroke problems, especially regarding gait.
- Other impairments, e.g. balance, interact with fitness to influence post-stroke problems and functional activity.

REFERENCES

Allied Dunbar National Fitness Survey, 1992. Main Findings. Sports Council and Health Education Authority, London.

Ainsworth, B.E., Haskell, W.L., Whitt, M.C., et al., 2000. Compendium of physical activities: an update of activity codes and MET intensities. Med. Sci. Sports Exerc. 32 (Suppl. 9), S498–S504.

Al Obaidi, S.M., Anthony, J., Al Shuwai, N., et al., 2004. Differences in back extensor strength between smokers and nonsmokers with and without low back pain. J. Orthop. Sports Phys. Ther. 34, 254–260.

Bassey, E.J., Short, A.H., 1990. A new method for measuring power output in a single leg extension: feasibility, reliability and validity. Eur. J. Appl. Physiol. Occup. Physiol. 60, 385–390.

Bernhardt, J., Chan, J., Nicola, I., et al., 2007. Little therapy, little physical activity: rehabilitation within the first 14 days of organized stroke unit care. J. Rehabil. Med. 39, 43–48.

Bohannon, R.W., 1992. Knee extension power, velocity and torque: relative deficits and relation to walking performance in stroke patients. Clin. Rehabil. 6, 125–131.

Boissy, P., Bourbonnais, D., Carlotti, M.M., et al., 1999. Maximal grip force in chronic stroke subjects and its relationship to global upper extremity function. Clin. Rehabil. 13, 354–362.

Brasil-Neto, J.P.M., de Lima, A.C.M., 2008. Sensory deficits in the unaffected hand of hemiparetic stroke patients. Cogn. Behav. Neurol. 21, 202–205.

Carin-Levy, G., Greig, C., Young, A., et al., 2006. Longitudinal changes in muscle strength and mass after acute stroke. Cerebrovasc. Dis. 21, 201–207.

Courbon, A., Calmels, P., Roche, F., et al., 2006. Relationship between maximal exercise capacity and walking capacity in adult hemiplegic stroke patients. Am. J. Phys. Med. Rehabil. 85, 436–442.

Cuoco, A., Callahan, D.M., Sayers, S., et al., 2004. Impact of muscle power and force on gait speed in disabled older men and women. J. Gerontol. A Biol. Sci. Med. Sci. 59, 1200–1206.

da Cunha Jr., I.T., Lim, P.A., Qureshy, H., et al., 2002. Gait outcomes after acute stroke rehabilitation with supported treadmill ambulation training: a randomized controlled pilot study. Arch. Phys. Med. Rehabil. 83, 1258–1265.

David, D., Regnaux, J.P., Lejaille, M., et al., 2006. Oxygen consumption during machine-assisted and unassisted walking: a pilot study in hemiplegic and healthy humans. Arch. Phys. Med. Rehabil. 87, 482–489.

Dawes, H., Collett, J., Ramsbottom, R., et al., 2004. Measuring oxygen cost during level walking in individuals with acquired brain injury in the clinical setting. J. Sports Sci. Med. 3(2), 76–82.

Dawes, H., Smith, C., Collett, J., et al., 2005. A pilot study to investigate explosive leg extensor power and walking performance after stroke. J. Sports Sci. Med. 4, 556–562.

Degens, H., Alway, S.E., 2006. Control of muscle size during disuse, disease, and aging. Int. J. Sports Med. 27, 94–99.

Eng, J.J., Dawson, A.S., Chu, K.S., 2004. Submaximal exercise in persons with stroke: test-retest reliability and concurrent validity with maximal oxygen consumption. Arch. Phys. Med. Rehabil. 85, 113–118.

Flansbjer, U.B., Downham, D., Lexell, J., 2006. Knee muscle strength, gait performance, and perceived participation after stroke. Arch. Phys. Med. Rehabil. 87, 974–980.

Gerrits, K.H., Beltman, M.J., Koppe, P.A., et al., 2009. Isometric muscle function of knee extensors and the relation with functional performance in patients with stroke. Arch. Phys. Med. Rehabil. 90, 480–487.

Greig, C.A., Savaridas, T., Saunders, D., et al., 2003. Lower limb muscle strength and power following 'recovery' from stroke. Age Ageing 32 (Suppl. 1), 34.

Harris, M.L., Polkey, M.I., Bath, P.M., et al., 2001. Quadriceps muscle weakness following acute hemiplegic stroke. Clin. Rehabil. 15, 274–281.

Hasegawa, R., Islam, M.M., Sung, C.L., et al., 2008. Threshold of lower body muscular strength necessary to perform ADL independently in community-dwelling older adults. Clin. Rehabil. 22, 902–910.

Hooker, S.P., Sui, X., Colabianchi, N., et al., 2008. Cardiorespiratory fitness as a predictor of fatal and nonfatal stroke in asymptomatic women and men. Stroke 39, 2950–2957.

Horstman, A.M., Beltman, M.J., Gerrits, K.H., et al., 2008. Intrinsic muscle strength and voluntary activation of both lower limbs and functional performance after stroke. Clin. Physiol. Funct. Imag. 28, 251–261.

Hsu, A.L., Tang, P.F., Jan, M.H., 2003. Analysis of impairments influencing gait velocity and asymmetry of hemiplegic patients after mild to moderate stroke. Arch. Phys. Med. Rehabil. 84, 1185–1193.

Karatas, M., Çetin, N., Bayramoglu, M., et al., 2004. Trunk muscle strength in relation to balance and functional disability in unihemispheric stroke patients. Am. J. Phys. Med. Rehabil. 83, 81–87.

Kelly, J.O., Kilbreath, S.L., Davis, G.M., et al., 2003. Cardiorespiratory fitness and walking ability in subacute stroke patients. Arch. Phys. Med. Rehabil. 84, 1780–1785.

Kim, C.M., Eng, J.J., 2003. The relationship of lower-extremity muscle torque to locomotor performance in people with stroke. Phys. Ther. 83, 49.

Kortebein, P., Symons, T.B., Ferrando, A., et al., 2008. Functional impact of 10 days of bed rest in healthy older adults. J. Gerontol. A Biol. Sci. Med. Sci. 63, 1076–1081.

Le Brasseur, N.K., Sayers, S.P., Ouellette, M.M., et al., 2006. Muscle impairments and behavioral factors mediate functional limitations and disability following stroke. Phys. Ther. 86, 1342–1350.

Lomaglio, M.J., Eng, J.J., 2005. Muscle strength and weight-bearing symmetry relate to sit-to-stand performance in individuals with stroke. Gait Posture 22, 126–131.

Mackay-Lyons, M.J., Makrides, L., 2002. Exercise capacity early after stroke. Arch. Phys. Med. Rehabil. 83, 1697–1702.

Maeda, A., Yuasa, T., Nakamura, K., et al., 2000. Physical performance tests after stroke: reliability and validity. Am. J. Phys. Med. Rehabil. 79, 519–525.

Malbut, K.E., Dinan, S., Young, A., 2002. Aerobic training in the 'oldest old': the effect of 24 weeks of training. Age Ageing 31, 255–260.

Michael, K., Macko, R.F., 2007. Ambulatory activity intensity profiles, fitness, and fatigue in chronic stroke. Top. Stroke Rehabil. 14, 5–12.

Nadeau, S., Arsenault, A.B., Gravel, D., et al., 1999. Analysis of the clinical factors determining natural and maximal gait speeds in adults with a stroke. Am. J. Phys. Med. Rehabil. 78, 123–130.

Narici, M.V., Maffulli, N., 2010. Sarcopenia: characteristics, mechanisms and functional significance. BMB 95, 139–159.

Newham, D.J., Hsiao, S.F., 2001. Knee muscle isometric strength, voluntary activation and antagonist co-contraction in the first six months after stroke. Disabil. Rehabil. 23, 379–386.

Ng, S.S., Hui-Chan, C.W., 2005. The timed up and go test: its reliability and association with lower-limb impairments and locomotor capacities in people with chronic stroke. Arch. Phys. Med. Rehabil. 86, 1641–1647.

Pang, M.Y.C., Eng, J.J., Dawson, A.S., 2005. Relationship between ambulatory capacity and cardiorespiratory fitness in chronic stroke. Chest 127, 495–501.

Patterson, S.L., Forrester, L.W., Rodgers, M.M., et al., 2007. Determinants of walking function after stroke: differences by deficit severity. Arch. Phys. Med. Rehabil. 88, 115–119.

Platts, M.M., Rafferty, D., Paul, L., 2006. Metabolic cost of over ground gait in younger stroke patients and healthy controls. Med. Sci. Sports Exerc. 38, 1041–1046.

Pohl, P.S., Duncan, P., Perera, S., et al., 2002. Rate of isometric knee extension strength development and walking speed after stroke. J. Rehabil. Res. Dev. 39, 651–658.

Puthoff, M.L., Nielsen, D.H., 2007. Relationships among impairments in lower-extremity strength and power, functional limitations, and disability in older adults. Phys. Ther. 87, 1334–1337.

Rantanen, T., Masaki, K., Foley, D., et al., 1998. Grip strength changes over 27 yr in Japanese-American men. J. Appl. Physiol. 85, 2047–2053.

Ryan, A.S., Dobrovolny, C.L., Smith, G.V., et al., 2002. Hemiparetic muscle atrophy and increased intramuscular fat in stroke patients. Arch. Phys. Med. Rehabil. 83, 1703–1707.

Saunders, D.H., Greig, C.A., Young, A., et al., 2008. Association of activity limitations and lower-limb explosive extensor power in ambulatory people with stroke. Arch. Phys. Med. Rehabil. 89, 677–683.

Shephard, R.J., 2009. Maximal oxygen intake and independence in old age. Br. J. Sports Med. 43, 342–346.

Shvartz, E., Reibold, R.C., 1990. Aerobic fitness norms for males and females aged 6 to 75 years: a review. Aviat. Space Environ. Med. 61, 3–11.

Skelton, D.A., Greig, C.A., Davies, J.M., et al., 1994. Strength, power and related functional ability of healthy people aged 65–89 years. Age Ageing 23, 371–377.

Skelton, D., Young, A., Walker, A., et al., 1999. Physical activity in later life: further analysis of the Allied Dunbar National Fitness Survey and the Health Education Authority National Survey of Activity and Health. Health Education Authority, London.

Suzuki, K., Imada, G., Iwaya, T., et al., 1999. Determinants and predictors of the maximum walking speed during computer-assisted gait training in hemiparetic stroke patients. Arch. Phys. Med. Rehabil. 80, 179–182.

Tanaka, S., Hachisuka, K., Ogata, H., 1998. Muscle strength of trunk flexion-extension in post-stroke hemiplegic patients. Am. J. Phys. Med. Rehabil. 77, 288–290.

USDHHS, 2008. Physical Activity Guidelines Advisory Committee Report. Centers for Disease Control and Prevention, Atlanta.

Wendel-Vos, G.C.W., Schuit, A.J., Feskens, E.J.M., et al., 2004. Physical activity and stroke. A meta-analysis of observational data. Int. J. Epidemiol. 33, 787–798.

Young, A., 2001. The health benefits of physical activity for a healthier old age. In: Young, A., Harries, M. (Eds.), Physical activity for patients: an exercise prescription. Royal College of Physicians, London, pp. 31–42.

Young, A., 1986. Exercise physiology in geriatric practice. Acta Med. Scand. Suppl. 711, 227–232.

Evidence for exercise and fitness training after stroke

5

David H. Saunders • Gillian Mead

INTRODUCTION

This chapter looks at the benefits of exercise and fitness training for stroke survivors in the context of 'why it should work' as well as discussing the evidence that suggests 'that it *does* work'.

'Exercise' (or 'exercise training') is defined as a subset of physical activity that is planned, structured, repetitive and performed deliberately to improve or maintain one or more components of physical fitness, which was defined in chapter 4 (p. 77). Most exercise training interventions are classified as either

93

cardiorespiratory (to increase cardiorespiratory fitness), resistance (to improve muscle strength and/or power) or mixed (a combination of both). A defining feature of any exercise training intervention is some form of progression in the training stimulus throughout the programme; for example, where the frequency, duration and/or the intensity of exercise sessions increases week by week. In the context of therapeutic interventions, exercise training is somewhat unusual in that it can confer functional and health benefits for people of any age even if already healthy, and can continue to do so in those who are already trained.

THEORETICAL BENEFIT OF EXERCISE

Why might exercise training be important for people post stroke? What benefits can they expect in terms of functional and psychosocial outcomes?

RATIONALE FOR FITNESS TRAINING IN PEOPLE WITH STROKE

The evidence presented in chapter 4 suggests that physical fitness is low after stroke and that there is scope for improving physical fitness. There is no biological reason why physical fitness after stroke cannot be increased by physical fitness training, providing the training is safe and feasible. If fitness is improved there are a range of potential benefits including increased participation in activities of daily living and improved muscle strength and power, all of which are of value to people with stroke. Exercise also provides a range of physical, social and psychological benefits that are not always dependent on fitness improvement.

PHYSICAL BENEFITS

The strength and nature of the associations between low fitness and post-stroke problems (chapter 4, p. 85) suggests that improving fitness may improve some common post-stroke problems.

Post-stroke physical activity and fitness are low, and these low levels are associated with common post-stroke functional limitations. Increased fitness and physical function could, in theory, also help with other post-stroke problems, such as reducing fatigue and the risk of falls and fractures, compensating for the increased energetic cost of the hemiparetic gait, reducing disability, and improving independence, quality of life and mood.

There are other potential benefits that may not be dependent on improvements in physical fitness. Physical therapies are known to promote structural brain remodelling (Gauthier et al. 2008) and this may improve post-stroke motor deficits. There is systematic review evidence that repetitive practice of some common day-to-day activities produces some modest improvements in mobility and activities of daily living in stroke patients (French et al. 2010). Therefore, participation in repetitive, task-related training may have functional benefits even if fitness is not improved.

PSYCHOSOCIAL BENEFITS

Exercising in a group with other people has been found to have psychosocial benefits in people with stroke (Carin-Levy et al. 2009, Patterson and Ross-Edwards 2009, Mead 2005). Self-reported benefits include social and motivational support gained by sharing the experience with others. Therefore, simply participating in exercise may be beneficial particularly where group activities are involved.

MORTALITY AND MORBIDITY

Exercise is known to be beneficial for people with a number of conditions which are risk factors for stroke or common co-morbid conditions associated with stroke. For example, systematic review evidence (p. 96) shows that exercise can lower blood pressure (Dickinson et al. 2006), improve vascular risk factors in people with obesity (Shaw et al. 2006) and type II diabetes (Thomas et al. 2006), reduce mortality in coronary heart disease patients (Jolliffe et al. 2000) and could benefit people with depression (Mead et al. 2008). Therefore, exercise and fitness training after stroke, particularly cardiorespiratory training, could reduce morbidity and mortality through secondary prevention of stroke and comorbid diseases.

These studies suggest that exercise training is not simply an intervention that is provided with the primary aim of improving fitness, but that it might have multiple other benefits after stroke.

RISKS AND HAZARDS

However, there may also be risks associated with exercise such as training-induced soft-tissue injuries, altered muscle tone, falls and vascular events. These risks need to be considered and managed in planning exercise programmes and are discussed in chapters 9 and 10.

EVIDENCE OF BENEFITS

There are different types of scientific study based on observation and experiment that provide empirical evidence. There is a hierarchy within these study designs that provides an increasing 'level of evidence'; that is, more trustworthy data which allows stronger recommendations to be made.

LEVELS OF EVIDENCE

Observational studies

Much of the data linking fitness and function in chapter 4 is from observational studies. These designs reveal associations between low fitness and post-stroke problems, but they do not prove that low fitness causes problems or that increasing fitness will alleviate problems. They do, however, allow one to *hypothesise* that increasing fitness may have benefits. However, to demonstrate that physical fitness training improves post-stroke problems, one needs to perform a randomised controlled trial.

Randomised controlled trials

These controlled study designs enable one to attribute any observed benefits of an intervention to the intervention itself, rather than other factors, such as type of patient recruited. Study participants, after assessment of eligibility and recruitment, but before the intervention to be studied begins, are randomly allocated to receive one or other of the alternative treatments. In the case of trials of fitness training, this might be either an exercise intervention (in addition to usual stroke care) or usual stroke care alone. After randomisation, the two (or more) groups of patients are followed up in exactly the same way. Thus any differences in outcomes at the end of the trial can be attributed to the intervention itself, in this case exercise.

Thus, randomised controlled trials (RCTs), particularly if they are large, provide a superior level of evidence about the effects to that of observational, uncontrolled studies. Generally, if clinical practice is to be changed, one needs robust evidence from RCTs. However, large trials of exercise – particularly after stroke – are difficult to carry out and, therefore, pooling the data from a number of studies is an effective way of taking stock of as much of the available evidence as possible; the mechanism to do this is provided by systematic reviews and meta-analyses.

Systematic reviews

The best level of evidence about the effects of an intervention such as exercise is provided by systematic review of RCT evidence. Systematic reviews are based on a specific question about a health-care intervention. Their rigorous methodology identifies and reduces bias (systematic error). Pooling data from a number of RCTs by meta-analysis increases statistical power (reducing random error) and can reveal consistent effects. Systematic reviews and meta-analyses produced by the Cochrane Collaboration (http://www.cochrane.org/) are subject to a process of continual updating and considered the least biased type of systematic review. The level of evidence provided by these reviews currently means they often make a substantial contribution to guiding health-care decisions and policy (see p. 104).

RANDOMISED TRIAL EVIDENCE

In this section, we introduce the **ST**roke: **A R**andomised **T**rial of **E**xercise or **R**elaxation (STARTER) trial (Mead et al. 2007). This is an example of how to design and perform a randomised trial of an exercise intervention. This trial controlled for the effects of social interaction by providing relaxation to the patients not allocated exercise, thereby allowing researchers to determine whether any beneficial effects of exercise were due to the exercise itself rather than the effects of social interaction. The intervention provided in STARTER was designed so that it could be delivered to groups of patients in the community setting.

STARTER was an exploratory trial which aimed to determine the feasibility of exercise training after stroke and to estimate how effective fitness training might be. It randomly allocated 66 participants, mean age 72 years, who had completed their stroke rehabilitation and who were able to walk without assistance from another person, to either fitness training or relaxation (control group). Both groups were held three times a week for 12 weeks. Both the exercise and relaxation (attention control) interventions were delivered in the same rehabilitation hospital by an advanced exercise professional three times a week (Monday, Wednesday, Friday) for groups of up to seven participants. A summary of the trial including the outcome measures is presented in Box 5.1. Details of the actual exercises are further described in chapter 10.

BOX 5.1 Randomised controlled trial – summary	
Participants	66 stroke patients
Intervention	Mixed training (group circuit training)
Comparison	Non-exercise attention control (relaxation)
Outcomes	Physical fitness
	Activity limitations
	Quality of life
	Mood

Content of the programme

During week 1, the instructor familiarised participants with techniques and equipment. At the start of each of the sessions the instructor measured blood pressure (as an additional safety check) and enquired whether the participants had fallen since the last session. Each session lasted 1 hour and 15 minutes (including 'tea-and-chat' after the interventions). Transport (minibus or taxi) was provided. Participants unable to attend every session of the 12-week programme were offered up to three additional 'catch-up' sessions.

The mode of exercise, initial exercise intensity and rate of progression were based on an exercise intervention designed to reduce falls in older frail people (Skelton et al. 2005) many of whom had had a previous stroke and community exercise sessions designed for the UK charity 'Different Strokes' (http://www.differentstrokes.co.uk/). Modifications to the intervention were made to meet the therapeutic aims of normalising body symmetry, anatomical alignment and muscle tone as much as possible during the training process. Further adaptations, e.g. inclusion of the stair climbing/descending exercise, were made by the study physiotherapist. Participants unable to perform or complete a particular exercise were given a shortened, modified or alternative task, i.e. the exercise was 'tailored' to the needs of individual patients (Chapter 10). Although we aimed for progression every 2–4 weeks, individuals not ready to progress (e.g. insufficient strength, endurance or technique) remained at their current prescription and only progressed when assessed by the instructor to be ready. The length of our exercise programme (12 weeks) was similar to previous studies in stroke participants at the time (Saunders et al. 2004).

Each session started with a warm-up to enhance circulation and mobility (15 to 20 minutes). The total duration of the exercise training increased from 15 minutes (week 1) to 40 minutes by week 12. Each session comprised a cardiorespiratory training component followed by a resistance training component.

Cardiorespiratory training

The cardiorespiratory training component involved a continuous 'circuit' of the following exercise stations:

- Cycle ergometry
- Raising and lowering an exercise ball of mass 1.4 kg and diameter 55 cm
- Shuttle walking
- Standing 'chest press' (against a wall)
- Stair climbing/descending (added after week 4).

All exercises were performed consecutively. During the transition between each circuit station, participants walked or marched on the spot to ensure continuous movement. The circuit duration increased from 9 minutes to 21 minutes by week 12. Cycling intensity was increased weekly by small increments in pedalling resistance and/or cadence, whilst maintaining a perceived rate of exertion in the range 13 to 16 (Borg 1982). Brisker efforts were encouraged during all cardiorespiratory exercises as participants became more familiar with the session. The endurance training ended with a graded cool-down and standing stretches.

Resistance training

The resistance training component comprised the following exercises:

- Upper back strengthening exercise (elastic resistance)
- Elbow extension, triceps brachii strengthening exercise (elastic resistance)
- Pole lifting exercise (weighted pole)
- Sit-to-stand exercise (body weight resistance).

All exercises progressed throughout the 12-week training programme. The upper back and triceps strengthening exercises were both performed whilst seated using elastic resistance training bands (Thera-Band™; red, green, blue and silver). Training progressed from four repetitions using a red band (lowest resistance) to 10 repetitions using a silver band (highest resistance). The pole lifting exercise was performed standing and progressing from four repetitions with a light pole (0.22 kg) to 15 repetitions with a heavier pole (3.6 kg). The sit-to-stand exercise (weight bearing evenly on both legs) progressed from four to 10 repetitions and became more difficult by introducing pauses during lowering into the chair, then increasing the frequency and duration of the pauses and increasing the angle of the knee bend and the upper body levers (i.e. the arms).

The resistance training ended with a gentle cool-down and flexibility exercises lasting 10 to 15 minutes. Box 5.2 provides a summary of the exercise training.

BOX 5.2 Exercise training summary	
Training type	Mixed cardiorespiratory and resistance training group circuit
Programme	12 weeks
Frequency	3 days per week
Intensity	Rating of perceived exertion 13–16 (6–20 scale)
Duration	15 min (week 1) increasing to 40 min (week 12)
Specificity	Task-related components; stair ascending/descending, chair rising and walking
Progression	Cycling intensity, exercise duration, repetition number, task complexity, resistance

Findings

A wide range of outcome measures were performed before the interventions, immediately after the interventions, then 4 months later to determine the extent to which any benefits were sustained longer term. Attendance at the classes was excellent, and compliance with individual exercises ranged from 94% to 99%. At 3 months 'role physical' (an item of the Short-Form 36 which measures domains of quality of life), timed up-and-go and walking economy were significantly better in the exercise group. By the final assessment 4 months after completing the interventions, 'role physical', was the only significant difference between groups. Role physical is an aspect of physical health which relates to the extent that people are able to perform physical activities. The lack of any difference in the other outcome measures suggests that, in order for benefits of training to be maintained, exercise training may need to be continued long term.

In conclusion, the STARTER trial demonstrated that this intervention was feasible, that attendance was high and that participants were able to comply with the majority of the individual exercises and safely participate in a varied programme of exercise training. In light of these findings the editors of this book support the recommendation in Box 5.3.

BOX 5.3 Recommendation

Until further evidence is available from other trials about the optimum exercise 'prescription', it would be reasonable to use the intervention developed for the STARTER trial when developing community-based services, as it is feasible for ambulatory stroke survivors who have completed their usual rehabilitation.

SYSTEMATIC REVIEW EVIDENCE

Trials of exercise after stroke have been examined in a number of systematic reviews that examine specific modes of exercise such as over-ground gait training (States et al. 2009), body-weight-supported treadmill training (Moseley et al. 2005) and circuit training classes (English and Hillier 2010). Mobility is often a key outcome of interest.

A Cochrane systematic review of physical fitness training after stroke published in 2009 demonstrated that cardiorespiratory training can improve walking (Saunders et al. 2009). This review was updated in 2010 (Brazzelli et al. 2011); all trials of exercise training after stroke, irrespective of other training variables (e.g. exercise mode, type of delivery), were included. A spectrum of outcome measures that spans the full range of plausible benefits that can arise from exercise were reported. This inclusive approach is probably the best current source of evidence available to take stock of the overall effects of exercise after stroke.

A comprehensive search was performed to locate all published RCTs examining exercise training after stroke (Brazzelli et al. 2011). RCTs were only included if they compared cardiorespiratory training, resistance training, or mixed training with no intervention, a non-exercise intervention, or usual care in stroke survivors. Trials were only included in this review where there was

BOX 5.4 Systematic review – summary of types of included randomised controlled trials	
Participants	Any stroke patient
Interventions	Cardiorespiratory training Resistance training Mixed training
Comparisons	No intervention Non-exercise control Usual care
Outcomes	Death and/or dependence Risk factors Adverse events Physical fitness Activity limitations Quality of life Mood

evidence of a progressive programme of exercise delivered with the intention of increasing fitness. The types of study included are summarised in Box 5.4.

In total 32 trials, involving a total of 1414 participants, met the search criteria:

- Cardiorespiratory training: 14 trials, 651 participants
- Resistance training: 7 trials, 246 participants
- Mixed training interventions: 11 trials, 517 participants

Most of these data relate to ambulatory stroke survivors in the chronic phase (more than 1 month) after stroke onset. Where possible, the data from trials reporting similar interventions and similar outcome measures could be pooled together in a meta-analysis.

An overview of the trial findings are shown in Table 5.1. In many instances diverse outcome measures and trial designs made data pooling difficult. There were few resistance training studies.

A noteworthy finding was that at the end of intervention the incidence of death (5/1414), cerebrovascular events (4/1414) and cardiovascular events (3/1414) was very low and was unrelated to the interventions.

Improvement in peak $\dot{V}O_2$ was the only beneficial modification to stroke risk factors. Most outcomes included in this review were either not examined, showed no significant change with training or were problematic to interpret due to risk of bias. However, sufficient data with consistent findings allow us to say something about the effects of training on physical fitness and activity limitation after stroke.

Effects on physical fitness

There is clear evidence that cardiorespiratory training can improve cardio-respiratory fitness in terms of both $\dot{V}O_2$ peak and maximum work capacity during cycle ergometry. The general pattern of findings among trials of resistance training suggests that muscle strength in a variety of muscle groups can be improved. Measures of fitness in mixed trials are fewer and less clear, but again they support the idea that these interventions have the potential to improve both domains of fitness.

Table 5.1 *Mobility outcomes*

Meta-analyses of RCTs examining the effects (mean difference and 95% CI) of cardiorespiratory training, resistance training or mixed training interventions on walking performance measures at the end of training and after a period of follow-up

Intervention	Walking outcome	End of intervention			End of follow-up		
		N (n)	Mean difference [95% CI]	Significance	N (n)	Mean difference [95% CI]	Significance
Cardiorespiratory training	MWS	7 (365)	8.66 m/min [2.98, 14.3]	P = 0.003	3 (186)	8.21 m/min [3.38, 13.05]	P = 0.0009
	PWS	4 (221)	4.68 m/min [1.40, 7.96]	P = 0.005	–	–	–
	6-MWT	4 (219)	47.1 m [19.4, 74.9]	P = 0.0009	2 (107)	69.3 metres [33.4, 105]	P = 0.0002
Resistance training	MWS	4 (104)	1.92 m/min [–3.50, 7.35]	NS	1 (24)	–19.8 m/min [–95.8, 56.2]	NS
	PWS	3 (80)	2.34 m/min [–6.77, 11.45]	NS	–	–	–
	6-MWT	2 (66)	3.78 m [–68.6, 76.1]	NS	1 (24)	11.0 m/min [–106, 128]	NS
Mixed training	MWS	–	–	–	–	–	–
	PWS	8 (397)	2.93 m/min [0.02, 5.84]	P = 0.05	3 (201)	–2.12 m/min [–4.85, 0.62]	NS
	6-MWT	3 (168)	30.6 m [8.90, 52.3]	P = 0.006	–	–	–

N (n), number of trials/participants; MWS, maximum walking speed; PWS, preferred or comfortable walking speed; 6-MWT, 6-minute walking test.

Evidence for exercise and fitness training after stroke

Effects on activity limitation

One of the most consistent findings of this review is that walking performance can be improved with exercise (Table 5.2). Meta-analyses show that after both cardiorespiratory training and mixed training performance improves in a range of walking performance tests and suggest that walking is both faster, and better tolerated. In contrast resistance training does not appear to have this effect on walking. The most likely reason for this relates to the specificity of the training response, that is where physical adaptations and benefits correspond closely to the types of movement and activity performed during training. Many of the cardiorespiratory and mixed training interventions included walking as an exercise mode.

Although the evidence shows that exercise can increase fitness ($\dot{V}O_2$ peak and strength) after stroke, this does not necessarily provide the mechanism for improved walking; walking performance could change as result of the 'repetitive practice' involved in walking. Such specificity effects can be seen in meta-analysis for the effect of cardiorespiratory training on maximum walking speed (Fig. 5.1); firstly, maximum walking over a short distance is unlikely to respond to improved cardiorespiratory fitness and, secondly, the only study to show no effect (Bateman et al. 2001) was also the only one containing no gait-oriented content of the intervention (cycle

Table 5.2	Overview of the range of benefits achievable after a programme of physical fitness training		
Outcomes	**Cardiorespiratory training**	**Mixed training**	**Resistance training**
Death	ns	ns	ns
Death or dependence	?	?	?
Risk factors	↑	?	?
Adverse events	↔	↔	↔
Physical fitness			
Cardiorespiratory fitness	⬆	↑	?
Musculoskeletal fitness	?	↔	↔
Activity limitations			
Global (disability) scales	↔	↔	?
Walking performance	⬆	↑	↔
Chair rising	↔	?	↔
Stair climbing	?	?	↔
Quality of life	↔	↔	↔
Mood	↔	↔	↔

⬆ Consistent benefit shown by more than one trial in meta-analysis.
↑ Some evidence of benefit in included trials.
↔ No significant or clear consistent benefit.
? No relevant trial data.
ns, not significant.

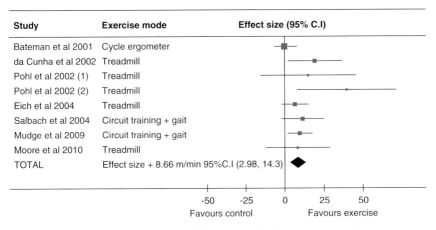

Study	Exercise mode	Effect size (95% C.I)
Bateman et al 2001	Cycle ergometer	
da Cunha et al 2002	Treadmill	
Pohl et al 2002 (1)	Treadmill	
Pohl et al 2002 (2)	Treadmill	
Eich et al 2004	Treadmill	
Salbach et al 2004	Circuit training + gait	
Mudge et al 2009	Circuit training + gait	
Moore et al 2010	Treadmill	
TOTAL	Effect size + 8.66 m/min 95%C.I (2.98, 14.3)	

-50   -25   0   25   50

Favours control   Favours exercise

FIG 5.1 Meta-analysis of seven trials (n=365) examining the effect of cardiorespiratory training interventions on maximum walking speed (m/min). The consistent pattern of positive effect sizes results in a significant pooled effect size (+8.66 m/min 95% CI [2.98, 14.3]).

ergometry). Whatever the underlying cause it is clear that specificity of walking training should be a key consideration for this 'patient-important' outcome.

A second basic principle of exercise training is that of reversibility, i.e. when training is stopped the benefits are reversed. Intriguingly, the data from this review suggest that improvements in speed and tolerance of walking after cardiorespiratory training persist and possibly even increase further after training is finished. It may be that improvements gained during training facilitate an increase in physical activity, in particular walking. This sustained increase in physical activity maintains physical fitness and maintains the gains in speed and tolerance of walking. This is an attractive prospect as it suggests that the 'cycle of detraining' (see Fig. 4.4, p. 88) can be broken.

In trials of mixed training the measures of gait performance may, however, be exaggerated. This is because, although all trials had a control group comparison, some did not expose those in the control group to any kind of intervention. The better designed trials exposed the control group to a non-exercise intervention to control for attention and factors such as increased physical activity getting to and from the training sessions (e.g. such as the STARTER trial, p. 96). When these confounded studies were excluded, the beneficial effects of exercise on gait are limited to cardiorespiratory training alone.

In summary, a comprehensive systematic review approach shows that the low fitness of stroke survivors can be improved. Interventions which include cardiorespiratory training improve how fast and how far people can walk. Improvements in gait are linked to task-specific cardiorespiratory training which involves walking/gait exercises and these may be sustained even after training has finished. Although exercise appears safe and feasible, there are too few other data to conclude whether exercise has wider benefits for people with stroke.

RELATED EVIDENCE

The RCT (p. 96) and systematic review evidence (p. 99) discussed has focused on exercise interventions alone. However, physical activity and exercise may be provided as one component within a complex intervention.

Complex lifestyle interventions may have a role in controlling risk factors and secondary stroke prevention. For example, a 12-month complex lifestyle intervention (Joubert et al. 2009) including smoking cessation, reduction in alcohol intake, maintenance of a recommended body mass index and taking exercise reduced vascular risk factors and caused increased physical activity in stroke survivors (n = 186).

Little is known about complex lifestyle interventions for stroke survivors. However, a complex lifestyle intervention is the foundation of cardiac rehabilitation and this is reflected in current recommendations (SIGN 2002). Since coronary heart disease and stroke are related, in that they share many of the same risk factors, this hints that this approach may have benefits for stroke.

TRANSLATING RESEARCH EVIDENCE INTO PRACTICE

Recommendations for exercise and physical activity after stroke do exist but these are generally modelled on those for healthy individuals and healthy elderly people rather than being based on controlled RCT and systematic review evidence (e.g. Gordon et al. 2004, Nelson et al. 2007).

Current clinical guidelines for stroke rehabilitation and management in the UK incorporate some recommendations for fitness training (Box 5.5).

BOX 5.5 Current fitness training recommendations

Department of Health/Vascular Programme/Stroke (National Stroke Strategy 2007)

'Rehabilitation – support to regain well-being – requires rehabilitation specialists and continuing support from a wide range of community-based services, such as exercise classes'

Royal College of Physicians Intercollegiate Stroke Working Party (2008)

'After stroke all patients should participate in aerobic training unless there are contraindications unrelated to stroke'

National Health Service Scotland (Better Heart Disease and Stroke Care Action Plan 2009)

'NHS Boards, through their stroke Managed Clinical Networks (MCNs), should continue to work with leisure industry representatives to make best use of the [Exercise and Fitness Training after Stroke] training course to improve access to exercise and fitness training for people with stroke in their area'

Scottish Intercollegiate Guidelines Network (SIGN) Guideline No. 118 (2010)

'Gait-oriented physical fitness training should be offered to all patients assessed as medically stable and functionally safe to participate, when the goal of treatment is to improve functional ambulation'

Guidelines are often influenced by systematic review evidence and the strength of recommendations is influenced by the level of evidence available (see p. 95). For example, the SIGN guideline for stroke (Guideline 118), which includes rehabilitation (Scottish Intercollegiate Guidelines Network 2010) includes a very simple statement about fitness training for gait; this is given a 'strong' recommendation as the evidence is derived from high-quality systematic review of studies showing a consistent effect.

Thus, the broad consensus is that exercise training after stroke should be implemented into the ongoing care of people after stroke (Gordon et al. 2004). However, the evidence base about the optimum exercise prescription and the optimum time for delivering exercise training is incomplete. With careful judgement, exercise professionals can design and deliver an exercise programme for stroke survivors, based on the available evidence, some common sense and extrapolation of knowledge from other diseases and patient groups.

Parts 3 and 4 of this book focus on how to implement the best available evidence into clinical practice for exercise professionals.

SUMMARY POINTS

THEORETICAL BENEFITS

- Participating in exercise may have a range of plausible effects after stroke, including:
  ○ Increased physical fitness and physical function
  ○ Psychosocial benefits
  ○ Reduced mortality/morbidity and secondary stroke prevention.
- Participating in exercise may have adverse events. However, these can be managed through careful screening, tailoring the intervention and monitoring.

EVIDENCE OF BENEFIT

- It is feasible and safe to participate in a variety of short-term fitness training after stroke; the incidence of death or serious adverse events is very low and unrelated to the interventions.
- There are insufficient data to assess the effects of:
  ○ Exercise on dependency, risk factors, quality of life and mood
  ○ Resistance training and mixed training.
- Cardiorespiratory training:
  ○ Improves cardiorespiratory fitness
  ○ Improves how fast and how far people can walk:
    – Benefits are specific to gait-oriented exercise modes
    – Benefits may be sustained after training finishes.
- Resistance training:
  ○ May improve muscle strength but the data are limited.
- Mixed training:
  ○ The few gait and functional benefits are difficult to attribute to the content of the mixed training interventions as these studies are often confounded.
- Training benefits are specific, that is they are likely to reflect the mode of training, e.g. gait training improves walking.
- Optimum exercise prescription in terms of type and dose has yet to be defined for people with stroke.

RELATED EVIDENCE

- Exercise training (or physical activity) may be combined with other lifestyle interventions.
- Complex lifestyle interventions may theoretically control risk factors and reduce incidence of secondary stroke, but there is little evidence to explore this concept.

TRANSLATING EVIDENCE INTO PRACTICE

- Clinical guidelines for stroke rehabilitation in the UK currently make statements recommending some aspects of exercise and these are based on systematic review evidence involving stroke survivors.
- Recommendations and guidelines need clinical and exercise professional judgement and experience in order to generate a tailored exercise prescription for individual stroke survivors.

REFERENCES

Bateman, A., Culpan, F.J., Pickering, A.D., et al., 2001. The effect of aerobic training on rehabilitation outcomes after recent severe brain injury: a randomized controlled evaluation. Arch. Phys. Med. Rehabil. 82, 174–182.

Borg, G.A., 1982. Psychophysical bases of perceived exertion. Med. Sci. Sports Exerc. 14, 377–381.

Brazzelli, M., Saunders, D.H., Greig, C.A., et al., 2011. Physical fitness training for stroke patients. Cochrane Database Syst. Rev. 11, CD003316: doi: 10.1002/14651858.

Carin-Levy, G., Kendall, M., Young, A., et al., 2009. The psychosocial effects of exercise and relaxation classes for persons surviving a stroke. Can. J. Occup. Ther. 76, 73–80.

Department of Health/Vascular Programme/Stroke, 2007. National Stroke Strategy. Department of Health, London.

Dickinson, H.O., Mason, J.M., Nicolson, D.J., et al., 2006. Lifestyle interventions to reduce raised blood pressure: a systematic review of randomized controlled trials. J. Hypertens. 24 (2), 215–233.

English, C., Hillier, S.L., 2010. Circuit class therapy for improving mobility after stroke. Cochrane Database Syst. Rev. 7, CD007513. doi:10.1002/14651858.

French, B., Thomas, L., Leathley, M., et al., 2010. Does repetitive task training improve functional activity after stroke? A Cochrane systematic review and meta-analysis. J. Rehabil. Med. 42, 9–14.

Gauthier, L.V., Taub, E., Perkins, C., et al., 2008. Remodeling the brain: plastic structural brain changes produced by different motor therapies after stroke. Stroke 39, 1520–1525.

Gordon, N.F., Gulanick, M., Costa, F., et al., 2004. Physical activity and exercise recommendations for stroke survivors: an American Heart Association scientific statement from the Council on Clinical Cardiology, Subcommittee on Exercise, Cardiac Rehabilitation, and Prevention; the Council on Cardiovascular Nursing; the Council on Nutrition, Physical Activity, and Metabolism; and the Stroke Council. Stroke 35, 1230–1240.

Intercollegiate Stroke Working Party, 2008. National Clinical Guideline for Stroke, third ed. Royal College of Physicians, London.

Jolliffe, J.A., Rees, K., Taylor, R.S., et al., 2000. Exercise-based rehabilitation for coronary heart disease. Cochrane Database Syst. Rev. 4, CD001800. doi:10.1002/14651858.

Joubert, J., Reid, C., Barton, D., et al., 2009. Integrated care improves risk-factor modification after stroke: initial results of the Integrated Care for the Reduction of Secondary Stroke model. J. Neurol. Neurosurg. Psychiatry 80, 279–284.

Mead, G.E., Greig, C.A., Cunningham, I., et al., 2007. Stroke: a randomized trial of exercise or relaxation. J. Am. Geriatr. Soc. 55, 892–899.

Mead, G.E., Morley, W., Campbell, P., et al., 2008. Exercise for depression. Cochrane Database Syst. Rev. 4, CD004366. doi:10.1002/14651858.

Mead, G., 2005. Exercise or relaxation after stroke? BMJ 330, 1337.

Moseley, A.M., Stark, A., Cameron, I.D., et al., 2005. Treadmill training and body weight support for walking after stroke. Cochrane Database Syst. Rev. 2, CD002840. doi:10.1002/14651858.

Nelson, M.E., Rejeski, W.J., Blair, S.N., et al., 2007. Physical activity and public health in older adults: recommendation from the American College of Sports Medicine and the American Heart Association. Med. Sci. Sports Exerc. 39, 1435–1445.

NHS Scotland, 2009. Better heart disease and stroke care action plan. The Scottish Government, Edinburgh.

Patterson, S., Ross-Edwards, B., 2009. Long-term stroke survivors' needs and perceptions of an exercise maintenance model of care. Int. J. Ther. Rehabil. 16, 659–669.

Saunders, D.H., Greig, C., Young, A., et al., 2004. Physical fitness training for stroke patients. Cochrane Database Syst. Rev. 1, CD003316. doi:10.1002/14651858.

Saunders, D.H., Greig, C.A., Mead, G.E., et al., 2009. Physical fitness training for stroke patients. Cochrane Database Syst. Rev. 4, CD003316. doi:10.1002/14651858.

Scottish Intercollegiate Guidelines Network (SIGN), 2002. Cardiac rehabilitation. SIGN Publication no. 57 edn, SIGN, Edinburgh.

Scottish Intercollegiate Guidelines Network (SIGN), 2010. Management of patients with stroke: rehabilitation, prevention and management of complications, and discharge planning, SIGN Publication no. 118 edn, SIGN, Edinburgh.

Shaw, K.A., Gennat, H.C., O'Rourke, P., et al., 2006. Exercise for overweight or obesity. Cochrane Database Syst. Rev. 4, CD003817. doi:10.1002/14651858.

Skelton, D., Dinan, S., Campbell, M., et al., 2005. Tailored group exercise (Falls Management Exercise – FaME) reduces falls in community-dwelling older frequent fallers (an RCT). Age Ageing 34, 636–639.

States, R.A., Pappas, E., Salem, Y., 2009. Overground physical therapy gait training for chronic stroke patients with mobility deficits. Cochrane Database Syst. Rev. 3, CD006075 doi:10.1002/14651858.

Thomas, D.E., Elliott, E.J., Naughton, G.A., 2006. Exercise for type 2 diabetes mellitus. Cochrane Database Syst. Rev. 3, CD002968. doi:10.1002/14651858.

Evidence for exercise and fitness training after stroke

Understanding and enhancing exercise behaviour after stroke

Marie Donaghy • Frederike van Wijck

CHAPTER CONTENTS

INTRODUCTION

The benefits of exercise after stroke described in chapter 5 should encourage stroke survivors to participate in an exercise programme to improve their health and wellbeing. Taking up exercise is an example of a health behaviour, which is a behaviour related to an individual's health status (Ogden 2004). However, taking up a health behaviour and maintaining this in the longer term is a well-known challenge for healthy people (Dugdill et al. 2005, Williams et al. 2007), and so it is reasonable to assume that is also likely to be a challenge for stroke survivors.

For example, in the STARTER trial (Mead et al. 2007) just over half the number of eligible patients indicated that they wished to participate, and some who initially agreed changed their minds. For those who did agree to participate, class attendance was excellent during the 12-week programme (chapter 5), indicating high levels of motivation. However, at the end of the trial, when the provision of formal exercise classes ceased, some of the participants did not continue to exercise.

These findings raise some interesting questions. Why do some people choose to participate in exercise and others don't? Why do some people who indicate a desire to participate in exercise change their minds? Why do people who participate in a programme of exercise training stop exercising once the programme has come to an end? Furthermore, since the benefits of exercise diminish when the training comes to an end (Mead et al. 2007), how can stroke survivors be encouraged to continue to be physically active beyond formal training programmes?

In this chapter, we will describe what we know about the barriers and motivators to exercising after stroke and explore theoretical concepts that describe and explain behaviour and behaviour change, in particular self-efficacy and the Transtheoretical Model (which includes stages of change). We will then explore how these concepts may apply to enhancing exercise behaviour amongst stroke survivors through techniques including motivational interviewing and goal setting. Finally, we will give exercise and health professionals some suggestions about how to use this information to help stroke survivors to start exercising and to continue exercising in the longer term.

BARRIERS AND MOTIVATORS TO EXERCISE

The evidence that shows benefits of physical fitness training for stroke survivors (chapter 5) has led to recommendations that exercise training should be provided as part of the post-stroke pathway (Best et al. 2010, Royal College of Physicians 2008, Scottish Government 2009, Scottish Intercollegiate Guidelines Network 2010). Participation in exercise may be perceived to be difficult by some stroke survivors, many of whom are sedentary (Shaughnessy et al. 2006). Sedentary behaviour patterns may arise as a direct result of the neurological effect of stroke (e.g. paresis which makes walking more difficult), or it may be that there are psychological barriers to exercise (e.g. fear of falling). Additionally, stroke survivors may not have been physically active prior to their stroke and so undertaking exercise training for the first time after a stroke may pose a considerable challenge. In addition to these personal barriers, there may be environmental barriers that reduce personal choice and impede participation. These may include inaccessible programmes, lack of community recreation facilities, transport difficulties, architectural barriers, system and policy barriers and social attitudes (Rimmer et al. 2000).

Although there are only a handful of small studies exploring barriers and motivators to exercise after stroke, these bring some important insights into the factors influencing exercise participation.

BARRIERS TO EXERCISE PARTICIPATION AFTER STROKE

One survey from North America with a group of 83 stroke survivors identified a number of barriers to exercise. The most commonly reported were: the cost of the programme (61% of respondents), lack of awareness of a fitness centre in their area (57%), no means of transportation (57%), no knowledge of how to exercise, whilst the least common barriers were lack of interest (16%), lack of time (11%) and concern that exercise would worsen their condition (1%) (Rimmer et al. 2008). Damush et al. (2007) conducted three focus groups with

13 stroke survivors recruited from an existing research study and found that the barriers preventing exercise participation were physical impairments resulting from the stroke, lack of motivation and lack of available facilities for exercise. Hammel et al. (2006), in a participatory action research study with 20 stroke survivors recruited from the community, identified both personal and environmental barriers; personal barriers related to physical and cognitive impairment including difficulty walking, fatigue and pain, motor impairments related to stroke, inattention and memory loss; environmental barriers included physical access, transportation and lack of social support. Robison et al. (2009) explored the barriers that prevented stroke survivors from returning to valued activities such as employment, domestic and social roles. Personal barriers were linked to physical and cognitive impairment, while environmental barriers included lack of adaptations to improve safety on entering or leaving the home, lack of social support and professional help.

MOTIVATORS TO EXERCISE PARTICIPATION AFTER STROKE

One qualitative study exploring the motivation of 29 stroke survivors, who were participating in a treadmill study (Resnick et al. 2008), highlighted the importance of personal goals (including increased ability in walking and stair climbing), physical benefits (feeling stronger, walking better and improved balance) and psychological benefits (including improvement in mood and the sense of independence). Another study demonstrated that social support from family, fellow stroke survivors and professionals facilitated exercise participation (Damush et al. 2007). Social and professional support and adaptability of the individual were also found to be helpful in resuming valued activities post stroke (Robison et al. 2009). An Australian qualitative study looked at the needs and perceptions of stroke survivors attending a 1 hour weekly exercise programme in the community. Ten stroke survivors in the chronic stage after stroke were interviewed. The findings suggest that a maintenance exercise class built confidence in participants, increased motivation and provided opportunity for both exercise participation and socialisation (Patterson and Ross-Edwards 2009).

RELEVANCE OF THIS KNOWLEDGE TO UNDERSTANDING EXERCISE PARTICIPATION

Although the studies described above were small, and some recruited patients from existing studies (and thus there may be inherent biases), the themes that emerge from this body of evidence include:

- The importance of barriers, both personal and environmental, that influence exercise participation. Personal barriers include fear of recurrent stroke, fatigue, pain and perceived lack of time, while environmental barriers include lack of access to suitable facilities and transport. Both types of barriers need to be considered when providing Exercise after Stroke services and setting up new services.
- The importance of social support in helping the stroke survivor to exercise. Thus, exercise and health professionals involved in Exercise after Stroke services may need to consider how best to involve family members and/or

carers in supporting the stroke survivor to exercise. Furthermore, exercising in a group with other stroke survivors is likely to enhance confidence and a sense of belonging; these positive experiences of exercising with other stroke survivors who were 'in the same boat' were also described in other studies (Carin-Levy et al. 2009, Mead 2009, Reed et al. 2010).

• Achievement of personal goals. These may include physical goals, e.g. improved walking, or return to work. Later in this chapter we will explore what we know about goal setting in stroke rehabilitation, and how to apply this to stroke survivors wishing to exercise.

OTHER POSSIBLE INFLUENCES ON EXERCISE BEHAVIOUR IN STROKE SURVIVORS

Exercise behaviour is complex (Biddle and Mutrie 2008) and whether stroke survivors engage in exercise or not will be influenced by their attitudes to exercise. These may be long-standing beliefs or beliefs that have changed as a result of the stroke. Their attitudes are likely to be influenced to some extent by the views of family, friends and professionals.

Whether we engage in or avoid physical activity is influenced by our knowledge, beliefs and feelings about exercise. This informs our attitude towards exercise participation; if our attitude is positive, we are more likely to engage in regular physical activity. Attitude can be defined as a psychological tendency to behave in a particular way. It is hypothetical and, like other psychological constructs such as personality and motivation, not open to direct observation. Attitudes can be inferred from verbal or non-verbal responses relating to feelings, beliefs and exercise behaviours. Exercise professionals could use carefully phrased questions to gain a better insight into individual stroke survivors' attitudes (e.g. how will exercise help you to do the things you want to do?) and confidence (self-efficacy) towards exercise participation (e.g. how confident are you that you will be able to do this exercise by yourself?).

THEORETICAL EXPLANATIONS OF EXERCISE BEHAVIOUR

Numerous theories and models have been developed to try and describe, explain and predict people's health behaviours (Connor and Norman 2005). Theories of health behaviour in general, and exercise behaviour in particular, have been applied by health and exercise psychologists as well as health promotion specialists to influence behaviour change in clinical and non-clinical populations for more than 30 years (Connor and Norman 2005). More recently, health-care professionals have used some of these theories to inform self-management interventions for people with long-term conditions (Jones 2006), for example in enhancing confidence or self-efficacy (Jones et al. 2009) and goal setting in the context of rehabilitation (Scobbie et al. 2009).

The theories introduced in this chapter have been selected for their relevance to stroke survivors as currently supported by the literature. However, because health and exercise psychology applied to stroke rehabilitation is a relatively new area of research, there are still many questions about how these theories apply to enhancing exercise behaviour after stroke.

SELF-EFFICACY

Self-efficacy is a psychological construct that has been defined as 'the belief in one's capabilities to organise and execute the course of action required to produce given attainments' (Bandura 1997, p. 3). It is a measure of confidence and is linked to a personal sense of control. If people believe that they can take action to solve a problem, they are more likely to do so and they will be more committed to the task (Bandura 1977). Self-efficacy includes holding a personal belief about the outcome of a particular behaviour or action and also the ability to make an accurate judgement on the skills required to carry out the behaviour. Self-efficacy beliefs are linked to the degree of effort put into achieving a task and to the perseverance to continue with the task in the face of adversity (Bandura 1997).

Four sources of information have been described that both appraise and enhance self-efficacy for any particular behaviour (Bandura 1997):

1. Performance accomplishments: successful performance of the behaviour is likely to increase self-efficacy, while repeated unsuccessful performance tends to lower self-efficacy, especially if this happens early on.
2. Vicarious experience: this refers to seeing others who are in a similar situation successfully perform the behaviour and comparing one's own performance to theirs.
3. Verbal persuasion: encouragement from others which demonstrates their belief that the person is capable of undertaking the behaviour.
4. Emotional arousal: self-efficacy in dealing with a task or situation is partially judged based on signs of stress. Reducing such symptoms and correcting their misinterpretation may enhance self-efficacy.

A recent systematic review and meta-analysis of 27 studies with 5501 healthy adults analysed interventions aimed at changing self-efficacy in the context of promoting lifestyle and recreational physical activity (Ashford et al. 2010). The findings showed that feedback in which a participant's performance was compared to that of others was the most influential component to increase self-efficacy related to physical activity. Also, interventions that incorporated vicarious experiences were more successful in this respect than ones that did not. Interestingly, verbal persuasion alone was insufficient to increase either self-efficacy or exercise behaviour.

How do the findings from this meta-analysis compare to other research in stroke? In two studies exploring stroke survivors' views on a community-based exercise scheme, participants commented positively on being in a stroke-specific group, which enabled them to learn from each other and compare their performance with that of others (Reed et al. 2010, Sharma et al. 2011). This suggests that stroke-specific exercise settings provide opportunities for vicarious learning, which may be instrumental in rebuilding self-efficacy. The finding that verbal encouragement alone was not sufficient echoes findings from a multinational randomised controlled trial with 314 stroke survivors; Boysen et al. (2009) found that repeated encouragement and verbal advice alone did not increase physical activity. Clearly, interventions to increase physical activity after stroke need to comprise more than just verbal support.

With the aim to increase perceived action control, Sniehotta et al. (2005) in a longitudinal study of 240 cardiac rehabilitation patients found that psychological interventions including detailed action plans, barrier-focused mental strategies and diary keeping resulted in more physical activity at follow-up, and better adherence to recommended levels of exercise intensity. Self-regulatory skills such as planning and action control also improved. The authors concluded that targeting self-regulatory skills can help post-rehabilitation cardiac patients to reduce behavioural risk factors and facilitate healthier lifestyle changes. These findings may well apply to stroke survivors, although this will require further research.

Psychological interventions for stroke survivors, based on the theory of self-efficacy, have been developed to increase confidence, facilitate recognition of personal efforts, enable goal setting and increasing exercise behaviour (Johnston et al. 2007, Jones et al. 2009, Jones and Riazi 2011, Shaughnessy and Resnick 2009). Support for the link between self-efficacy and exercise behaviour was found by Shaugnessy et al. (2006). Their survey of 312 stroke survivors found that self-efficacy and outcome expectations (i.e. beliefs that certain outcomes will be produced by personal action) were positively linked to reported exercise behaviour. Additionally, those who had exercised before their stroke were more likely to participate in regular exercise post stroke, while doctor's recommendations influenced participation. However, taken together, these factors only explained 33% of the total variance in reported exercise behaviour, suggesting that there must be other factors that predict exercise participation after stroke.

The influence of self-efficacy on outcomes after stroke and the effectiveness of self-management strategies based on self-efficacy were examined in a systematic review by Jones and Riazi (2011). A total of 18 studies with 1418 participants investigated the influence of self-efficacy on rehabilitation outcomes, indicating that self-efficacy impacts on quality of life, mood, independence in activities of daily living, as well as aspects of physical functioning such as walking. A total of four studies with 343 participants explored the effectiveness of self-management strategies, based on self-efficacy theory. Only two randomised controlled trials were included, so the findings need to be interpreted with caution. Although there was some support for self-management strategies based on self-efficacy principles, many questions still remain, including the best way to deliver such interventions to stroke survivors (e.g. group-based or individual).

Self-efficacy is a critical determinant of self-regulation, a term described by Bandura (1986) as an individual's evaluation of their own actions against identified expectations or desires, which allows them to modify their future behaviour. Based on this function, it will be important to establish people's view of what they want to achieve and what they think they can achieve. For example, a stroke survivor may be motivated to exercise to improve their walking, if they perceive a discrepancy between their current abilities and what they would like to achieve. However, their motivation may be dampened if they don't perceive themselves as being able to achieve an improvement. Motivational interviewing is one technique that exercise professionals might want to use to establish stroke survivors' views and enhance their self-regulatory skills. This technique is described later in the chapter.

TRANSTHEORETICAL MODEL (INCORPORATING STAGES OF CHANGE)

Taking up a health behaviour such as exercise is easier said than done (just think about those New Year resolutions to go to the gym!). Based on earlier research on smoking cessation (DiClemente et al. 1985), we now have a much better appreciation that initiating a health behaviour is not like flicking a switch, but a process of change.

The transtheoretical model was constructed in an attempt to explain the dynamics of behavioural changes, synthesising ideas from other social cognitive models into one comprehensive, multi-layered 'supra' structure (DiClemente et al. 1985). The Transtheoretical Model presents three key ideas:

- First, behaviour change is seen as a dynamic process that occurs in the following *stages*:
  - Pre-contemplation: this stage is characterised by a lack of awareness of risk, and an absence of any intention to change; e.g. a stroke survivor is not aware of the risks of their sedentary behaviour and has no intention to become more physically active.
  - Contemplation: this stage is characterised by an intention to change behaviour, but an absence of actual action; e.g. the stroke survivor is considering exercise, but has not actually started exercising.
  - Preparation: This stage is characterised by some action, however this is insufficient to meet a specific target; e.g. the stroke survivor has attended a few exercise classes, but is not meeting the recommendation of 3 x 1 hour per week (Best et al. 2010).
  - Action: people in this stage have successfully stuck to their intended behaviour for 6 months; e.g. the stroke survivor has undertaken 3 x 1-hour exercise sessions per week for 6 months.
  - Maintenance: people in this stage have continued to meet their targets for more than 6 months; e.g. the stroke survivor has maintained class attendance for more than 6 months or has introduced regular physical activity into their daily routine, sufficient to meet the recommendation. Relapse can occur at any stage, as can be seen in Figure 6.1.
- Second, it is suggested that progress through these stages is driven by a series of 10 *processes* specific to particular stages, including 'consciousness raising' (receiving information on how exercise may help, how exercise classes can be accessed), 'counter-conditioning' (using the positive aspects of exercise to counter fears and anxieties about future health) and 'stimulus control' (controlling situations that may trigger dropping out from the exercise class). Other processes include 'warning of risk' (receiving information on risks of exercise and how these can be reduced), 'caring about consequences' (discussing how one feels about exercising), 'increasing health alternatives' (increasing physical activity in everyday activities), 'understanding benefits' (belief that participation in exercise is possible), 'helping relationships' (eliciting social support for exercise

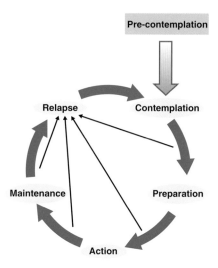

FIG 6.1 An illustration of the cyclical stages of behaviour change from the Transtheoretical Model. Relapse can occur at any point in the cycle of change.

participation), 'environmental re-evaluation' (learning about physical activity opportunities in the community), and 'reinforcement management' (rewarding yourself for physical activity or receiving a reward from others).

- Third, the notion that weighing up the advantages of change ('pros') against the disadvantages ('cons') can help people to successfully change behaviour. For example, the stroke survivor who considers that they will improve their walking and feel better by exercising regularly is more likely to want to start exercising than the stroke survivor who feels that they would probably get tired from exercising regularly. Earlier on, we cautioned that the intention to exercise is not the same as actual exercise behaviour. One of the strengths of this stage theory is that it distinguishes between the motivational stages and the action stages. During the motivational stage, the stroke survivor might demonstrate the intention to participate in exercise based on self-beliefs, taking account of risk perceptions, outcome expectancies and perceived self-efficacy. In the action stages, the exercise must be planned, initiated and maintained and relapses managed.

The Transtheoretical Model is one of the most researched models when assessing stages of engagement and it has been used for exercise counselling, guiding people through individual interventions at each stage and has been well received by health-care professionals. It may help health or exercise professionals to target their intervention. For example, providing a sheet with exercises is likely to be appropriate when a stroke survivor is in the Preparation stage, but counterproductive when they are still in the Contemplative stage.

In summary, this section has presented an introduction to the concept of self-efficacy and one landmark health behaviour theory that has been used by health-care professionals with a range of populations and different health behaviours. Research indicates there is some value in using these concepts and theories to explain and predict health behaviour and to inform interventions, although further examining their application to increasing exercise participation in stroke survivors and long-term management of stroke will be required.

APPLYING THEORY TO PRACTICE

Exercise and health-care professionals can use the findings from research on the barriers and motivators to exercise and interventions based on the theory of self-efficacy to develop a range of techniques to facilitate stroke survivors' engagement and participation in exercise. A summary of these techniques is provided in Box 6.1. Some of these may be familiar and easy to apply, whilst others (e.g. challenge ambivalence, teasing out the issues that prevent the stroke survivor from changing their behaviour) may require some further practical training.

Motivational interviewing is a technique that has been linked to increasing intrinsic motivation, self-efficacy and self-regulatory skills. In a meta-analysis that included 119 studies relating to substance use (tobacco, alcohol, drugs, marijuana) and health-related behaviors (diet, exercise, safe sex), motivational interviewing produced statistically significant results in the small effect range, suggesting that this was a useful counselling approach for facilitating behaviour change (Lundahl et al. 2010).

It is an approach that is used in health promotion to facilitate behaviour change in a number of lifestyle areas, e.g. smoking cessation, alcohol and drug rehabilitation, as well as exercise participation in healthy people and people with chronic heart disease (e.g. Hardcastle et al. 2008). Motivational interviewing techniques provide exercise and health-care professionals with an approach that allows the stroke survivor to express their feelings and beliefs about exercise and support them in their decision-making. Following motivational interviewing, we will provide a synopsis of goal setting, which can be used to set more specific targets, once a person has decided to become more physically active.

MOTIVATIONAL INTERVIEWING

Motivational interviewing has been defined as a collaborative person-centred form of guiding to elicit and strengthen motivation for change (Miller and Rollnick 2009). It is a useful approach where people know what they want to achieve, but are prevented from achieving it because they are trapped in a cycle of negative thinking on why they cannot achieve it. The concept of motivational interviewing arose out of work with problem drinkers (Miller and Rollnick, 1991) and it was then transferred to facilitate areas of lifestyle change, such as taking up exercise in people with chronic heart conditions as well as people with diabetes who have been advised to exercise.

The approach taken in motivational interviewing is one of guiding by communicating in a partner-like relationship. The overall goal is to increase motivation by encouraging an evaluation of views, expectations and behaviours, challenging

BOX 6.1 Encouraging physical activity after stroke: applying health behaviour theory

- Provide information about stroke and recovery from stroke. This will allow the stroke survivor to consider the seriousness of the event and the risk of a further stroke.
- Provide information regarding the benefits of exercise including the risks associated with remaining sedentary versus the risks associated with participating in exercise.
- Ask the stroke survivor how they feel about exercise and what they believe they are capable of doing in regard to exercise participation.
- Explore with the stroke survivor how confident they feel about their ability to successfully participate in an exercise programme.
- Ask them about their previous experiences in regard to what makes them confident or not confident about participating in exercise.
- Discuss with them what action they would like to take to improve their confidence. This may include: speaking with other stroke survivors, observing an exercise class, testing out their own capabilities by undertaking a supervised exercise session.
- Explore what it is they would like to achieve in relation to improving their physical activity and function and what they think they can achieve and how.
- Ask about barriers to exercise and what is stopping them participate.
- Find out what they consider to be social and environmental impediments and facilitators to achieving their goals.
- Challenge ambivalence, teasing out the issues that prevent the stroke survivor from changing their behaviour.
- Discuss the importance of change to enable the stroke survivor to be the person they want to be – in regard to physical activity and function.
- Undertake problem-solving exercises with them to enable them to overcome perceived or actual barriers.
- Discuss what they can do to facilitate participation in physical activity, e.g. seek a referral to an exercise class from the doctor or physiotherapist, find out what is offered in their local area, involve family or friends in making arrangements for transport.
- Find out from them what they can do routinely to increase exercise participation, e.g. making a point of going out for a short walk most days of the week.
- Provide feedback regarding exercise participation and discuss how rewards can be used to increase motivation.
- Encourage stroke survivors to use a diary that records their exercise sessions and where they can document other information, for example costs and benefits of exercise, targets achieved, actions taken to overcome barriers.
- Discuss relapse from exercise participation and how this can be managed. Encourage the stroke survivor to come up with strategies that are meaningful to them.

ambivalence, so that change arises from within and is not imposed. Key aspects of the approach can be summarised as follows:

- The health or exercise professional learns about the stroke survivor's perspective, beliefs and values, finding out what works best for them.
- The motivation to change comes from the individual and is not imposed – direct persuasion will not work.

- The style of communication is facilitatory, using open-ended questions to challenge where appropriate, providing affirmation of the person's intentions, reflecting on actions and decisions taken in order to support the person's beliefs that they can achieve success.
- The 'readiness ruler', using a scale of 0–10, can be used to explore with individuals their readiness to change. This scale is a longitudinal representation of the stages of change. The lower numbers indicate not ready to change, the higher numbers indicate ready for change[1]. A score of 5 or above suggests that they are considering changing. Using open-ended questions, clients are asked how important the change is to them, and how confident they are in achieving the change. Their answers can be probed and challenged on why they see themselves at certain points on the scale, helping them challenge their own beliefs and attitudes, in order to manage their ambivalence and to make their own decisions.

The underlying principles of motivational interviewing include:

1. Effective listening: hearing what the individual is saying and seeking to understand the person's feelings and expectations without making any judgements.
2. Importance of change: through discussion the importance of change is highlighted in regard to the discrepancy between how the person wants to be and how he or she is currently feeling in regard to his or her function, health, family and happiness. For example, when the individual sees how engaging with exercise may help overcome the discrepancy between where they are now in regard to their function and where they want to be, this is more likely to influence decisions to change.
3. Flow with resistance: for example, resistance to change may arise where the stroke survivor and the exercise professional see the problem and/or solution differently. Motivational interviewing avoids confrontation and looks for opportunity where the resistance can be re-framed, involving the person actively in problem solving.
4. Support self-efficacy: a general goal of motivational interviewing is to enhance the individual's confidence to cope with obstacles and to be successful.

The approach taken by exercise and health-care professionals when applying any of the techniques should be one of partnership working, including active listening (see chapter 7), allowing the stroke survivor to express their feelings and beliefs about exercise and supporting them in their decision making. Open-ended questions are used to confirm, challenge or reflect on what has been said when discussing exercise participation. It is important to explore what the stroke survivor thinks will work best for them, be non-judgemental and when discussing barriers and motivators to participation, always look to the stroke survivor to come up with solutions.

The case study in Box 6.2 serves to illustrate how theory can inform practice by applying some of the techniques listed in Box 6.1.

[1]Note that Price et al. (1999) found that stroke survivors may have difficulty using 'rulers' of this type; hence exercise professionals would need to take care explaining the ruler, and check for inconsistency in responses as an indication of whether this method is suitable for the individual.

Understanding and enhancing exercise behaviour after stroke

BOX 6.2 Case study

Joan is a 59-year-old school teacher who had a right hemispheric stroke resulting in left mild hemiparesis. Prior to her stroke, Joan spent her leisure time watching television or going to the theatre with friends. She has never been keen on sports or physical activity, preferring to use her car rather than walk or take public transport. Joan now wants to improve her walking and knows that joining an exercise class will help her do this, but lacks confidence in her ability to succeed. Joan is able to walk around the house and short distances outside. Joan has recently retired from teaching and feels she now has time to participate in regular exercise.

She arranges to meet with David, an exercise professional, to discuss how to get started. David explores with Joan how physically fit she is at the moment and how fit she wants to be in the future. Joan talks about her current levels of physical activity which include washing, dressing, cooking, some light housework and the occasional outing in the car to visit friends. Joan discusses with David the risk factors for having a further stroke if she remains inactive. For Joan the recognition that exercising five times a week may reduce the risk of her having another stroke, as well as improving her walking, reinforces her motivation and intention to change her sedentary lifestyle to one that includes regular exercise. David explores with Joan what she perceives will be possible barriers to exercise, he listens carefully, probing into what she thinks she will be able to do and what she sees as being difficult. Joan highlights fatigue as a barrier; she says that she worries she will get breathless and will not have the energy to keep going in an exercise class. David asks her why she thinks this may happen, and explores what situations she has been in previously when this has happened, and what the worst possible outcome might be if she goes to an exercise class.

Following this discussion, Joan re-appraises her worry of not being able to continue to exercise in class. Based on the evidence that she only gets breathless going up flights of stairs and the re-assurance from David that class participants work within their own levels of aerobic effort, she now feels less anxious about her ability to take part in the exercise class. David asks Joan about how ready she feels to start the class and her confidence that she will continue to attend. Joan explains that she has never participated in an exercise class but that she did find the exercises given to her by the physiotherapist while in hospital very helpful. Joan demonstrates in the ensuing discussion that her motivation and intention is high to start exercising, but that her confidence about being successful and enjoying the programme is still low. David suggests that she comes along to meet people in the class so that she can speak to them about their experience before she decides to commit herself to attending. Joan does this and finds people's experiences re-assuring. She thinks 'well if they can do it and they have had a stroke, then I can do it'. Comparing herself to other stroke survivors and seeing similarities in what 'they can and cannot physically do' increases Joan's confidence that she will be able to undertake the exercise programme.

At the next face-to-face session, David explores with Joan anticipated barriers (e.g. transport – how she will get to the class, cost of attendance) and how these will be resolved if they arise. They also discuss coping strategies and how Joan can get back on track if she has any setbacks. Joan is shown how to keep a weekly diary in which she can note the exercise sessions she has attended and how she felt before and after them. They also discuss how benefits (e.g. ability to walk further, feelings of wellbeing) and losses (e.g. time commitment and financial cost of attendance) could be noted weekly and feelings of optimism in regard to continuing with the exercise. Joan starts the class 2 weeks later.

GOAL SETTING

Motivational interviewing can be helpful in encouraging an individual to take up a health behaviour such as exercise, or to become more physically active in general. Once they have indicated to be ready, goal setting can be used to identify more specific milestones, chart progress and increase self-efficacy.

Background

Goal setting can be defined as 'the identification of and agreement on a behavioural target which the patient, therapist or team will work towards over a specified period of time' (Royal College of Physicians 2008, p. 37). Goal setting was developed several decades ago, originally in the context of organisational psychology with a view to explain and optimise performance (Locke and Latham 2002). It has since been applied to other areas and is now a well-established component in the fields of sport and exercise (Schmidt and Wrisberg 2008), while its integration into rehabilitation is a more recent development. Goal setting has been included in a range of clinical guidelines for stroke (Royal College of Physicians 2008, Scottish Intercollegiate Guidelines Network 2010), although the evidence base is still being developed. Goal setting can be used to enhance an individual's motivation and engagement with their rehabilitation or training programme, increase adherence, evaluate progress, improve multidisciplinary teamwork and ultimately improve outcomes (Levack et al. 2006, Wade 1999).

A number of different theories underpin goal setting (Playford et al. 2009), with social cognitive theory comprising the concept of self-efficacy being most frequently cited (Scobbie et al. 2009). The concept of self-efficacy, which was introduced earlier in this chapter, refers to the confidence an individual has in their own abilities to undertake a particular action (Bandura 1997). Combined with expectations about the outcome of a particular action (i.e. outcome expectancies), self-efficacy is thought to influence an individual's motivation to set their own goals and their determination to pursue these goals in the face of obstacles.

A recent theoretical framework for goal setting and action planning in rehabilitation was proposed by Scobbie et al. (2011). This identified four key components: goal negotiation (in which patients appraise their current situation and explore which issues they would like to address), goal setting (in which general intentions are translated into specific goals that can be evaluated), planning (in which specific actions on how the goal will be achieved are identified, as well as coping strategies for overcoming any barriers or set-backs) and, finally, appraisal and feedback (in which progress is assessed and implications for further action are considered). This promising theoretical framework will now need to be evaluated empirically to ascertain its effectiveness in actual practice.

Evidence for goal setting with stroke survivors

What is the evidence supporting goal setting? Despite the broad support for goal setting in clinical practice (Royal College of Physicians 2008, Scottish Intercollegiate Guidelines Network 2010), guidance on implementing goal setting (Turner-Stokes 2009), and a substantial body of literature on goal setting in general (e.g. Levack et al. 2006), the actual body of research on goal setting with stroke survivors in particular is small, with few good quality studies (Rosewilliam et al. 2011). One study indicated that formal goal setting can help stroke survivors clarify goals in relation to self-care ability, and improve their perceived ability in self-care (Folden 1993). Whether this perceived improvement translated into actual improvement was not explored, however. Another study suggested that active participation in goal setting helped participants to remember their goals better, made them feel more involved and manage more tasks compared to a group that did not participate in goal setting (Wressle et al. 2002). However, this was not a randomised controlled trial and differences between the two groups may have confounded the findings. More rigorously designed studies are needed to examine the actual impact of goal setting on adherence and outcomes in rehabilitation (Levack et al. 2006).

Other studies have explored the experiences of goal setting by stroke survivors, their carers and health-care professionals. Stroke survivors who participated in a community-based exercise and education scheme valued the exercise and goal-setting components, which were seen as key elements in helping them to adapt to life after stroke and rebuild their confidence (Reed et al. 2010). A study exploring experiences of an exercise referral scheme also suggested that participants felt that the scheme had given them confidence to become more active outside the formal exercise sessions (Sharma et al. 2011). However, a number of barriers to active engagement in the goal-setting process were also experienced, which will be discussed below.

It is important to be aware of potential differences in goal setting between professionals and stroke survivors, in terms of the types of goals set and the assessment of goal attainment. Stroke survivors tend to be more optimistic, articulate hopes and set more general, long-term goals (e.g. 'getting back to golf'), while health-care professionals may set more short-term, specific goals (e.g. to be able to walk with one stick for 10 meters with supervision only in 2 weeks' time) (Laver et al. 2010, Lawler et al. 1999, Wressle et al. 1999). Stroke survivors tend to compare their goal attainment with their pre-stroke status, while health-care professionals tend to compare with more recent performance (Wressle et al. 1999), which may result in stroke survivors judging their goal attainment to be lower than health-care professionals (Reid and Chesson 1998). Finally, health-care professionals tend to have more favourable opinions about the level of collaboration with stroke survivors in the goal-setting process than stroke survivors themselves (McAndrew et al. 1999). Health and exercise professionals need to be aware of these potential differences in goal setting, which may impact on their professional relationship with the stroke survivor (Mew and Fossey 1996). However, a collaborative goal setting process may facilitate a discussion between the stroke survivor and the exercise professional and help come to agreed goals.

Current areas of expert agreement in goal setting (and some gaps)

A range of methods to set goals has been proposed, although there is no single agreed methodology (Playford et al. 2009). An expert consensus meeting broadly agreed on the following principles for goal setting in rehabilitation:

- Goals should have a time frame: short-term goals should link to specific objectives; intermediate goals should be defined at the level of activity; and, finally, long-term goals should capture the stroke survivor's broader aims in terms of participation in life roles. (For definitions of 'activity' and 'participation', the reader is referred to the World Health Organization International Classification of Functioning, Disability and Health 2001.) It is important that the connections between short-term, intermediate and long-term goals be made clear to the stroke survivor.

- Goal setting should be person-centred: i.e. it should be a collaborative process in which the whole person is considered (i.e. not just their impairments and disabilities but also their aspirations, motivation, concerns, needs and social circumstances) and in which a deeper understanding of the person's issues and agreement on their management is sought.
- Goals are generally recommended to be SMART (i.e. specific, measurable, ambitious, relevant and time-limited), although there are different interpretations of what each of these letters means (Playford et al. 2009, Wade 2009). For example, there is debate on whether the 'A' should stand for 'ambitious' or 'achievable', with the consensus that goals do not necessarily have to be achievable, as long as there is a possibility that they can be achieved.

Barriers and motivators to goal setting

The main motivators to goal setting are the perceptions of health-care professionals that stroke survivors are more motivated, that their input has more impact as goal setting helps to focus on targets that are meaningful, and overall more holistic, person-centred rehabilitation (Leach et al. 2010, van de Weyer et al. 2010). The next chapter in this book will provide a very clear example of how a specific, concrete yet ambitious goal inspired an individual stroke survivor (i.e. to take his daughter down the aisle at her wedding) to increase his physical activity.

However, there are a number of barriers to person-centred goal setting in the context of stroke rehabilitation (Leach et al. 2010, Rosewilliam et al. 2011). These include factors associated with the stroke survivor, the health-care professional as well as the organisation:

- Stroke survivors may not feel able to participate in goal setting for a number of different reasons: they may not feel ready, they may be unfamiliar with goal setting, or may not have enough knowledge about stroke recovery to be able to set targets (Laver et al. 2010). They may have cognitive impairments or a lack of insight in their situation. Stroke survivors with executive dysfunction may find it difficult to set realistic goals, while communication difficulties may also be a barrier. Furthermore, some stroke survivors may find it difficult to set goals because they have not yet come to terms with the aftermath of their stroke, or may suffer from depression. Together, these factors mean that the level of participation by stroke survivors in their own goal setting can be low, particular amongst people over 85 years and those with a lower level of education (Almborg et al. 2008). Exercise and health-care professionals should be aware of these potential barriers to goal setting to enable stroke participants to take part in goal setting in a meaningful way.

- Barriers to goal setting associated with health-care professionals include a lack of expertise and/or confidence in setting goals, and difficulty in consistently explaining the meaning of therapy goals as well as how they relate to the person's own goals. In addition, some health-care professionals perceive themselves to fully involve patients in goal setting, although their patients do not always share this view (McAndrew et al. 1999).
- Organisational barriers may include a lack of staff training and/or time. It is important for managers to appreciate that goal setting requires skill on behalf of the health or exercise professional, as well as resources.

These barriers can be overcome through education however; e.g. training staff in goal setting and communication, mentoring less experienced staff, and educating stroke survivors about recovery and the goal-setting process.

In summary, goal setting is an integral part of rehabilitation and exercise training. Despite the broad support for this process and the considerable body of literature, there are still many questions about optimal methods for goal setting with stroke survivors. In particular, there is little guidance on the best methods to involve stroke survivors with executive dysfunction, cognitive and/or communication impairment in this process. Further research needs to be undertaken to identify goals that stroke survivors wish to achieve from physical activity interventions, identify barriers to goal attainment in the context of physical activity after stroke, and strategies for how these may be overcome. Furthermore, it is important that exercise and health-care professionals teach stroke survivors how to set their own goals, monitor their own progress, obtain regular feedback and adjust their activity where necessary, to enable them to enjoy a more independent, active lifestyle in the long term.

SUMMARY POINTS

- There are challenges to stroke survivors being able to increase levels of physical activity and maintain these over the longer term.
- The uptake and maintenance of long-term physical activity is likely to be influenced by stroke survivors' motivation to participate, self-efficacy, confidence in predicting successful outcomes from exercise, beliefs about benefits and barriers, as well as self-regulatory skills.
- Social cognitive theories provide a framework from which certain self-regulatory techniques can be applied to facilitate self-efficacy, motivation, intention, engagement in an exercise training programme after stroke and maintenance of this activity, as well as abilities to cope with barriers and set-backs.
- Motivational interviewing can enable the stroke survivor to deal with ambivalence, increase self-efficacy, establish readiness to change, develop self-regulatory skills and set appropriate goals. Exercise professionals can use these techniques to facilitate stroke survivors' participation in exercise.

- Goal setting can be used to help stroke survivors clarify their personal targets related to physical activity, enhance their motivation and self-efficacy and monitor their progress. This has the potential to re-build confidence, enhance personal goal attainment and encourage stroke survivors to attempt other activities outside any formal exercise classes.

REFERENCES

Almborg, A.H., Ulander, K., Thulin, A., et al., 2008. Patients' perceptions of their participation in discharge planning after acute stroke. J. Clin. Nurs. 18, 199–209.

Ashford, S., Edmunds, J., French, J.P., 2010. What is the best way to change self-efficacy to promote lifestyle and recreational physical activity? A systematic review with meta-analysis. Br. J. Health Psychol. 15, 265–288.

Bandura, A., 1986. Social foundations of thought and action: a social cognitive theory. Prentice Hall, Englewood Cliffs, NJ.

Bandura, A., 1977. Self efficacy: toward a unifying theory of behavioural change. Psychol. Rev. 84, 191–215.

Bandura, A., 1997. Self-efficacy: the exercise of control. Freeman, New York.

Best, C., van Wijck, F., Dinan-Young, S., et al., 2010. Best practice guidance for the development of exercise after stroke services in community settings. Edinburgh University, Edinburgh. Available online at http://www.exerciseafterstroke.org.uk/ (accessed 08.09.2011).

Biddle, S.J.H., Mutrie, N., 2008. Psychology of physical activity: determinants, well-being and interventions, second ed. Routledge, Oxon.

Boysen, G., Krarup, L.H., Zeng, X., et al., 2009. ExStroke Pilot Trial of the effect of repeated instructions to improve physical activity after ischaemic stroke: a multinational randomised controlled clinical trial. BMJ 339, b2810.

Carin-Levy, G., Kendall, M., Young, A., et al., 2009. The psychosocial effects of exercise and relaxation classes for persons surviving a stroke. Can. J. Occup. Ther. 76, 73–76.

Connor, M., Norman, P., 2005. Predicting health behaviour: research and practice with social cognition models. Open University Press, Maidenhead.

Damush, T.M., Plue, L., Bakas, T., et al., 2007. Barriers and facilitators to exercise among stroke survivors. Rehabil. Nurs. 32, 253–260.

DiClemente, C.C., Prochaska, J.O., Gibertini, M., 1985. Self-efficacy and the stages of self-change of smoking. Cognit. Ther. Res. 9, 181–200.

Dugdill, L., Graham, R.C., McNair, F., 2005. Exercise referral: the public health panacea for physical activity promotion? A critical perspective of exercise referral schemes: their development and evaluation. Ergonomics 48, 1390–1410.

Folden, S.L., 1993. Effect of a supportive-educative nursing intervention on older adults' perceptions of self-care after a stroke. Rehabil. Nurs. 18, 162–167.

Hammel, J., Jones, R., Gossett, A., et al., 2006. Examining barriers and supports to community living and participation after a stroke from a participatory action research approach. Top. Stroke Rehabil. 13, 43–58.

Hardcastle, S., Taylor, A., Bailey, M., et al., 2008. A randomised controlled trial on the effectiveness of a primary health care based counselling intervention on physical activity, diet and CHD risk factors. Patient Educ. Couns. 70, 31–39.

Jones, F., 2006. Strategies to enhance chronic disease self-management: how can we apply this to stroke? Disabil. Rehabil. 28, 841–847.

Jones, F., Mandy, A., Partridge, C., 2009. Changing self-efficacy in individuals following a first time stroke: preliminary study of a novel self-management intervention. Clin. Rehabil. 23, 522–533.

Jones, F., Riazi, A., 2011. Self-efficacy and self-management after stroke: a systematic review. Disabil. Rehabil. 33, 797–810.

Laver, K., Rehab, M.C., Halbert, J., et al., 2010. Patient readiness and ability to set recovery goals during the first 6 months after stroke. J. Allied Health 39, e149–e154.

Lawler, J., Dowswell, G., Hearn, J., et al., 1999. Recovering from stroke: a qualitative investigation of the role of goal setting in late stroke recovery. J. Adv. Nurs. 30, 401–409.

Leach, E., Cornwell, P., Fleming, J., et al., 2010. Patient centered goal-setting in a subacute rehabilitation setting. Disabil. Rehabil. 32, 159–172.

Levack, W.M., Taylor, K., Siegert, R.J., et al., 2006. Is goal planning in rehabilitation effective? A systematic review. Clin. Rehabil. 20, 739–755.

Locke, E.A., Latham, G.P., 2002. Building a practically useful theory of goal setting and task motivation: a 35-year odyssey. Am. Psychol. 57, 705–717.

Lundahl, D., Tollefson, D., Gambles, C., et al., 2010. A meta-analysis of motivational interviewing: twenty five years of empirical studies. Res. Soc. Work Pract. 20, 137–160.

McAndrew, E., McDermott, S., Vitzakovitch, S., et al., 1999. Therapist and patient perceptions of the occupational therapy goal-setting process: a pilot study. Phys. Occup. Ther. Geriatr. 17, 55–63.

Mead, G., Greig, C.A., Cunningham, I., et al., 2007. STroke: A Randomised Trial of Exercise or Relaxation (STARTER). J. Am. Geriatr. Soc. 55, 892–899.

Mead, G.E., 2009. Exercise after stroke. Editorial. BMJ 339, 247–248.

Mew, M.M., Fossey, E., 1996. Client-centred aspects of clinical reasoning during an initial assessment using the Canadian Occupational Performance Measure. Aust. Occup. Ther. J. 43, 155–166.

Miller, W., Rollnick, S., 1991. Motivational interviewing: preparing people to change addictive behavior. Guilford Press, New York.

Miller, W.R., Rollnick, S., 2009. Ten things that motivational interviewing is not. Behav. Cognit. Psychother. 37, 129–140.

Ogden, J., 2004. Health psychology: a textbook, third ed. Open University Press, Maidenhead.

Patterson, S., Ross-Edwards, B., 2009. Long term stroke survivors' needs and perceptions of an exercise maintenance model of care. Int. J. Ther. Rehabil. 16, 659–669.

Playford, E.D., Siegert, R., Levack, W., et al., 2009. Areas of consensus and controversy about goal setting in rehabilitation: a conference report. Clin. Rehabil. 23, 334–344.

Price, C.I.M., Curless, R.H., Rodgers, H., 1999. Can stroke patients use visual analogue scales? Stroke 30, 1357–1361.

Royal College of Physicians, 2008. National clinical guideline for stroke, third ed. Intercollegiate Stroke Working Party, Royal College of Physicians, London.

Reed, M., Harrington, R., Duggan, A., et al., 2010. Meeting stroke survivors' perceived needs: a qualitative study of a community-based exercise and education scheme. Clin. Rehabil. 24, 16–25.

Reid, A., Chesson, R., 1998. Goal attainment scaling. Is it appropriate for stroke patients and their physiotherapists? Physiotherapy 84 (3), 136–144.

Resnick, B., Michael, K., Shaughnessy, M., et al., 2008. Motivators for treadmill exercise after stroke. Top. Stroke Rehabil. 15, 494–502.

Rimmer, J.H., Rubin, S.S., Braddock, D., 2000. Barriers to exercise in African American women with physical disabilities. Arch. Phys. Med. Rehabil. 81, 182–188.

Rimmer, J.H., Wang, E., Smith, D., 2008. Barriers associated with exercise and community access for individuals with stroke. J. Rehabil. Res. Dev. 45, 315–322.

Robison, J., Wiles, R., Ellis-Hill, C., et al., 2009. Resuming previously valued activities post-stroke: who or what helps? Disabil. Rehabil. 31, 1555–1566.

Rosewilliam, S., Roskell, C.A., Pandyan, A., 2011. A systematic review and synthesis of the quantitative and qualitative evidence behind patient-centred goal setting in stroke rehabilitation. Clin. Rehabil. 25, 501–514.

Scobbie, L., Dixon, D., Wyke, S., 2009. Goal setting and action planning in the rehabilitation setting: development of a theoretically informed practice framework. Clin. Rehabil. 25, 468–482.

Scobbie, L., Dixon, D., Wyke, S., 2011. Goal setting and action planning in the rehabilitation setting: development of a theoretically informed practice framework. Clin. Rehabil. 25, 468–482.

Schmidt, R.A., Wrisberg, C.A., 2008. Motor learning and performance. A situation-based learning approach, third ed. Human Kinetics, Champaign, IL.

Scottish Government, 2009. Better heart disease and stroke care action plan. Scottish Government, Edinburgh. Available online at http://www.scotland.gov.uk/ Publications/2009/06/29102453/11 (accessed 08.09.2011).

Sharma, H., Bulley, C., van Wijck, F., 2011. Experiences of an exercise referral scheme from the perspective of people with chronic stroke: a qualitative study. Physiotherapy. doi.org/10.1016/j. physio.2011.05.004.

Shaughnessy, M., Resnick, B.M., Macko, R.F., 2006. Testing a model of post-stroke exercise behaviour. Rehabil. Nurs. 31, 15–21.

Shaughnessy, M., Resnick, B.M., 2009. Using theory to develop an exercise intervention for patients post stroke. Top. Stroke Rehabil. 16, 140–146.

Scottish Intercollegiate Guidelines Network, 2010. Guideline 118: Management of patients with stroke: rehabilitation, prevention and management of complications, and discharge planning:a national clinical guideline. Scottish Intercollegiate Guidelines Network (SIGN), Edinburgh. Available online at: http://www.sign.ac.uk/guidelines/ fulltext/118/index.html (accessed 08.09.2011).

Sniehotta, F.F., Scholz, U., Schwarzer, R., et al., 2005. Long term effects of two psychological interventions on physical exercise and self regulation following, coronary rehabilitation. Int. J. Behav. Med. 12, 244–255.

Turner-Stokes, L., 2009. Goal attainment scaling (GAS) in rehabilitation: a practical guide. Clin. Rehabil. 23, 362–370.

van De Weyer, R.C., Ballinger, C., Playford, E.D., 2010. Goal setting in neurological rehabilitation: staff perspectives. Disabil. Rehabil. 32, 1419–1427.

Wade, D.T., 1999. Goal planning in stroke rehabilitation: Why? Top. Stroke Rehabil. 6, 1–7.

Wade, D.T., 2009. Goal setting in rehabilitation: an overview of what, why and how. Clin. Rehabil. 23, 291–295.

Williams, N.H., Hendry, M., France, B., et al., 2007. Effectiveness of exercise-referral schemes to promote physical activity in adults: systematic review. Br. J. Gen. Pract. 57, 979–986.

Wressle, E., Eeg-Olofsson, A.M., Marcusson, J., et al., 2002. Improved client participation in the rehabilitation process using a client-centred goal formulation structure. J. Rehabil. Med. 34, 5–11.

Wressle, E., Oberg, B., Henriksson, C., 1999. The rehabilitation process for the geriatric stroke patient – an exploratory study of goal setting and interventions. Disabil. Rehabil. 21, 80–87.

Communication: getting it right

Sheena Borthwick • Marie Donaghy

CHAPTER CONTENTS

INTRODUCTION

Good communication is an essential aspect of delivering exercise programmes for stroke survivors. It includes interpersonal communication between the exercise professional and the stroke survivor attending the class, members of the stroke survivor's family and health-care professionals. Communication is a complex process; whether it is a brief social chat or an exchange of complex instructions, specific skills such as listening, speech, language, gestures and cognitive skills (memory and attention) are used frequently and effortlessly. Some stroke survivors will not notice any change in their communication, whilst, for others, effortless communication may no longer be possible. Furthermore, cognitive skills may be impaired which may slow down the processing of auditory or visual information.

The specific types of communication problems that frequently occur as a direct result of stroke include aphasia and dysarthria. Communication disability persisting after stroke is relatively common and unfortunately the impact of this disability often stretches much further than may be expected because stroke survivors with communication difficulties experience low self-esteem, loss of social confidence and feelings of stigmatisation (Dickson et al. 2008). Overcoming the challenges that communication disability brings requires an awareness of the complexities of communication, the influence of the environment and a willingness to engage in a partnership with the individual to overcome some of the hurdles.

The environment has a strong influence on communication (Howe et al. 2008). This includes both the physical environment with its space and acoustics, and the social environment. The social environment refers to the opportunity to communicate prior to, during and following exercise sessions. The expectations, beliefs and values of both the exercise professional and the stroke survivor will influence the social environment. Good communication is therefore important to facilitate a shared understanding of the potential benefits and barriers of engaging in the exercise programme, and to agree with the stroke survivor the goals, content and processes of the exercise programme.

The purpose of this chapter is to increase awareness of the factors influencing communication, to describe some of the more common communication disorders experienced after stroke and to introduce the principles underpinning good communication that will assist in creating the right social environment for both exercise professionals and stroke survivors.

DEMONSTRATING EFFECTIVE COMMUNICATION SKILLS

WHAT IS COMMUNICATION?

Communication could simply be described as a process of giving and receiving information. It is a shared activity involving two or more people covering a range of activities such as engaging in social greetings, giving instructions, negotiating agreements, expressing opinions and discussing world events. The information exchange occurs in different contexts, informal and formal, and where the balance of power and control may be shared equally or held by one or more of the participants. However, this description fails to recognise the complexities of how and why we communicate with each other and does not take into account that people are individuals who see things differently.

HOW DO WE COMMUNICATE?

Communication can be both verbal and non-verbal. The expressions 'It's not what she said, it's the way she said it' or 'Actions speak louder than words' demonstrate this. The term non-verbal communication could be interpreted as any form of communication not involving spoken or written words; however, this is not strictly true as non-verbal messages often accompany verbal expression (Hargie and Dickson 2004).

Non-verbal communication can serve several purposes; it can:

- Completely replace speech, e.g. where the chosen method to communicate is sign language or a simple signal or gesture across a busy room.
- Complement speech by emphasising some aspects of the message, e.g. showing emotion and pointing and gesturing to clarify points.
- Contradict the spoken word, e.g. body language that suggests another message. These non-verbal behaviours can be deliberate such as when

using sarcasm or humour. However, behaviours can also be outwith personal control, e.g. blushing or tensing, and therefore revealing the true message.

- Control the initiation and turn taking in conversation, e.g. eye contact acts as a signal for when to listen and when to talk.

Utilising all the available modes of communication (Fig. 7.1) and being aware of one's own non-verbal communication is important when establishing effective working relationships with stroke survivors.

In practice, the most appropriate modes of communication should be selected that suit the context and individual stroke survivor's needs in order to deliver an effective exercise programme. In addition to interaction with stroke survivors, contact should be maintained with those referring into the service and there should be close liaison with other members of the multidisciplinary team such as physiotherapists, occupational therapists and speech and language therapists. Different contexts may seem most suited to a particular mode of communication, e.g. written service information leaflets. However, ensuring the exercise service is truly accessible requires a flexible approach where information is provided in a suitable format for the stroke survivor after establishing their abilities and preferences.

USING ACTIVE LISTENING

Communication requires both encoding or sending of signals and decoding or receiving of signals. Passive listening itself is not always sufficient. Actively listening is when attention to the message being conveyed is demonstrated and thought processes are applied to assimilate the information.

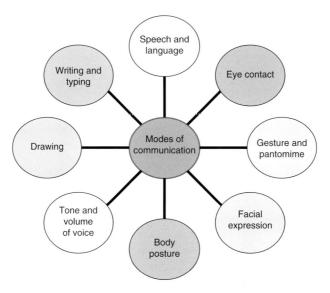

FIG 7.1 Diagram showing the many different modes of communication.

Active listening involves the following:

- Considering what the person is actually meaning by attending to the words, body language and tone of voice to extract the real message.
- Considering the full implication of the information, e.g. is it expected or unusual?
- Using and providing feedback as the communication progresses, i.e.:
  ◦ Being aware of one's own non-verbal signals
  ◦ Using paraphrasing or recapping to ensure a shared understanding
  ◦ Responding with empathy
  ◦ Providing encouragement to elaborate with appropriate questioning and prompting.

Health-care professionals are likely to receive training to understand the components and benefits of their communication practices (Parry and Brown 2009).

Communication skills can be improved with practice, and the effect this has on working relationships and the experience for stroke survivors attending an exercise programme can be self-monitored.

APPRECIATING INDIVIDUAL DIFFERENCES

Stroke survivors attending an exercise programme come with a range of different cultural and socio-economic backgrounds. Differences in language, customs and religions all have the potential of causing misunderstandings, unless respect is given to these differences. This can be established by listening carefully to what is being said, learning about the person's customs, observing and being sensitive to cultural differences. When English is not the first language, it is important to ensure that instructions can be followed or, where necessary, that a professional interpreter or health-care advocate is present.

It is important to establish the views of the stroke survivors attending the class with regard to how they view their stroke, their recovery and any concerns they may have about participating in an exercise programme. Following stroke, the way a person sees themselves may be threatened by the impact of the stroke and subsequent impairment and disability. A stroke survivor may try to maintain the sense of the self they were before the stroke. This may be observed in conversations related to their physical ability such as *'this is not how I walk. ... having to use a stick, I normally walk 6–8 miles at the week-end without any problem'*; or relating to cognitive ability *'I am usually a quick thinker, my job requires me to make a lot of decisions and my memory for people's faces and recalling past events I have been told is remarkable'*.

Others will succumb to feelings of loss and despair focusing on the change in their abilities and coming to a different view of the self which may or may not be reinforced by family and friends. This may be observed in conversations, e.g. *'I am having difficulty walking with the weakness in my right leg, it just keeps giving way. I don't envisage that I will ever walk again'* or *'I used to have a good memory but not now…my memory is really poor and I struggle to remember the day of the week'*.

By appreciating these individual differences, we learn to understand that for some people optimism and hope is important, whilst for others pessimism, grief reactions and intense awareness of functional losses result in a revised view of themselves. The importance is in recognising these differences and providing communication that acknowledges and accepts these individual views.

COMMUNICATION DISABILITY AFTER STROKE

It is common to experience an impaired ability to communicate after stroke; however, communication and disability are not often words people associate together. If asked to describe a disability, there is a tendency to focus on the physical abilities of an individual and this has led to some of the organisations that work with those with communication disability to describe it as a 'hidden disability'. Certainly it is often not immediately apparent when you meet someone that they have a communication difficulty, and this can produce an additional hurdle where the listener is taken by surprise and feels unprepared or lacks awareness of how to help the situation.

The communication disability may be temporary but a significant proportion of stroke survivors will have life-long symptoms which present in many different ways and with differing severity. There are many areas of the brain involved in communication, such as areas involved in processing an auditory signal, recognising a written word, attaching meaning to the signal or controlling the muscles of articulation, breathing and voice. Figure 7.2 shows a cognitive model representing the different layers in speech production with their associated communication disorders.

Given the complexity of communication, it is not surprising that there are diverse presentations; however, it is possible to group the impairments into three main categories. Understanding the type of communication disorder is

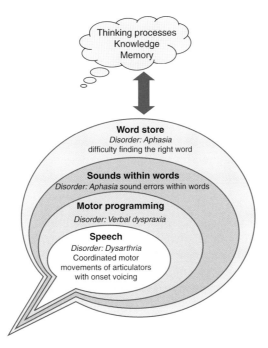

FIG 7.2 A cognitive model representing the layers in speech production with associated communication disorders.

the first step in supporting that individual to overcome the communication barriers that are likely to occur.

MOTOR SPEECH DISORDERS

Motor speech disorders occur when there is difficulty in planning or executing a motor movement essential for speech. Articulation requires precise, coordinated movements of the jaw, lips, tongue, soft palate and larynx, all supported with controlled breaths to give volume to the voice. If there is disruption to the innervation of any of the muscles of articulation, the result will alter the quality of the speech. Dysarthria is the term used to describe a motor speech disorder. There are a number of types of dysarthria depending on the type of stroke; however, they all will affect the person's production of speech and as a result one may find it difficult to interpret what they are saying. The severity of dysarthria can vary from minor imprecise articulation or slurred speech to someone with a complete inability to produce any sounds or intelligible words where they are reliant on alternative means of communication (e.g. writing or electronic communication aids). When someone presents with dysarthria, there is no reason to presume that they have difficulty understanding your speech or that they have been intellectually impaired. Unfortunately, however, a negative reaction from others is one of the most disabling aspects of living with dysarthria and can have a serious detrimental effect on the individual's confidence in any social situation.

LANGUAGE DISORDERS

Language is an agreed symbolic system by which we convey meaning. In this case we are using our shared knowledge of the written English language, but this information could have been presented in many languages, spoken, signed or passed on using some yet uncharted code (assuming both parties have knowledge of the system). The brain processes language by interpreting and attaching meaning to the learned symbols. The language processing areas of our brain are located in the left hemisphere for the majority of right handed people and some left handed people, and damage in these areas results in a disorder known as aphasia. It is estimated that as many as 30% of people having their first stroke will experience symptoms of aphasia (Engelter et al. 2006). Aphasia is sometimes referred to as dysphasia and at one time dysphasia was the term used to indicate a less severe disorder, but this distinction was not always helpful. Symptoms of aphasia vary greatly and can present across all communication modalities, e.g. understanding and producing spoken language, reading and writing, signing and interpreting symbols. The severity of impairment will also differ across these modalities and, therefore, finding out and working with the individual's strengths is vital to maximise success in communication.

People with aphasia are likely to have been working with a speech and language therapist during their recovery from stroke. A recent Cochrane systematic review on speech and language therapy for aphasia after stroke states that '*The primary aim of speech and language therapy in aphasia management and rehabilitation is to maximise individuals' ability to communicate*' (Kelly et al. 2010,

p. 2). Therefore the focus of therapy will have been not only on spoken communication, but also in establishing any effective means of communication. Although the person with aphasia will be the expert in their own condition, they will need all their communication partners to support them and adapt to their specific communication needs.

When working with a stroke survivor with aphasia, the exercise professional will need to be aware that there may be difficulty both understanding and expressing language in any given modality. Being aware of what works best for that particular stroke survivor is the key to overcoming the communication barriers.

COGNITIVE COMMUNICATION DISORDERS

Aphasia and dysarthria are the main disorders of communication experienced after stroke; however, there are many more symptoms that can persist after stroke, which can have an adverse effect on successful communication. Some of these disorders are more obvious, e.g. a stroke survivor warns their exercise professional that their memory is very poor after their stroke and it is rapidly clear that they need to take written notes to compensate. Other presentations may be quite subtle and can sometimes be misinterpreted. There has been increasing research into communication disorders experienced after right hemisphere stroke and this has led to an increased awareness of the role of the non-dominant hemisphere in processing language. The following list describes some of the changes that have been observed after stroke. Unlike with aphasia and dysarthria, it is possible that the individual will have quite limited awareness of these changes themselves, but family and friends who know them well are often more distressed by their changed and occasionally challenging behaviour:

- Difficulty understanding emotional content (e.g. failure to react to the emotional response of someone they are talking to).
- Difficulty using and understanding facial expression and intonation (e.g. communicating with a very 'flat' (i.e. expressionless) face and monotonous voice).
- Difficulty in following the rules in conversation (e.g. talking over other people and not allowing others to talk).
- Difficulty in making inferences (e.g. making very literal interpretations of what is being said and therefore unable to appreciate humour, sarcasm or complex information).

These are just a few examples and one can appreciate that it is often very difficult to avoid making personal judgements about individuals who are presenting with what we often consider rude or inappropriate responses to our well-intentioned attempts at social interaction. In these cases it is important to work on establishing rapport whilst being aware of these more subtle aspects of communication disability.

IMPACT OF A COMMUNICATION DISABILITY

Understanding how a communication disability could impact on the individual's ability to access, participate and maintain an exercise programme may be the primary concern; however, having an understanding of the wider implications of living with a communication disability will help the exercise professional to appreciate some of the initial anxieties and perhaps reluctance that may be exhibited in the initial sessions. Personal experiences consisting of other's reactions to attempts at communication contribute greatly to increasing or decreasing a person's confidence and willingness to engage in new situations and relationships.

Researchers have studied the impact of living with persisting aphasia (Parr et al. 1997), hoping to inform and influence the services that aim to offer rehabilitation and support for stroke survivors. Research into the impact of dysarthria has shown that even relatively mild speech impairments can have significant effects on aspects of everyday life (Dickson et al. 2008). When exploring the potential changes in communication ability for a stroke survivor, it is important to consider:

- Their ability to communicate in familiar and potentially new situations
- How these changes have impacted on their role in life and maintaining autonomy
- How this has affected their participation in work and leisure activities
- How these changes are affecting their psychological wellbeing.

For some stroke survivors, practical concerns around overcoming barriers in communication may mean they are reluctant to attempt new situations (Case study 1; Box 7.1) but for others it may well be low self-esteem and confidence that act as barriers (Case study 2; Box 7.2).

BOX 7.1 Case study 1: Barriers to communication after stroke

Stewart, a 56-year-old, medically retired financial advisor, had a left middle cerebral artery ischaemic stroke over 1 year ago. Stewart has aphasia and, although he has made a reasonable physical recovery from his stroke, he now regrets not having spent more time focusing on his fitness. Before his stroke he occasionally played a game of golf, but he has refused to go back to the golf club indicating to his wife that he could not cope with the social circle.

Stewart doesn't like taking part in conversations with more than two people as he cannot follow the rapid flow of conversation, tends to have to switch off and feels this is socially unacceptable. Although he can contribute to a conversation, his speech is slow and disjointed and he needs time to plan his response. He often makes errors and gets frustrated trying to correct his words. About reading, Stewart says, 'reading. . . .yeah. . .great. I can. . . . .slow you know. No hurry and yes I get it!'

He prefers to get written information as this backs up his understanding.

Stewart's wife has suggested he take a place at an Exercise after Stroke class, but he is not sure how to make the first step. He doesn't want to be dependent on his wife, who would take time off work to accompany him, as this makes him feel helpless. The telephone is not an option for Stewart and he is hoping the receptionist will be understanding, and that there will be no written forms to be completed. Then there is the process of explaining his difficulties. Stewart has built up his confidence to try the programme and hopes the exercise professionals understand his communication difficulties.

> **BOX 7.2 Case study 2: Barriers to communication after stroke**
>
> Anne is a 62-year-old widow. Her main enjoyment before her stroke was her regular trips with the local walking club. She has now been discharged home and has made a good recovery, but is acutely aware that her speech sounds slurred.
>
> *'They will think I have been hitting the bottle. It's the look people give you. Yesterday the girl in the bakery was so rude. She pulled a face and I felt like walking out of the shop. Of course it made my speech so much worse. It is difficult to control my emotions after this stroke, I can easily feel like I am about to cry. I hate the sound of my own voice, it just isn't me. I would really like to build up my stamina to get back to keeping up with my walking friends but I am very nervous about going to the exercise class as you never know how people will react when you start to talk.'*

IDENTIFYING POTENTIAL COMMUNICATION BREAKDOWN

Information from the referring health-care professional or multidisciplinary team that works with the stroke survivor, as well as from the initial pre-exercise assessment with the exercise professional (chapter 8), can help to identify any potential barriers to communication. Acknowledging any reported or observed difficulties is important as a first step in communicating with individual stroke survivors, as this demonstrates that the exercise professional is aware and willing to work with the person to minimise any barriers (see Box 7.3). Asking whether there are any modes of communication that are more difficult and thinking about how to adapt one's own communications are ways of ensuring that any communication needs are supported.

DEVELOPING SKILLS TO OVERCOME THE BARRIERS IN COMMUNICATION

The UK communication disability network known as Connect is an organisation that has undertaken extensive research into the experiences of individuals with communication disability. It provides a source of advice to services on how to improve their services for people with post-stroke communication disorders (Parr et al. 2006). According to this guidance, consideration should be given to:

- Written documentation used by the service, e.g. information leaflets, appointment letters and registration forms, giving consideration as to how suitable these are for individuals with language disorders.
- Personal interactions, including social interaction, interviews and providing instruction during classes.
- The environment, considering the effect of noise, privacy and the welcome received.

Anxiety about getting communication right can exist for both parties and it is important to remember that this will not always happen instantly. The most effective resources to remember are giving time and showing a willingness to keep trying. Attempts at communication do not need to be perfect for successful transfer of information to take place (see Box 7.4).

BOX 7.3 Overview of possible barriers to delivering and receiving information

Barriers to delivering effective communication

- Failure to acknowledge individual and cultural differences
- Giving too much or too little information
- Giving the wrong or conflicting information
- Lack of clarity in speech or inappropriate rate of speech
- Using a language that is not shared
- Failing to support the verbal message with appropriate body language
- Using an inappropriate tone of voice
- Failing to focus on the needs or interests of the listener
- Making inappropriate assumptions
- Failure to take into account the presence of a communication disability
- Failure to utilise alternative modes of communication

Barriers to receiving information

- Distraction with noise, thoughts
- Failure to actively listen
- Information too complex to understand
- Misinterpreting the verbal and non-verbal messages
- Inattention or poor attention span
- Personal bias or making judgements about the information or the speaker
- Interruptions and failing to let the speaker finish
- Visual impairments
- Hearing impairments
- Failure to take into account the presence of a communication disability
- Failure to acknowledge alternative modes of communication

BOX 7.4 Work hard to understand

An example showing that communication does not need to be perfect for successful transfer of information to take place.

At fsirt tihs may look lkie nonesne, but yuor biran wntas to mkae snese of thsee wrods and you have lkliey raed tihs wtihuot a porbelm.

Wrods dno't hvae to be precceft to be udrensootd.

Preparation can include finding out what helps and putting this into action. The following are strategies that are often found helpful. The exercise professional should, wherever possible:

- Avoid distraction, ensuring he/she gives and receives full attention.
- Give lots of time to respond rather than rushing on to the next point.
- Check if the stroke survivor wants gaps in communication to be filled in, but should not assume this is the case.
- Avoid pretending that he/she has understood; honesty is the best policy.
- Accept and encourage any method of communication rather than demanding speech.

- Recap occasionally and check that the communication partners have understood each other.
- Be positive, patient and prepared to repeat where necessary.
- Demonstrate empathy and understanding of any signs of stress, frustration or low mood.

In this chapter the authors emphasise that communication skills can be improved by acknowledging that people have different perspectives, cultural backgrounds and views of the world that we need to respectfully listen to and understand. Communication disabilities are diverse, ranging from minor cognitive or speech impairment to complex change and inability to communicate through speech. For some stroke survivors there will be no change in self-perspective and/or no communication difficulties. Some will adapt to change utilising the communication abilities that remain intact. For others their self-esteem and confidence may be severely impaired. Whatever the communication challenges, exercise professionals can optimise their interactions by taking a person-centred approach, trying out the strategies in this chapter, reflecting on the results and sharing their successes with colleagues.

SUMMARY POINTS

- Communication disability is common after stroke and has an impact on both the individual and those they want to communicate with.
- Communication is a complex process and therefore difficulties present in many different ways.
- You can develop your skills as an effective communicator and help to minimise the difficulties with communication in a person-centred way.
- The experience individuals have in communicating with staff will determine their future participation, engagement and attitude towards the service.

REFERENCES

Dickson, S., Barbour, S., Brady, M., et al., 2008. Patients' experiences of disruptions associated with post stroke dysarthria. Int. J. Lang. Commun. Disord. 43, 135–153.

Engelter, S.T., Gostynski, M., Papa, S., et al., 2006. Epidemiology of aphasia attributable to first ischaemic stroke: incidence, severity, fluency, etiology and thrombolysis. Stroke 37, 1379–1384.

Hargie, O., Dickson, D., 2004. Skilled interpersonal communication, fourth ed. Routledge, London.

Howe, T.J., Worrall, L.E., Hickson, L.M.H., 2008. Interviews with people with aphasia: environmental factors that influence their community participation. Aphasiology 22, 1092–1120.

Kelly, H., Brady, M.C., Enderby, P., 2010. Speech and language therapy for aphasia following stroke. Cochrane Database Syst. Rev 5, CD000425. doi:10.1002/14651858.

Parr, S., Byng, S., Gilpin, S., 1997. Talking about aphasia. Open University Press, Buckingham.

Parr, S., Pound, C., Hewitt, A., 2006. Communication access to health and social services. Top. Lang. Disord. 26, 189–198.

Parry, R.H., Brown, K., 2009. Teaching and learning communication skills in physiotherapy: what is done and how should it be done? Physiotherapy 95, 294–301.

One stroke survivor's journey

John Brown

8

The purpose of this chapter is to share one stroke survivor's experience of returning to exercise following a stroke. Being physically active and engaging in sport had been a lifetime habit for John, and his motivation and determination to return to the gym was high. This will not always be the case; other stroke survivors participating in exercise following stroke may need to change their behaviour to reap the benefits of improved fitness and increased mobility (see chapter 6). John's story gives us an insight into some of the highs and lows and the milestones reached.

John's experience has helped shape the content of the only UK course for exercise professionals on stroke. We are indebted to him for sharing his experiences with exercise professionals and tutors undertaking the Register of Exercise Professionals Level 4 course on exercise after stroke. Names have been changed to provide anonymity to the health professionals involved in John's care.

JOHN'S STORY

I have always been enthusiastic about keeping fit. My wife would probably say I'm obsessive! During my Diploma of Education year I opted for Physical Education as my second teaching subject, so at the end of it I was qualified to assist with it in school. I was once told by one of Her Majesty's Inspectors that I was unique in Scotland, being the only Principal Teacher of English to be teaching games.

I played my last game of rugby just before my 50th birthday and after my 'retirement' from the game would spend 3 hours a week in the gym and swim

141

50 to 60 lengths once a week. We also enjoyed holidays walking in the Lake District or Perthshire, so you could say that January 21st 1997 was something of a surprise to me!

STROKE AND HOSPITAL REHABILITATION

It was a Tuesday evening and my wife, Audrey, and I had decided to go to the gym as usual. The fitness room was relatively quiet. I climbed on an exercise bike, set my programme and started pedalling. Audrey, meanwhile, was on the treadmill. After a few minutes, I felt stiffness in my right calf. Thinking it no more than that I pedalled faster. The feeling moved slowly up my right side, my vision began to blur and when I tried to call to Audrey the words wouldn't come. Two others helped me down from the bike and laid me on mats. The doctor arrived and diagnosed a stroke. It was 6 months before my daughter's wedding.

The ambulance came and I was taken to hospital. By the time I'd reached the hospital my voice had returned, though it was pitched several octaves higher. I had various tests and then spent 3 days in a general medical ward until a bed became available in the stroke ward. During my second day I had my first meeting with James Carter, the Senior Physiotherapist, who, when he learned of the July wedding, was adamant that he would have me walking my daughter down the aisle. I had never thought otherwise.

My 9 weeks of treatment got off to a most inauspicious start. I'd noticed sharp pain behind my right knee and, after an ultrasound scan, it was diagnosed as a deep venous thrombosis, so I was given a large dose of warfarin and put on a heparin drip for 1 week. This was most frustrating as it meant postponing the start of physiotherapy. However, 2 weeks later I'd reached the first benchmark of standing unaided for 10 seconds.

My daughter flew from Chicago to see me over Valentine's Day weekend and when I said goodbye to her I promised I'd reach the last objective, walking 10 metres, for her birthday on March 1st. I did. I had now been in rehabilitation for about 5 weeks and I was able to get out of bed and into my wheelchair unaided. I could also walk a little and stand up in the shower, so I thought discharge must be coming. At the end of the first week in March, James Carter suggested the 24th as my 'release' date, which was ideal as it was the start of the Easter holidays and Audrey and I would have a fortnight to work out a routine before she went back to school. I had a home visit with my physiotherapist and an occupational therapist on March 13th and on Sunday 24th Audrey picked me up and took me home. I had spent 9 weeks in the stroke ward.

IMPORTANT FIRST STEPS

The next 2 weeks at home were important. I needed to show Audrey I could cope at home alone. I still needed considerable help showering, drying and dressing. Walking up and down stairs too was tiring. However, the 2 weeks gave us enough time to establish a routine and, when Audrey's new term began, I felt confident about being left in the house on my own. There were just over 3 months until the wedding so I began the work needed to enable me to walk my daughter down the aisle. I knew this was not going to be straightforward as her wedding was being held in Dirleton Castle, a very old castle which had restricted access for people with mobility problems! I began by walking up and down the living room until I'd almost worn a path in the carpet. I had two falls; on both occasions I turned too quickly, caught my right foot in the pile and over I went. I crawled to an armchair, dragged myself onto my knees and then onto my feet and continued walking. I was still apprehensive about walking outdoors as our pavements were rather uneven, but I had to make a start. I decided to make the post box, 20 yards down our street, my first goal. I did the trip daily for a week or two then I increased the distance, until I could manage 50 to 100 yards. During this time I had also been attending bi-weekly physiotherapy sessions at the hospital, so by July I was able to walk over the moat bridge and climb the wooden steps at the castle. I even shuffled around the dance floor that evening.

In my physiotherapy, my balance and limb strengthening were paramount, but I was also given what I thought were rather meaningless tasks such as turning over cards from a pack or undoing knots in a long piece of string, but I realised how useful they'd been when, in September, I tied my shoelace for the first time in 9 months! However, shirt sleeve buttons were proving more difficult and I would get angry and frustrated at not being able to manage them.

BROADENING HORIZONS AND TACKLING FRUSTRATIONS

As August ended, Brenda, my community physiotherapist, said I'd soon need only a weekly visit, and that in a week or two she would allow me to use the exercise bike. On my third visit she helped me onto the bike; 5 minutes later she was helping me off as I was looking a little pale. I was exhausted, but happy; it was another small step along the road to near normality.

I used the bike each week and also went up to the Sports Centre for my 5 minutes on a Sunday. I tried swimming again, but it was more stopping myself from drowning than swimming. However, by November I could 'doggy-paddle' a width and my bike time was increasing.

My social life was also improving. I had joined the local Chest Heart & Stroke Scotland club, a friend took me for a weekly coffee, and I was now a member of the local Probus Club. Audrey and I visited the cinema and we shopped, both of which required using my wheelchair, but I was having as normal a life as possible. My walking distance was increasing, I could manage a hundred yards and more without difficulty, I was able to use my right hand to hold a spoon and, if I supported it with my left, raise a wine glass – half-full!

In January 1998 it was suggested my physiotherapy be reduced to a monthly session, and then, when I went in February, I was told that, as there had been no marked deterioration in my progress, I could end the sessions. I felt a mixture of emotions; while I was pleased to finish, I was also sad that the friendship and trust I had found there was over.

So I decided that my next goal would be to regain my driving licence.

In early February I underwent a driving assessment in a rehabilitation hospital centre. My peripheral vision and speed of reaction were found to be normal so I drove round the grounds of the hospital in an automatic car.

I tended to over-compensate at corners, otherwise I had no problems and was told there was no reason why I could not drive, so I informed the Driver and Vehicle Licensing Agency, had a lesson with a British School of Motoring Instructor for the Disabled, and in May took delivery of a new car. Now I could take Audrey to the cinema!

Although I was making decent progress physically, and things seemed to be going well, there were still occasions when I would grow very angry at not being able to do something relatively trivial, such as placing objects on shelves. As it was Audrey who bore the brunt of my anger, I decided something needed to be done about it. I was still visiting my doctor monthly and I discussed the problem with him. He suggested I see a volunteer counsellor who did some work at the surgery. I agreed, and during our first few meetings we just talked about my stroke and the progress I'd made since surviving it. Having someone else to talk to made an enormous difference and we were soon setting non-physical targets. Rosalind, my counsellor, wanted me to be a little more independent as far as money and shopping were concerned, so I began to visit the local supermarket alone and also to practise my signature so that I would be able to do simple things such as signing cheques. I had been so focused on physical rehabilitation that I had neglected the ordinary things and my sessions with Rosalind certainly helped a great deal.

She also introduced me to a Community Care worker, Brian, who was involved in a local mental care project; Brian offered to collect me on Monday mornings and take me to the pool or gym. It seemed a good deal, and on occasional Wednesdays we'd take a trip to the cinema. This involvement with people outside of my family was of real benefit to me.

We had 2 months of using the car before we were off to Chicago in July to celebrate Jenny and Jon's first wedding anniversary. While we were in the USA we also spent a few days in Washington DC with Jenny's in-laws, and this visit proved to be very significant in my rehabilitation process. Her mother-in-law had arranged for me to see a physical therapist who had written a book on stroke rehabilitation and on July 17th I had my 'consultation'. After an hour and a half of extreme physical exercise I was told that if I could stay for a year I might be jogging at the end of it. I was astonished. I knew I'd improve but not to such an extent, so when we returned home I used Yellow Pages and selected, quite at random, a private physiotherapy clinic in Edinburgh. I went regularly over the next 2 years.

Initially we worked on correcting my gait, as I had fallen into the habit of hitching my right hip, and I also needed help with my right shoulder, which was still painful and I found it difficult to raise my right hand above my head. I was given exercises to do at home and also told to practise such mundane things as shaving and teeth brushing with my right hand. It was also suggested that I try aquarobics where I could exercise and the water would bear my weight. I found myself in a class with fifteen or sixteen ladies, but I always stood in the front right hand corner of the pool to avoid distractions!

I was also continuing my work in the gym, and later, during my regular physiotherapy visits, I asked whether a yoga class might help. It seemed a good idea so I began beginners' classes. I found some of the poses hard to begin with, but enjoyed the relaxation and breathing, and gradually was able to stretch my muscles further.

In June 1998, I read an article in the 'Different Strokes' magazine about a device called a 'functional electrical stimulator', which had been developed in a Salisbury hospital and which was a walking aid designed for stroke survivors with drop foot. Using an electrical impulse, it caused a heel strike with the affected foot thus making walking less tiring. I told my general practitioner about the article and he referred me for an assessment. My wife and I travelled to Birmingham for this and then to Salisbury for a fitting. We had to return to Salisbury 5 weeks later to see if we had been able to use it and whether it had been of benefit. I still wear it for longer walks, and over the last 10 years or so have walked distances of up to 7 miles when we have revisited the Lake District.

In September 1996, before my stroke, Audrey and I had started ballroom dancing lessons so we would be able to manage a turn around the floor at the wedding. My stroke had curtailed these lessons somewhat, but the dance club had kept our places open and we resumed normal service in September 1999. My balance has been helped by dancing and, although some of the turns can be tricky, I can usually 'improvise' without it being too noticeable.

That year I also began voluntary work in a local primary school. I had mentioned my wish to do something worthwhile with some of my spare time to a neighbour, who was a member of staff, and a few days later was contacted by the Head Teacher. I spent 10 years of thursday mornings there listening to reading and talking about books and language, including punctuation and grammar, with small groups of Primary 4 to 7 pupils. I had left my previous teaching post so suddenly that I felt I needed to try to do a little more. The school roll never exceeded 75 pupils and I thoroughly enjoyed my decade with them. I gave up last summer having passed the official retiral age by a number of years.

So, in addition to my regime in the gym, I have my dancing from September to May with one or two tea dances in the intervening period, yoga once a week, a bridge club during the winter months, plenty of gardening in the summer and the cinema fairly regularly. I also manage to help out with a few household chores: I can dust and use the hoover, and am also able to do a little ironing. Two months of the year, usually in the Spring and the Autumn, are spent visiting in the USA and we try to have a few days walking somewhere in Britain on a regular basis.

ONGOING CHALLENGES

Although the past 13 years have been very much an onward journey, there are, nevertheless, still difficulties. My right shoulder still gives me some pain, and I do have remedial massage on it every 2 months or so. The massage loosens the joint and eases some of the fibrous tissue around it.

I am still prone to mood swings and can be short-tempered on occasions. I know this is happening and have to step back and look at my behaviour. I am also much more emotional than I was before my stroke; I find it hard to listen to some pieces of music or watch some film scenes without a lump in my throat. However, although I was concerned about this early in my recovery, I have come to realise that this is simply a result of my stroke and I let the tears come.

CURRENT GYM PROGRAMME

I try to manage a workout in the gym for an hour two or three times a week, though it's more likely to be two these days. I will spend 10 minutes on the rowing machine and then 10 minutes on the treadmill as cardiovascular exercise. Then I will complete 10 repetitions on most of the weights machines, the weights varying according to the muscle group being worked. After that I continue with a number of stretching and strengthening exercises on the mat. I use a number of yoga exercises for some of the former, and a medicine ball for the latter. As my strength and stamina improved over the years I changed my targets, but as age has begun to catch up with me I have 'modified' these. I have reduced my target on the rowing machine from 2000 metres to 1800 and the weights by 5 kg.

The gym work is still very important to me, and I do feel the strenuous exercise improves my feeling of general wellbeing, as well as allowing me an extra glass of wine in the evening!

KEY MESSAGES

- Physical activity and sport were an important part of my life from an early age. This lifetime habit gave me confidence that I could return to regular exercise and the motivation to continue to achieve my plans and goals – even at times when my mood was very low. For others where exercise and sport has not been a lifetime habit it is likely that following rehabilitation will require greater levels of support to help them engage in appropriate physical activities that they will enjoy.
- My story highlights that recovery can continue over a long period of time and that participation in physical activity can continue to provide benefits to stroke survivors, despite the changes with getting older that are occurring at the same time.
- I have given examples of the support and actions that I found useful to cope with emotional and everyday activities that had become difficult for me, which included sessions with a counsellor.
- Family support is important in getting back to activities previously enjoyed. For me, this included ballroom dancing and going to the cinema. I acknowledge that stroke survivors and their families will enjoy a range of different leisure pastimes and that their health, social and financial circumstances may facilitate or prevent people from returning to the things that they previously enjoyed doing. It is likely that compromises will have to be made in deciding appropriate plans and goals.
- The exercise routine outlined provides me with the right balance of aerobic, strength and flexibility that I require to maintain my fitness. I recommend that individuals seek support from an exercise professional or physiotherapist to ensure that the programme is designed to take account of their particular needs.

EDITORS' COMMENT

The voice of the stroke survivor is extremely important to health and exercise professionals. Through their words we can gain an understanding of recovery, the milestones, what helps to motivate and what works best and for whom. While scientific evidence and randomised controlled trials are crucial to providing the best treatment interventions for short- and long-term survival, we need to understand how best to enable stroke survivors to continue with their own recovery and self-care. John's story is one of many stories we have heard over the years, each one bringing a unique insight into the impact of stroke and exercise after stroke on people's lives. It has highlighted that stroke recovery can last for many months and years, and that exercise can play a crucial role in facilitating recovery and improving quality of life after stroke.

PART 3
PRACTICAL APPLICATIONS OF EXERCISE AND FITNESS TRAINING AFTER STROKE

PART CONTENTS

Preparing for exercise after stroke

9

John M.A. Dennis • Catherine S. Best •
Susie Dinan-Young • Gillian Mead

CHAPTER CONTENTS

INTRODUCTION

Clinical guidelines generally recommend that exercise training should be provided as part of the post-rehabilitation care of stroke survivors. This is because much of the evidence about the effectiveness of exercise comes from trials which provided exercise training *after* usual stroke care had been completed (chapter 5). Some stroke services may wish to integrate exercise training into usual stroke rehabilitation and, whilst it is highly plausible that exercise training may be of benefit at this stage in the patient journey, the evidence base is less strong. This may change as new trials are published.

This chapter will detail the preparatory processes, undertaken by both health-care and exercise professionals, before a stroke survivor commences exercise and fitness training. We are assuming that exercise is provided in community settings, and delivered by an exercise professional, who may have come from one of the professional backgrounds mentioned in chapter 2.

One of the central recommendations is that patients should be formally *referred* to exercise services, just as they might be referred to other services. This means that the referrer provides important clinical information to the exercise professional or physiotherapist delivering the exercise. In the UK, exercise referral schemes have been available in the community for many years now, and there are established referral routes in and out of the services (Department of Health 2001). In the UK, Exercise after Stroke services are being developed using the well-established exercise referral pathways for people with coronary heart disease and those who have had a fall.

EXERCISE REFERRAL ROUTES INTO THE EXERCISE AFTER STROKE SERVICE

People who have had a stroke can access Exercise after Stroke services, either after discharge from stroke rehabilitation or from primary care.

REFERRAL FROM STROKE REHABILITATION

People who have recently had a stroke and have undergone a period of rehabilitation should be referred as a part of, or immediately following, discharge from inpatient or outpatient physiotherapy. If exercise has been included as part of rehabilitation, the physiotherapist will have important information on individual stroke survivors' responses to exercise and the duration and intensity of training that can be tolerated. This information is very important for the exercise professional who will be delivering exercise in the community setting. For this reason, the ideal referral route into an Exercise after Stroke service is from a physiotherapist who has worked with the patient on aspects of their physical fitness.

REFERRAL FROM PRIMARY CARE

The other main route into Exercise after Stroke services is for stroke survivors already discharged from secondary health-care services. All health professionals who come into contact with stroke survivors should address the issue of exercise along with other lifestyle factors which are important for secondary stroke prevention. Health professionals should address personal, social and environmental barriers to exercise (see chapter 6). Referral to an Exercise after Stroke service should be made wherever possible. People who had a stroke some time ago or did not receive inpatient treatment should access Exercise after Stroke services through their general practitioner (GP) or other appropriate health professional, e.g. practice nurse (delegated by the GP), community physiotherapist, stroke specialist nurse or occupational therapist.

PROCESS OF REFERRAL TO AN EXERCISE AFTER STROKE SERVICE

Based on an extensive scoping project to identify Exercise after Stroke services in Scotland and existing guidelines for exercise referral schemes (Best et al. 2010), we developed a referral pathway for people after stroke (Fig. 9.1). More information is given about each stage in the following sections.

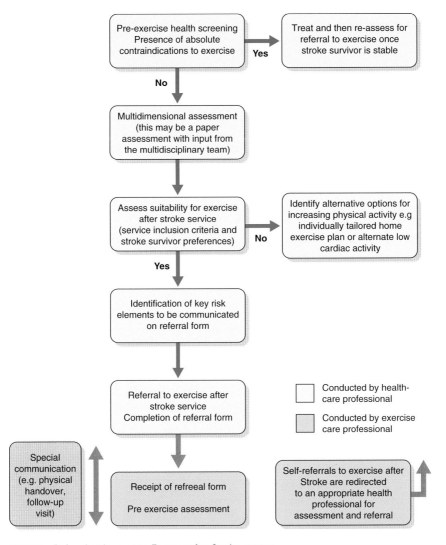

FIG 9.1   Referral pathways into Exercise after Stroke services.

PRE-EXERCISE ASSESSMENTS

Pre-exercise assessment by a health professional prior to referral to an Exercise after Stroke service has four elements:

1. Screening for absolute contraindications for exercise: to identify people who should not be exercising due to unstable medical conditions.

2. Multidimensional assessment: to give the exercise professional a global picture of the individual stroke survivor's medical and functional status.
3. Local Exercise after Stroke inclusion criteria: to ensure a match between the stroke survivor and the Exercise after Stroke session.
4. Risk assessment and management: to highlight areas of the multidimensional assessment that require specific tailoring of the exercise intervention in order to ensure the maximum possible benefit from exercise.

The four elements are described in detail below as separate processes for the sake of clarity; however, in practice there is a great deal of overlap between these elements and they will usually all be completed within a single assessment session.

SCREENING FOR ABSOLUTE CONTRAINDICATIONS FOR EXERCISE AFTER STROKE

The referring health professional will determine whether there are any absolute contraindications to exercise after stroke. These absolute contraindications are based on the most recent ACSM guidelines for exercise testing (ACSM 2010) and also absolute contraindications for exercise training in vulnerable older patients (Dinan 2001). Note that the absolute contraindications are mainly due to unstable heart disease (Box 9.1).

BOX 9.1 Absolute contraindications to Exercise after Stroke

- Recent electrocardiogram changes suggesting significant ischaemia, recent myocardial infarction (within 2 days) or other acute cardiac event
- Unstable angina
- Uncontrolled cardiac dysrhythmias causing symptoms or haemodynamic compromise
- Symptomatic severe aortic stenosis
- Uncontrolled symptomatic heart failure
- Acute pulmonary embolism or pulmonary infarction
- Acute myocarditis or pericarditis
- Suspected or known dissecting aneurysm
- Acute systemic infection, accompanied by fever, body aches or swollen lymph glands
- Extreme obesity, with weight exceeding the recommendations or the equipment capacity (usually >159 kg [350 lb])
- Uncontrolled visual or vestibular disturbances
- Recent injurious fall without medical assessment
- Known inability to comply with exercise sessions

Based on American College of Sports Medicine absolute contraindications to exercise testing (ACSM 2010), and the absolute contraindications to exercise training in vulnerable older patients (Dinan 2001).

MULTIDIMENSIONAL PRE-EXERCISE ASSESSMENT

The long-term effects of stroke are varied and wide-ranging so the exercise professional will need an overview of the stroke survivor's residual neurological impairments (chapter 1) as well as any other post-stroke problems, co-morbidities and medication (chapter 3), so that the exercise programme can be tailored to the needs of individual stroke survivors. Once absolute contraindications to exercise have been excluded, the health professional should proceed to the multidimensional assessment, which should cover all domains shown in Box 9.2. Most of this information would be available from the stroke

---

BOX 9.2 Multidimensional pre-exercise assessment

This information should be transferred to the exercise professional, once absolute contraindications to exercise have been ruled out, and the stroke survivor has given written informed consent to be referred. (For an example of the content of a referral form see Box 9.3.)

- General medical and stroke medical history
- Information on any co-morbidity that might contraindicate or restrict exercise, e.g. ischaemic heart disease, heart failure, respiratory disease, poor circulation, uncontrolled epilepsy, joint replacements, etc.
- Medications and how these may restrict exercise ability
- Pain status: stroke-related (central or shoulder), musculoskeletal or other
- Joint active and passive range of motion (particularly with relation to the risks associated with subluxation or poor control in shoulder movement – a common source of post stroke pain)
- Problems with muscle tone
- Motor control: coordination of joint stability, strength and power, protective reactions, movement involving single and multiple body segments, and functional activities
- Balance both in static and dynamic situations and recovery responses
- Gait (walking ability), addressing both neurological and biomechanical aspects of gait. Ideally, this should include different variations of gait (i.e. slow, fast, backward and side-stepping, turning, managing obstacles and stair climbing) in different environments (i.e. rough and smooth ground, flat ground and slopes, different lighting and noise conditions)
- Visuospatial problems, difficulties with body schema awareness
- Functional abilities history and direct observations of functional tasks related to activities of daily living
- Compensatory overuse of less affected side
- Activity history including current physical activity status, interests, preferences, means and readiness to exercise. This indicates that the stroke survivor has agreed with the referring party that they are ready to exercise, are motivated enough to attempt a programme, and able to attend the intended exercise programme times
- Communication: the stroke survivor's ability to understand and follow instructions and to communicate with the exercise instructor, including the presence of aphasia and/or dysarthria (see chapter 3)
- Cognition: the presence of memory impairment, executive dysfunction, impaired insight or dementia, may require adapted communication strategies to allow the individual to participate or require the involvement of a communication assistant

survivor's medical records. This type of assessment is labelled 'multidimensional' as one health professional may not be able to complete all relevant sections. If this is the case, input from other members of the multidisciplinary team or primary care team should be sought where necessary. This information must be communicated to the exercise professional in appropriate terminology. Each service will need to design its own form according to local requirements. An example of a referral form that was developed by the NHS Greater Glasgow and Clyde therapeutic exercise working group is shown in Box 9.3.

The health professional needs to be cognisant of the ACSM list of *relative* contraindications to exercise testing, including left main coronary stenosis, moderate stenotic valvular heart disease, electrolyte disturbance, systolic BP >200 mmHg or diastolic BP >110 mmHg at rest, tachydysrhythmia or bradydysrhythmia, hypertrophic cardiomyopathy or other forms of outflow tract obstruction, neuromuscular or musculoskeletal or rheumatoid arthritis that are exacerbated by exercise, high-degree atrioventricular block, ventricular aneurysm, uncontrolled metabolic disease, chronic infections and mental or physical impairment leading to inability to exercise adequately (ACSM 2010). If the patient has any of these relative contraindications, the health professional must consider how best to manage these problems. The health professional and exercise professional should also discuss whether it is safe to start exercise, or whether exercise should be deferred until these problems have been optimally managed. Some degree of clinical judgement may be required. For example, in our STARTER trial, we did not allow patients to start the exercise programme if their blood pressure exceeded >180 mmHg systolic or >100 mmHg diastolic, and we asked their GP to review antihypertensive medication. Patients were allowed to start the exercise programme once their blood pressure was lower than this limit (Mead et al. 2007).

LOCAL EXERCISE AFTER STROKE SERVICE INCLUSION CRITERIA

The health-care professional will assess the stroke survivor's suitability for an exercise service. Box 9.4 gives an example of Exercise after Stroke service inclusion criteria. The emphasis of this part of the process is on inclusion. The inclusion criteria are not a repetition of the absolute contraindications to exercise. Instead, they describe characteristics of stroke survivors who are appropriate for referral into a particular service. This is based on the stroke survivor's clinical and functional characteristics, the type of exercise that will be provided and the level of expertise of the exercise professionals.

RISK ASSESSMENT AND MANAGEMENT BY REFERRING HEALTH-CARE PROFESSIONAL

Risk assessment concerns the evaluation and stratification of the type and level of risk of an adverse event to a stroke survivor during or immediately following exercise. Risk management concerns the ongoing adaptations that are made to minimise this risk. The most significant risks to stroke survivors from participating in exercise are from cardiac events, falls and fractures, although these are all rare.

BOX 9.3 Exercise referral information

1. Name
2. Address
3. Date of birth
4. Telephone number
5. General practitioner details
   - Name
   - Address
   - Telephone and fax number
6. Next of kin and contact details
7. Health problems
   - Cardiac history – including left ventricular function and any associated heart failure
   - Others, e.g.:
     - Respiratory history
     - Multiple sclerosis
     - Osteoarthritis
     - Rheumatoid arthritis
     - Falls history
     - Fracture history
     - Back pain
     - Joint replacement
     - Osteoporosis
     - Diabetes
     - Epilepsy
8. Stroke history
   - Time since stroke/date of stroke
   - Functional levels post stroke
   - Chronic fatigue
   - Hearing impairment
   - Visual impairment
   - Cognitive/perceptual impairment
   - Use of aids (e.g. walking aids)
9. Medication
10. Has attended National Health Service Rehabilitation Service?
    - Name and location of service
    - Dates
    - How many exercise sessions attended
    - Relevant tests completed and results
    - Blood pressure
    - Agreed training heart rate
11. Personal exercise considerations and limitations:
    - Tone/spasticity
    - Contractures
    - Poor balance/strength
    - Splinting
    - Difficulty moving on/off equipment
    - Ability to self-monitor/pace self
    - Readiness to exercise
    - General physical activity levels (current and pre-stroke)
    - Access to transport

BOX 9.4 Example Exercise after Stroke inclusion criteria

- Able to sit in any seat independently (time unlimited)
- Able to mobilise more than 5 m with or without a walking aid, independently or supervised
- In cases where the stroke survivor has aphasia, communication strategies in place to allow participation
- Tinetti balance and gait score minimum 12/28

The current available evidence suggests that the benefits of exercise outweigh the risks for the general population and for stroke survivors. For this reason, risk assessment should not be construed in a negative sense, raising fears about the participation of stroke survivors in exercise and resulting in individuals being excluded from Exercise after Stroke services. Rather, the process should focus on the more positive aspects with the aim of enabling stroke survivors to safely participate in exercise.

The health professional contributes to the ongoing risk assessment and stratification process by providing clear information (about the nature and severity of the stroke survivor's primary conditions and any co-morbidities, medications, impairments and activity limitations). This enables the exercise professional to continue the assessment process in relation to the proposed exercise programme for the individual. This information also enables the exercise professional to adapt and tailor the exercise programme (type, intensity, duration, positioning, etc.) and to put in place safety procedures and/or equipment to manage the risks identified for each individual.

As mentioned in chapter 3, there is considerable co-morbidity with stroke and cardiac disease. It is estimated that around 75% of stroke survivors have co-morbid heart disease (Roth 1993) and that between 20% and 40% of stroke survivors will test positive for silent cardiac ischaemia (Adams et al. 2003). In people with known coronary heart disease, the primary cause of death after exercise is ventricular fibrillation. Nevertheless, the overall risk from exercise is low, even in people with coronary disease, as in cardiac rehabilitation programmes (where exercise is tailored to minimise risk) cardiac arrests occur at a rate of 1 in 12 000 to 15 000 in people with cardiac disease (Zipes and Wellens 1998).

The American Heart Association (AHA) recommends that graded exercise testing with electrocardiac monitoring is a prerequisite to referral for exercise (Gordon et al. 2004) because up to 75% of stroke survivors will have underlying coronary artery disease which may be 'silent'. However, exercise testing itself may carry risks (e.g. many stroke survivors will not have sufficient balance or strength to undergo conventional treadmill testing), and other testing protocols (e.g. arm cycle ergometry) may not be practical. Treadmill exercise testing protocols have been developed and validated for stroke survivors with gait impairments (Ivey et al. 2011). The AHA suggests that, if an exercise test cannot be performed for practical reasons, lighter intensity exercise should be prescribed. However, the Scottish Intercollegiate Guidelines Network (2002) guidelines for ischaemic heart disease suggest that, for most clients, clinical risk stratification based on history, examination and resting electrocardiogram combined with a functional capacity test, such as a shuttle walking test or a 6-minute walking test, will be sufficient. Exercise testing and echocardiography is recommended only for high-risk clients.

Our recommendation is that treadmill exercise testing is not essential prior to referral to Exercise after Stroke services. A functional test such as the 6-minute walk, in combination with detailed referral information, is usually sufficient.

Once the absolute contraindications to exercise have been ruled out for a stroke survivor, then assessment of cardiac risk level should be a clinical decision. Factors to be considered include those listed as the American College of Sports Medicine's (2010) relative contraindications to exercise testing and Scottish Intercollegiate Guidelines Network Guideline 57 (2002). The cardiac risk factors that must be considered include those listed in Box 9.5.

Where any of these signs and symptoms or other indications of cardiac disease are present, this should be communicated clearly to the exercise professional in the referral documentation. It may be necessary for the health professional to optimise the medical management of these conditions before the stroke survivor begins the exercise programme. For example, if the stroke survivor is experiencing angina at low levels of exercise, then anti-anginal medication needs to be reviewed, and consideration given for the need for further investigation and treatment.

BOX 9.5 Cardiac risk factors to be evaluated

- History of myocardial infarction complicated by heart failure, cardiogenic shock and/or complex ventricular arrhythmias
- Tachyarrhythmias or bradyarrhythmias
- High degree atrioventricular block
- Angina or breathlessness occurring at a low level of exercise
- Cardiomyopathy
- Moderate stenotic valvular heart disease
- Complex ventricular ectopy
- Left main coronary artery stenosis

The other key risk for stroke survivors undertaking exercise is from falls and fractures. In the Cochrane review of circuit class therapy to improve mobility after stroke, only two of the six trials reported adverse events during therapy (English and Hillier 2010). There were a total of nine falls in the intervention groups compared with three in the control groups (English and Hillier 2010). The authors attributed this to the fact that balance is systematically challenged during circuit therapy. None of the falls was serious but the risk of falls from participation in exercise should be carefully evaluated and session design measures (e.g. adaptations to pace, transitions between exercises and direction changes) introduced to minimise this risk for stroke survivors. The health professional should assess whether there is a risk of falls or fractures and it should be remembered that this is usually in the context of a group of stroke survivors. This is a clinical decision based on factors such as a history of falls, evidence of impaired balance or vision, osteoporosis, or prescription of psychoactive medication. The Falls

Management Exercise (FaME) trial (Skelton et al. 2005) demonstrated that an exercise intervention for older people at risk of falling could be delivered safely and effectively (with no falls during the intervention). Thus, exercise can be delivered safely for these groups, but the exercise professional needs to be aware of the stroke survivor's risk for falls in order to tailor the intervention effectively.

The risk assessment highlights areas of the multidimensional assessment that require particular attention and tailoring of the exercise programme for the individual stroke survivor (see chapter 10).

Following the risk assessment, health professionals should engage stroke survivors in a discussion of the relative risks of exercise versus inactivity and the benefits of exercise so that stroke survivors can make an informed decision on whether to be referred to an Exercise after Stroke service. The health professional should also explore with the stroke survivor how to recognise new symptoms that might indicate that a part or the whole of the exercise programme was, in some way, unsuitable for them. For example, stroke survivors with osteoarthritic knees should be taught to recognise and respect an increase in pain, stiffness or swelling; stroke survivors who experience a severe increase in their habitual level of resting muscle tone, should be instructed to consult the exercise professional about the problem and only continue to exercise if the exercise can be appropriately tailored to resolve the problem (Young and Dinan 2005). At this time, it is recommended that written informed consent should be sought and obtained for a referral for exercise.

This section completes the four elements of the pre-exercise assessment process conducted by the health professional.

BARRIERS AND MOTIVATORS TO EXERCISE AFTER STROKE

The majority of community-dwelling stroke survivors are inactive (Rand et al. 2009, Moore et al. 2010). As chapter 6 explained, initiating exercise and maintaining this in the long term is a challenge, even for people with no health conditions. The optimum methods for promoting physical activity after stroke are not known as this is a relatively new research area. However, repeated advice to be more active is probably not sufficient to change behaviour after stroke (Boysen et al. 2009). To enable stroke survivors – where appropriate – to enjoy the benefits of a more physically active lifestyle, it is necessary to explore individual physical, psychosocial and environmental barriers to exercise (Damush et al. 2007, Gordon et al. 2004, Mead 2009).

Where stroke survivors are reluctant to engage in group exercise, other options for increasing activity levels should be explored. Health professionals should consider the presence of depression, as this may be a barrier to taking up a new physical activity programme. Ideally, most ambulatory stroke survivors will be recommended to join an Exercise after Stroke programme.

An indication of the individual's barriers and motivators to exercise should be included in the referral documentation, as this information is invaluable for the exercise professional receiving and using the referral as the basis for an individually tailored programme, as will be explained in chapter 10.

The following processes will ensure the appropriate allocation of responsibilities between the health professional, the exercise professional and the Exercise after Stroke service and include:

- Formal referral from a health-care professional (as described above and listed in Box 9.6)
- Transfer of responsibility
- Transfer of information.

BOX 9.6 Key responsibilities of the referring health professional

- To assess the stroke survivor for absolute contraindications for exercise
- To complete a multidimensional assessment which will include: identifying **pathologies** that are present, and ensuring that they (and their medications) are accurately and clearly communicated to the exercise professional
- To highlight any way these may influence the **safety or comfort of everyday physical activity**, e.g. susceptibility to angina or postural hypotension
- To identify the most **appropriate form of exercise** for the individual (for most stroke survivors this will be an Exercise After Stroke service) – based on current relevant evidence and clinical reasoning, local Exercise After Stroke service inclusion criteria and personal preferences of the stroke survivor
- To identify any key risk elements for exercise that emerge from the multidimensional assessment, e.g. risk of falls, cardiac events, prescribed medications that will affect response to exercise. These may need to be optimally managed before the stroke survivor starts to exercise, and tailoring of the exercise may be needed for individual stroke survivors
- To educate the stroke survivor in the **early recognition of symptoms** which might indicate that a part or the whole of the exercise programme was, in some way, unsuitable to them at that time. For example, people with osteoarthritic knees should be taught to recognise and respect an increase in pain, stiffness or swelling; stroke survivors who experience a severe increase in their habitual level of resting muscle tone, etc., should be instructed to consult the exercise professional about the problem and only continue to exercise if the exercise can be appropriately tailored to resolve the problem/adverse effect
- To communicate that any problem, e.g. worsening pain in arthritic knee, should be discussed with the exercise professional and the GP or referring health professional (Young and Dinan 2005)

ALLOCATION OF RESPONSIBILITIES FOR THE STROKE SURVIVOR

Once it has been agreed by the GP or physiotherapist that the stroke survivor is suitable to be referred for supervised exercise (i.e. pre-exercise health screen and multidimensional assessment including risk assessment completed) and that the proposed exercise professional and exercises and programme are appropriate, the responsibility for the design and delivery of the exercise programme and the monitoring of the stroke survivor's response to the exercise passes to the exercise professional (Department of Health 2001). In the UK, the GP remains responsible for the overall management of each patient's care programme (Department of Health 2001).

The allocation of responsibility to the fitness sector includes the owner or manager of the fitness facility where the session takes place. The responsibilities of the fitness centre operator are to ensure that there are adequate systems in place to support the process of patient referral (secure records/confidentiality, etc.) and – importantly – to ensure the exercise professionals are properly qualified.

In the UK, all exercise professionals delivering exercise to people after stroke should be qualified according to the National Occupational Standards laid down by SkillsActive (www.skillsactive.com) and should be on the Register of Exercise Professionals at the Level 4 Exercise after Stroke category. In other countries, different qualifications may exist, but the same principles apply, i.e. the exercise professional should be sufficiently experienced to design, deliver and progress exercise for this patient group, and have the required qualifications and experience to meet the conditions of their insurance cover.

TRANSFER OF INFORMATION

Written, informed consent should be sought from the stroke survivor before referral and transfer of information. Exercise after Stroke services must have procedures and supporting documents to ensure an adequate transfer of relevant medical information to the exercise professional from the referrer.

An example of the domains included in the referral form developed in NHS Greater Glasgow and Clyde for those already screened and who have no absolute contraindications for exercise is shown in Box. 9.3. Referral forms need to be designed according to local needs.

THE ROLE OF THE EXERCISE PROFESSIONAL IN PREPARING FOR EXERCISE AFTER STROKE

PRE-EXERCISE ASSESSMENT

Before joining the first exercise session, each stroke survivor should have a half-hour appointment with the exercise professional for pre-exercise assessment, information exchange and, where appropriate, some exercise induction. Extra time should be allowed when scheduling this pre-exercise session for people who are new to the service, to accommodate practicalities, such as getting through sports centre reception, finding a locker, etc. Chapter 10 will cover in detail how to design an exercise programme for individual stroke survivors.

MANAGING RISKS FOR STROKE SURVIVORS

Exercise professionals play a crucial role in risk assessment, stratification and management. In the context of exercise after stroke, risks arise from the following three main sources:

1. The facility
2. The equipment
3. The people, activities and level of supervision.

Each of these sources of risk will be detailed below.

The facility

Space

Access to the building and the exercise area, as well as the area itself, needs to be assessed for risks of tripping or falling. Making sudden changes of direction to avoid equipment or walls could cause loss of balance and a fall.

Floor surface

It is essential that this be a non-slip surface and it should be checked for evidence of other factors which could make it slippery, e.g. dust or water. It is likely that a number of activities may occur in this space, so it may be necessary to brush the floor before each session. Floor surfaces should also be checked for loose tiles, broken or loose floor panels and any uneven surfaces. Where there is a risk, it is the exercise professional's responsibility to decide whether adequate controls can be instigated to enable the session to take place.

Windows

Opening windows can present a hazard in warm weather, especially where participants are likely to use walls for balance. Checks should be made that open windows do not present an obstruction.

Temperature

Low temperatures reduce coordination and muscle power and could increase susceptibility to falls. The temperature of the room should be comfortable.

Lighting

Ensure good but not harsh lighting and avoid 'deep' shadows or bright lights shining on floor surfaces. Where shadows are present, someone with impaired vision may see a step where there is none or, worse, fail to see an obstacle, misjudge a movement and therefore experience a fall.

Equipment

Objects

All equipment must be checked for damage and correct set-up. Obstacles to be stepped onto should have a non-slip base and be totally stable. Care should be taken when using exercise steps that these have been correctly set up and that any removable top is firmly in place. Mats can provide different surfaces to walk over when balance skills and confidence are adequate, but should be checked for non-slip backing and any damaged edges.

The layout and positioning of the equipment may present a hazard, perhaps for those entering the room or wishing to access chairs. Consequently, equipment must be set up to ensure that less confident participants are not forced to negotiate various obstacles before they are confident.

Although the programme is movement-based, there should be chairs provided for those who require seated alternatives or rest periods. Chairs should be checked for stability and safety.

Handrails

Less confident individuals should be able to hold onto a handrail or other solid object. Given that this may have to take considerable weight, it should be tested prior to each session. Avoid using doors as a support.

Footwear

Slippers, sandals and loose-fitting shoes may all contribute to a trip. Thick-soled trainers reduce proprioceptive feedback and often cause a trip because of the thickness of the sole and the ease of 'catching' on steps and 'sticking' to certain floor surfaces. Laced, thin-soled shoes with a moderate height (1.5 to 3 cm) non-slip heel are recommended.

Spectacles

Bifocal and varifocal lenses are widely used and require extra care on stairs, exercise steps or circuit layouts using different levels. It is safer to have single lens glasses so that the stairs cannot be viewed out of focus through reading lenses. Even if people have worn them for many years, the ageing nervous system is less able to quickly adapt between different foci. It is useful to remind participants that a correct posture will also enhance the efficiency of any type of lens, i.e. keeping the head and neck erect and only looking down with the eyes.

PEOPLE, ACTIVITIES AND THE LEVEL OF SUPERVISION

The greatest risks probably occur from the activities which participants are asked to perform and the level of supervision of these activities. The ratio of supervision to participant will depend, ultimately, on the functional abilities and disabilities within the group. The safety and effectiveness of the session will rest with the skill of the exercise professional, who will use his/ her expertise and observation to control and challenge participants. Adequate staff training is consequently an essential control measure.

The checklist in Figure 9.2 summarises the key points that should be checked every session and provides a way of recording these on a weekly or monthly basis. More columns can be added to locate the record in a single document.

GROUP EXERCISE FORMAT

Another element in the preparation for exercise is choosing the format of the session. There is evidence that group circuit training is effective in improving functional outcomes after stroke (Wevers et al. 2009). As mentioned in chapter 6, stroke survivors report benefits from the social aspect of the group (Carin-Levy et al. 2009, Reed et al. 2010). Group exercise is likely to be more cost effective (English et al. 2007); more specific evidence will be available on completion of an on-going trial of circuit training (van de Port et al. 2009). Where possible and appropriate, Exercise after Stroke services should therefore be delivered in a group format rather than individual gym sessions. Individual sessions and home exercise booklets can help to supplement the group sessions (see chapters 10 and 13).

Session checklist

Session _____ Date _____

Venue _____

Carried out by _____

Facility	
Floor surfaces – sounds and clean	
Handrail – secure	
Windows – no obstruction	
Temperature – adequate	
Equipment	
Ice packs accessible	
Blankets available	
Obstacles – steps checked for set up	
Mats – non-slip	
Positioning of equipment	
Chairs – stable and safe	
Systems and organisation	
Alarm/ phone working	
Emergency action plan in place	
All staff trained in Emergency Operating Procedures	
Specific individual needs accommodated	
Medical history available and all participants screened	
Emergency contact numbers available	
Further comments:	

FIG 9.2 Example of a risk-assessment proforma for exercise and fitness training after stroke.

SUMMARY POINTS

- Stroke survivors must be formally referred to an Exercise after Stroke service by a health-care professional.
- Stroke survivors must be screened for contraindications to exercise, and then undergo a multidimensional assessment. This will be undertaken by the referring health-care professional.
- The exercise professional should assess the stroke survivor and then design an appropriate exercise programme, ensuring that risks have been identified and management plans put into place.
- The exercise professional is responsible for the stroke survivor's welfare while undertaking the exercise programme.
- Ongoing responsibility for the stroke survivor's health lies with his/her GP.

Adams, R.J., Chimowitz, M.I., Alpert, J.S., et al., 2003. Coronary risk evaluation in patients with transient ischemic attack and ischemic stroke: a scientific statement for healthcare professionals from the Stroke Council and the Council on Clinical Cardiology of the American Heart Association/American Stroke Association. Stroke 34, 2310–2322.

American College of Sports Medicine (ACSM), 2010. Guidelines for exercise testing and prescription, eighth ed. Lippincott Williams & Wilkins, Philadelphia, PA.

Best, C.S., van Wijck, F., Dennis, J., et al., 2010. Models of service delivery for exercise after stroke. Cerebrovasc. Dis 29 (S2).

Boysen, G., Krarup, N.H., Zeng, X., et al., 2009. ExStroke Pilot Trial of the effect of repeated instructions to improve physical activity after ischaemic stroke: a multinational randomised controlled clinical trial. BMJ 339, b2810.

Carin-Levy, G., Kendall, M., Young, A., et al., 2009. The psychosocial effects of exercise and relaxation classes for persons surviving a stroke. Can. J. Occup. Ther. 76, 73–76.

Damush, T.M., Plue, N., Bakas, T., et al., 2007. Barriers and facilitators to exercise among stroke survivors. Rehabil. Nurs. 32, 253–260.

Department of Health, 2001. Exercise referral systems: A national quality assurance framework. Department of Health, London. Available online at: http://www.dh.gov.uk/prod_consum_dh/groups/dh_digitalassets/@dh/@en/documents/digitalasset/dh_4079009.pdf.

Dinan, S., 2001. Delivering an exercise prescription for vulnerable older patients. In: Young, A., Harries, M. (Eds.), Physical activity for patients: an exercise prescription. Royal College of Physicians, London, pp. 53–70.

English, C., Hillier, S.N., 2010. Circuit class therapy for improving mobility after stroke. Cochrane Database Syst. Rev. 7, CD007513. doi:10.1002/14651858.

English, C.K., Hillier, S.N., Stiller, K.R., et al., 2007. Circuit class therapy versus individual physiotherapy sessions during inpatient stroke rehabilitation:

a controlled trial. Arch. Phys. Med. Rehabil. 88, 955–963.

Gordon, N.F., Gulanick, M., Costa, F., et al., 2004. Physical activity and exercise recommendations for stroke survivors: an American Heart Association scientific statement from the Council on Clinical Cardiology, Subcommittee on Exercise, Cardiac Rehabilitation, and Prevention; the Council on Cardiovascular Nursing; the Council on Nutrition, Physical Activity, and Metabolism; and the Stroke Council. Circulation 109, 2031–2041.

Ivey, F.M., Ryan, S.A., Hafer-Macko, C.E., Macko, R.F., 2011. Stroke. In: Saxton, J.M. (Ed.), Exercise and chronic disease. An evidence-based approach. Routledge, London, pp. 56–91.

Mead, G., Greig, C.A., Cunningham, I., et al., 2007. STroke: A Randomised Trial of Exercise or Relaxation (STARTER). J. Am. Geriatr. Soc. 55, 892–899.

Mead, G.E., 2009. Exercise after stroke. BMJ 339, b2795.

Moore, J.N., Roth, E.J., Killian, C., et al., 2010. Locomotor training improves daily stepping activity and gait efficiency in individuals poststroke who have reached a 'plateau' in recovery. Stroke 41, 129–135.

Rand, D., Eng, J.J., Tang, P.F., et al., 2009. How active are people with stroke? Use of accelerometers to assess physical activity. Stroke 40, 163–168.

Reed, M., Harrington, R., Duggan, A., et al., 2010. Meeting stroke survivors' perceived needs: a qualitative study of a community-based exercise and education scheme. Clin. Rehabil. 24, 16–25.

Roth, E.J., 1993. Heart disease in patients with stroke: incidence, impact, and implications for rehabilitation. Part 1: Classification and prevalence. Arch. Phys. Med. Rehabil. 74, 752–760.

Scottish Intercollegiate Guidelines Network, 2002. Guideline 57: Cardiac rehabilitation. SIGN, Edinburgh.

Skelton, D.A., Dinan, S., Campbell, M.G., et al., 2005. Tailored group exercise (Falls Management Exercise) reduces falls in community dwelling older frequent fallers (an RCT). Age Ageing 34, 636–639.

van de Port, I.G.N., Wevers, N., Roelse, H., et al., 2009. Cost-effectiveness of a structured progressive task-oriented circuit class training programme to enhance walking competency after stroke: the protocol of the FIT-Stroke trial. BMC Neurol. 9, 43 doi:10.1186/1471-2377-9-43.

Wevers, N., van De Port, I., Vermue, M., et al., 2009. Effects of task-oriented circuit class training on walking competency after stroke: a systematic review. Stroke 40, 2450–2459.

Young, A., Dinan, S., 2005. Active in later life. BMJ 330, 189–191.

Zipes, D.P., Wellens, H.J.J., 1998. Sudden cardiac death. Circulation 98, 2334–2351.

Designing and delivering an exercise and fitness training programme for stroke survivors

10

John M.A. Dennis • Sara Wicebloom-Paul •
Bex Townley • Susie Dinan-Young

CHAPTER CONTENTS

INTRODUCTION

Stroke survivors can benefit from improved physical fitness, function and quality of life through appropriate design and delivery of exercise and fitness training.

The design of evidence-based, safe and effective exercise programmes for stroke survivors requires a specialised skill set, informed by ongoing professional development in stroke and its treatment, as well as the rapidly developing evidence base and best practice guidance on stroke and exercise.

There is a distinct difference between providing routine 'aerobic fitness' programmes for people without a significant disability, and exercise and fitness training programmes for stroke survivors. Firstly, the exercise programme must be *adapted* for stroke in general (e.g. longer warm up and cool down, the integration of seated endurance exercises in between walking training sections). Secondly, the variables of the exercise training programme (i.e. the frequency, intensity, duration and exercise technique) must be *tailored*, or specifically adjusted, to the needs of each individual stroke survivor, taking any co-morbidities into consideration.

Designing exercise and fitness training for stroke survivors must take into account the rehabilitation and functional training approaches applied by physiotherapists (and other therapists) in the field of stroke rehabilitation. Through therapy-based adaptation and tailoring strategies, exercise professionals are able to provide programmes that (i) accommodate individuals with often complex pathology and functional challenges, (ii) reduce risks, (iii) maintain and progress (wherever possible) any functional and fitness gains made in the therapy setting and (iv) facilitate long-term self-management of physical activity.

The aim of this chapter is to outline the fundamental principles involved in the design of safe and effective exercise and fitness training programmes for stroke survivors and to explore the special considerations that must be taken into account. A key theme is the adaptation and tailoring of exercise programmes to suit the individual with stroke, while achieving the broad aims of improving physical fitness and functional activity levels.

The approach presented here is based on a combination of evidence, including the STARTER trial (Mead et al. 2007), the Cochrane systematic review discussed in chapter 5 (Brazzelli et al. 2011, Saunders et al. 2004, 2009), best practice from the fields of exercise and physiotherapy, as well as published recommendations drawn from national documents including the Best Practice Guidelines for community-based Exercise after Stroke services (Best et al. 2010).

RISK ASSESSMENT AND MANAGEMENT

Safety first

'Safety first' has to be the starting point when designing a progressive exercise programme for stroke survivors (Dinan and Dennis 2010). This is due to the complex, multiple and often variable difficulties that stroke survivors may experience, and to the inherent underlying cardiac risk present in a significant portion of the stroke population, as highlighted in chapter 9. Assessing risks and adjusting exercise to the individual takes into consideration individual factors (including clinical, physiological, psychological and age-related), exercise-related and environmental factors that may increase the risk of an injury or adverse event during exercise. Risk assessment, stratification and management are crucial for safe, effective session design and for the progression of exercise.

Prior to commencing an exercise programme

Chapter 9 detailed the risk assessment procedures that need to be completed for stroke survivors prior to their enrolment in an exercise programme. A risk management plan should have been agreed with the referring health professional in advance for predictable adverse events that might occur in an exercise session. This plan needs to take into account any medical problems. For example, in stroke survivors with diabetes, agreement needs to be reached about the dose of insulin prior to exercise and the management of hypoglycaemia in response to exercise.

Exercise professionals need to be aware that stroke survivors may take medication, not only for secondary stroke prevention but also for co-morbidities (chapter 3). They need to know the effects and potential adverse effects of all these medications on the stroke survivor's ability to exercise safely (chapter 9). Detailed information about drugs and their side effects can be found in the British National Formulary.

This chapter starts from the point where these full risk assessment procedures have been completed by both the referring health-care professional and the exercise professional, and the responsibility for the design and delivery of the exercise programme as well as the monitoring of the individual's response to the exercise has been passed to the exercise professional.

Prior to each session

Prior to each session, the exercise professional needs to assess the risks associated with the individual stroke survivor, the exercise programme, as well as the equipment and the facility, to ensure compliance with local regulations. Each element of the risk assessment described in chapter 9, to be undertaken before a stroke survivor starts an exercise programme, also needs to be checked before each exercise session. The nature of the post-stroke fluctuations in health and functional capacity and the likelihood of 'off' days (e.g. due to fatigue, poor motivation, depression) make it necessary for the exercise professional to check on and gather information from individual stroke survivors prior to each session. The exercise professional needs to ask each individual whether there has been any change in their medical condition, or anything else that has happened since the previous session that might impact on their safety. Resting heart rate is often taken and blood pressure as required, depending on local protocol. If the stroke survivor enters a session feeling unwell, or with new symptoms that might impact on their safety, the exercise professional must recommend that the stroke survivor does not exercise, but seeks medical advice prior to resuming exercise. This should only occur once the individual has been given permission by their general practitioner (GP).

Ongoing monitoring of participants

Exercise professionals should continually monitor performance and anticipate having to tailor exercises for individual stroke survivors. They should ensure that stroke survivors initiate each exercise safely. For example, a carefully staged approach is required for a stroke survivor with hemiplegia when mounting an exercise bike (Fig. 10.1). Exercise professionals should also monitor the stroke survivor's response (including tone) to strengthening/endurance exercises, whether the stroke survivor is undertaking exercises and performing movement patterns safely and effectively.

Exercise professionals must be able to recognise the signs and symptoms that require stroke survivors to be signposted back to their GP or other appropriate health professional. Chapter 3 covered the common co-morbidities that the exercise professional needs to be aware of and the possible approaches to their emergency management; additional recommendations on emergency situations are provided below.

Any deterioration in the stroke survivor's functional and/or medical status, including deterioration in performance beyond reasonable expectation, aggravation or worsening of an existing condition or identification of new symptoms or signs, should instigate a discussion with, and referral back to the referring health-care professional for further assessment before continuing with their exercise programme. If a stroke survivor becomes unwell during a session with symptoms such as dizziness, chest pain or excessive breathlessness, the exercise must be terminated and first aid administered if necessary. One should consider the possibility of a further stroke, cardiac event, infection or other condition. A further stroke or transient ischaemic attack would normally manifest itself with a sudden deterioration in neurological symptoms, e.g. sudden worsening of pre-existing weakness of a limb, or new neurological symptoms if the stroke affects a different part of the brain. In this case, emergency procedures need to be followed (see below).

Participants should have their risks re-assessed regularly, e.g. midway and at the end of the programme, alongside their goals and other reviews. These reviews need to be undertaken on an individual basis; for some it will involve asking questions about perceived changes in performance, for others it may include more formal assessment.

Check-up at the end of each session

At the end of each session, the exercise professional should check how the stroke survivor is feeling. If there is undue fatigue, or muscle ache that might be a direct result of exercise, this should be taken into account at the

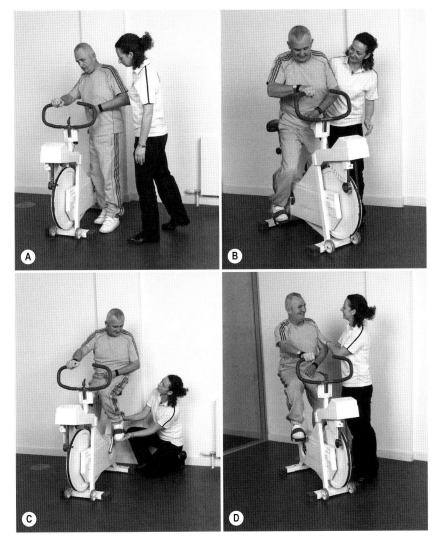

FIG 10.1 (A) Mounting cycle: note approach from non-affected side. (B) Mounting cycle: note non-affected foot on pedal. (C) Mounting cycle: note assisting affected foot onto pedal. (D) Mounting cycle: final position.

next session, e.g. the exercise professional may decide not to progress the exercise, or may reduce the intensity or number of repetitions.

EMERGENCY PROCEDURES

Acute medical problems may occur in any person at any time, irrespective of whether they are exercising or not, and unrelated to the stroke or their co-morbidities. Should an acute medical event (medical emergency) arise, by UK law the exercise professional should defer to the duty first-aider in the building. The duty first-aider must either call for an emergency ambulance or advise the stroke survivor to seek advice from their

173

GP before returning to the session with the GP's permission to continue with exercise. A Health and Safety Executive approved accident/incident report form must be completed by the duty first-aider with details of the incident and all advice/actions taken. Full guidance on the procedures required by law can be found within the Health and Safety (First-Aid) Regulations (1981). Exercise professionals working in other countries should follow the national and local health and safety regulations for that country.

Each exercise location will have its own operational policy for management of emergencies – including medical and other emergencies, e.g. fire. Exercise professionals should familiarise themselves with the legal framework for emergency procedures in their place of work before commencing at that location. All health, safety and emergency requirements must be conscientiously and regularly checked and all required procedures must be followed. All first aid equipment and emergency links must be operational, e.g. an on-site telephone and a designated staff member should be available for the duration of the session and, ideally, to assist with access to and from the session. In addition to the emergency plan, Box 10.1 provides other examples of the requirements that should be in place. These may vary across different services and countries, but in the authors' opinion these are the minimum requirements. Box 10.2 lists emergency procedures for Exercise after Stroke services, which may vary in different countries.

BOX 10.1 Health and safety requirements for exercise and fitness training after stroke services

- All staff should have first aid training in order to assess and manage incidents
- All staff must be trained appropriately in cardiopulmonary resuscitation
- All staff should be trained in manual handling to be able to assist if a fall has taken place. Also, if specialist lifting equipment is available, all staff should be familiar with its use
- There should be an alarm/immediate phone access in the facility to summon additional help
- An emergency plan should be in place

BOX 10.2 Emergency procedures for Exercise after Stroke Services

- Contact the emergency services and apply usual first aid and resuscitation as required
- If new symptoms of stroke/cardiac condition arise, contact the emergency services
- Return to exercise is not permitted until the general practitioner/other appropriate health professional has reviewed the case and acknowledges the appropriateness of resuming exercise

It is essential that the exercise professional integrates achievable health and functional aims within the goals of each individual. The stroke survivor's goals should be discussed with them prior to planning the exercise programme and integrated wherever possible – so long as they do not compromise safety.

Other reasons to engage the stroke survivor in the exercise programming process are to promote a sense of ownership of the programme, enhance self-efficacy, self-management and adherence to exercise in the longer term, as described in chapter 6. Each exercise session should incorporate each of the programme aims listed below, and one or more of the stroke survivor's own goals. One way to do this is by ensuring that the fitness progressions are clearly working towards both programme and personal goals.

The primary aim of each exercise session should be:

- To improve all components of physical fitness (see below), with priority given to cardiovascular endurance, functional muscle strength and endurance in order to achieve optimum health and functional gain, while promoting psychosocial wellbeing.

Secondary session aims should include the following:

- To improve the performance of specific everyday functional activities of daily living (ADLs) and instrumental activities of daily living (IADL) with an emphasis on normalising posture, movement and function.
- To promote achievement of the stroke survivor's specific short- and long-term personal goals as well as more general health and functional outcomes.
- To enhance self-efficacy and self-management in relation to physical activity.

IMPROVING COMPONENTS OF FITNESS

In general, health-related exercise programmes should aim to include the following components of physical fitness (ACSM 2010):

- Cardiovascular endurance
- Muscular strength
- Muscular endurance
- Flexibility
- Body composition
- Motor skills and coordination (i.e. agility, coordination, balance, power, reaction time and speed).

For ambulant stroke survivors, evidence indicates that the three fitness components that need to be prioritised are cardiovascular/cardiorespiratory endurance, muscle strength and muscle endurance (chapters 4 and 5). This is not to say that the other components should not feature in the programme, but rather that the cardiovascular, muscle strength and endurance components should be the focus. However, any gains in these fitness components must be able to support the ability to undertake daily functional activities. For many ambulant stroke survivors, problems with balance, coordination and limited range of movement affect their ability to undertake such activities. Thus, in the context of exercise and fitness training after stroke, cardiovascular/cardiorespiratory endurance, muscle strength and endurance all need to be trained in the context of functional activities. Exercise professionals should have a clear understanding of the rationale for each exercise in terms of how this targets the components of fitness, relates to functional activities and each individual's goals.

Whilst body composition is included as a component of physical fitness in the ACSM terminology (2010), it is not considered here as a factor in the design process, but rather as a programme outcome.

CARDIOVASCULAR ENDURANCE

As discussed in chapter 4, cardiorespiratory fitness (or 'aerobic fitness') is the central capacity of the circulatory and respiratory systems to supply oxygen, together with the peripheral capacity of skeletal muscle to utilise oxygen. Any rhythmic, aerobic, continuous activity involving the large muscle groups that is maintained for a prolonged period of time, increases heart rate and the return of blood to the heart, can improve cardiovascular fitness.

Stroke survivors are known to have generally lower levels of cardiovascular fitness compared to healthy age-matched controls, which impacts on health and everyday life (Saunders et al. 2009; chapter 4). This considerable shortfall in fitness needs to be addressed by appropriate strength and endurance training.

The design of the cardiovascular training component must therefore include exercises that use the large muscle groups, as these create the main demand for increased cardiac activity. Only if an individual has no use of large muscle groups at all (e.g. due to paralysis) is it possible to gain a minimal improvement in aerobic fitness by using muscles not usually deemed important in this type of training. In addition, given the specificity of training principle (see below), if the exercise programme aims to improve functional daily activities, it needs to simulate those same activities.

Cardiovascular fitness after stroke can be improved through exercise programmes that include walking (Brazzelli et al. 2011, Saunders et al. 2009). The authors suggested that other modalities should also be considered, depending on the individual's functional capacity and goals. As stroke survivors make certain physical fitness and functional gains, a wider range of exercise opportunities may be appropriate, e.g. walking, cycling, swimming (Figs 10.2 and 10.3).

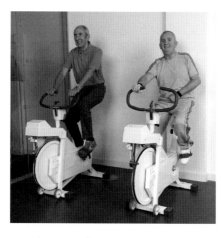

FIG 10.2 Cardiorespiratory endurance: cycling.

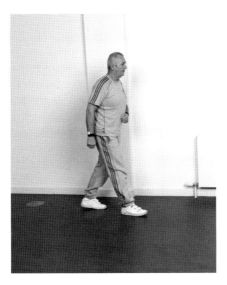

FIG 10.3 Cardiorespiratory endurance: walking.

A key consideration when designing a programme for cardiovascular fitness is to address balance and coordination impairments. This can be achieved by including some dynamic endurance activities (e.g. side stepping, knee-to-hand) and by selecting exercise modalities that enhance safety. Box 10.3 provides an example of how a cardiovascular endurance exercise can be tailored for an individual stroke survivor with balance difficulties and muscle weakness.

BOX 10.3 Example of tailoring a cardiovascular endurance exercise for an individual stroke survivor

A 'step-up' exercise (Figs 10.23 and 10.24) is a good example of an aerobic exercise; however, eliciting a cardiovascular response on this exercise may be hampered by poor dynamic balance coupled with muscle weakness. In this case, the exercise professional should consider offering more support or an alternative targeted exercise that requires less balance (e.g. forward/backwards weight transfer with upper limb support for balance on a level floor), which may enable a more fluid and rhythmical movement pattern.

If the stroke survivor is demonstrating asymmetry of trunk posture (e.g. shortening on one side of their trunk while completing a more strenuous exercise like the step-up), then balance is more likely to be at risk due to a lateral shift in their centre of gravity. This can be counteracted by prompting the stroke survivor to correct their posture, by adding a tailored corrective side stretch prior to and at the end of the exercise (Fig. 10.7), or by altering it to a bilateral exercise, such as sit to stand or squat with their back supported against the wall.

MUSCULAR STRENGTH, POWER AND ENDURANCE

Muscle strength is the maximum force or torque that can be generated by a specific muscle or muscle group (chapter 4). The higher the resistance during a strength exercise, the lower the number of repetitions achievable. Health-related weight training typically features 6–12 repetitions, competitive weight lifting features 2–5 repetitions until a maximal contraction is required, which is progressed to just one repetition for Olympic weight lifting. Chapter 4 explained the correlations between levels of muscular strength and the ability to undertake everyday activities (Kraemer and French 2005, Saunders et al. 2008). For example, hip flexor and knee flexor/extensor strength of the affected leg are key factors in walking performance and in negotiating stairs (Flansbjer et al. 2006, Le Brasseur et al. 2006).

Applying the exercise science concepts underpinning health-related weight training to exercise after stroke requires additional knowledge and skills to ensure the approach takes account of any possible muscle tone abnormalities and underlying cardiac pathology. It should also be consistent with the principles of skill acquisition and strengthening used in exercise and therapy settings, e.g. training should ideally match everyday functional activities to enhance functional gain (Skelton et al. 1994, 1995, Skelton and McLaughlin 1996). This is because strength training, like any form of training, is highly specific. An example is a bench press (lying down), which does not functionally match pushing a heavy door open with one arm (standing). Box 10.4 and Figures 10.4 and 10.5 provide other examples of how a muscular strength exercise could be tailored to an individual stroke survivor.

When designing the strength element of a training programme for stroke, the focus is on improving performance of functional movement patterns and activities involving both sides of the body. These training activities, therefore, need to reflect the specific movement patterns, including movement speed and postural changes, of actual functional activities. An exercise such as the 'pole raise', which reflects taking an object from a low to a higher level (e.g. a table to a shelf) and vice versa while encouraging postural symmetry, is an example of a useful exercise for training this functional task (Fig. 10.5).

BOX 10.4 Example of tailoring a muscular strength exercise for an individual stroke survivor

In the STARTER trial (Mead et al. 2007), an upper limb strengthening exercise might be the standing 'ball raise'. This exercise is designed to improve lifting capacity and core stability while maintaining an active base of support.

A stroke survivor with increased upper limb tone may need to alter their hand position on the ball to accommodate their lack of supination (i.e. bringing their palm upwards) or use a smaller ball (Fig. 10.26).

For a stroke survivor with balance impairments, the ball raise exercise may need to be undertaken with a smaller ball and/or in a seated position.

Meanwhile, the key aim of utilising large upper limb muscle groups (e.g. shoulder flexors and triceps) remains intact which, as part of an 'active rest' cycle within the cardiac based circuit, is important as heart rate is not allowed to fall significantly.

Alternatively, as part of the strengthening section of the exercise session, an elasticated resistance band can be used to strengthen upper limbs in a similar pattern.

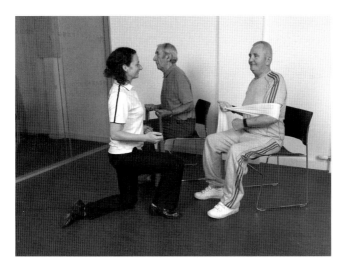

FIG 10.4 Exercises requiring grip must be tailored to prevent increased tone, e.g. 'upper-back strengthener'.

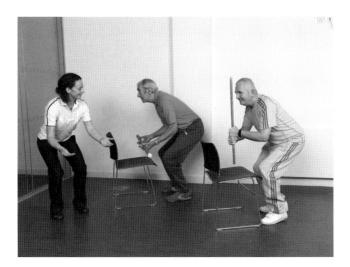

FIG 10.5 'Pole raise' strengthening exercise with tailored option.

For stroke survivors, improving weakness and reduced function in their affected arm often features on their list of goals, particularly if this is related to activities such as holding a dog lead, carrying shopping or getting dressed. The potential for improvements in arm function varies, and depends on the initial level of impairment (Nakayama et al. 1994), type of stroke, time since stroke and rehabilitation received. As chapter 5 has shown, evidence indicates that strength gains are achievable, even in affected limbs – as long as there is no paralysis (Duncan et al. 2003).

A key consideration for stroke survivors must be to limit any adverse increases in muscle tone through inappropriate application of force. For example, forcing the execution of a stretching exercise or using a weight in the hand of the affected side in a severely affected upper limb to increase range of movement in that limb is contraindicated due to the risk of permanent joint damage. The shoulder is particularly at risk of injury after stroke, as the shoulder joint may sublux (dislocate) when any muscle weakness or muscle imbalance is present, which can have long-lasting pain and functional deficits as a result (chapter 3). Any significant manual stretching should only be administered under direct guidance/supervision of a suitably qualified health professional. It is reasonable, however, for the stroke survivor to actively self-stretch tight or 'tonal' muscle groups, either by using their intrinsic opposition muscle groups of that limb, or by using active assisted exercises (e.g. clasping hands and gently stretching forward to achieve biceps/brachialis lengthening; Fig. 10.6). In active self-stretching, the stroke survivor is in control of their own movement within a pain-free range, and the exercise professional should monitor closely that this remains within an agreed range of movement, pre-determined by information from the referring health-care professional.

Maximal or near maximal muscular contractions, such as those required to lift extremely heavy weights, are *not recommended*, as they often lead to a stroke survivor altering their posture inappropriately to complete the action, regardless of the loss of correct form. This can lead to poor posture and an increase in abnormal tone which can affect subsequent function and increase the risk of injury (e.g. a fall, back or joint injury). Maximal effort against high resistance is also associated with a decreased venous return and an elevation in arterial blood pressure. These adverse effects can be exacerbated if the resistance exercises are incorrectly performed, such as by holding the breath during the movement, causing an acute increase in blood pressure due to the physiological mechanism known as the Valsalva manoeuvre (Brooks 1997). Therefore, whilst carefully prescribed, cautiously progressed and closely monitored weight training has been shown to be beneficial in restoring function after stroke, heavy and intense weight training is contraindicated.

Once sufficient baseline strength and postural stability is achieved, the stroke survivor is likely to feel more confident to try out new exercises. However, the fundamental recommendations and cautions mentioned previously remain, and the exercise professional should continue to monitor and provide guidance on the selection and performance of appropriate strength exercises.

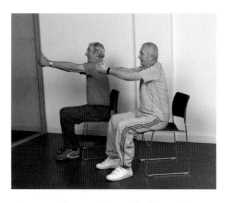

FIG 10.6 Active self-stretching: seated arm and upper back stretch.

Muscular power output is defined as the greatest rate of work achieved during a single, fast, resisted contraction (chapter 4). It is the ability to combine the fitness components of strength and speed to produce a movement under load at a given speed. Getting activities done faster is usually not a priority for stroke survivors, but improving function often is. Chapter 4 explained the relationship between muscle power and function, e.g. knee extensor power, particularly on the affected side, is the most important factor predicting comfortable walking speed and stair climbing (Le Brasseur et al. 2006).

Finally, with regards to training muscle endurance after stroke, the exercise professional should focus on improving efficiency of movement so that a particular function may be achieved with less energy expenditure. 'Normalising movement' is the remit and concern of the physiotherapist, but the exercise professional's priority is to ensure that repetitive movement is sustainable without increasing compensatory patterns or hypertonia. In fact, repetition of pain-free movement may help to increase range of movement by reducing soft tissue thixotropy. Where there is hypertonia (chapter 3), repetition of pain-free movement should be encouraged whenever possible (Axelson 2005, Lakie and Robson 1988, Vattanslip et al. 2000).

FLEXIBILITY

Flexibility is the ability to move a given joint through its range of movement. A joint that lacks full range of movement is more prone to injury and can create limitations in daily functioning, such as dressing and walking or reaching to shelves. A joint that is too flexible may be unstable and therefore also prone to injury, particularly to the soft tissue surrounding the joint, e.g. the shoulder (chapter 3).

While there is some variation in the views about the relevance of stretch exercises in the warm up for general populations, expert consensus in all clinical populations recommends that warm up stretching (i.e. short, not developed and performed at the end of the warm up) is essential for those who have had a stroke. Although there is a lack of research, experience suggests that it appears to help stroke survivors to familiarise themselves with their current range of movement (remembering that this may vary considerably between sessions) and to prepare for physical activity (Fig. 10.7).

Stretching activities should be performed only once the muscles are warm, due to the improved viscosity within the joint capsule and pliability (thixotropy) of the muscle tissue (Lakie and Robson 1988). A key consideration when providing a warm up for stroke survivors is that paresis, increased tone (hypertonia) and lower levels of physical activity all reduce intramuscular blood flow. This means that cardiac demand is reduced, and increasing intramuscular blood flow will take longer than normal. Following exercise, blood flow from vasodilatation, increased heart rate and muscle pumping activity, combined with increased muscle pliability and temperature, are likely to increase.

Improving functional flexibility (i.e. the flexibility required for the execution of functional tasks/ADLs) is the aim, which is best achieved with structured, controlled movements through full available pain-free range that mimic functional tasks (e.g. reaching to dry your back). Controlled, active range of movement exercises are advised during the warm up. In the cool down, longer,

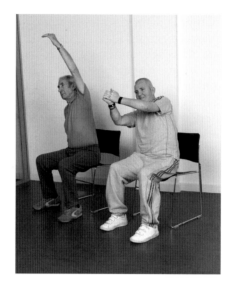

FIG 10.7 Seated side stretch.

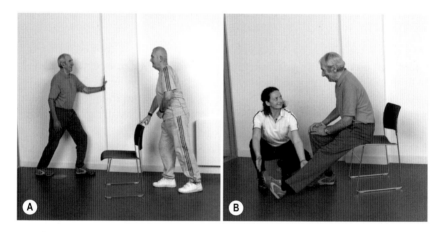

FIG 10.8 Calf stretch performed (A) standing and (B) seated.

supported, 'developmental' stretches held at full range are used to develop flexibility, ideally performed 2–3 times consecutively, when soft tissue is at its warmest and most pliable (Fig. 10.8). Evidence underpinning stretching in neurological rehabilitation is patchy, however. A Cochrane systematic review showed no clinically relevant effects of stretching on joint mobility in people with neurological conditions (including stroke) who already had, or were at risk of developing, contractures (Katalinic et al. 2010).

MOTOR SKILLS AND COORDINATION

Motor skills and coordination relate to the ability to recruit muscle activity effectively and to time movements correctly, in terms of both speed and sequence, to complete a functional task (e.g. reach and grasp an object). Most people are probably familiar with the following two common coordination tests: (i) pointing your finger towards a point in space (usually the tester's finger) and then to your nose with eyes open and then closed, and (ii) walking heel to toe on a line with eyes open then with eyes closed. Both of these tasks require appropriately timed neuromuscular recruitment of the right intensity to produce a smooth and appropriately paced movement with the required accuracy.

Motor skills can be divided into two groups: gross and fine. Gross motor skill, involving larger body movements, is required for balance, including the maintenance of both static posture (e.g. sitting or standing) and dynamic posture (e.g. maintenance of the body in an upright orientation while walking), as well as for the multitasking inherent in daily life (e.g. walking and carrying an object). Fine motor skills are required for smaller actions, such as taking hold of the handlebars of a bike, writing or threading a needle.

Each functional movement can be broken down into several components in order to produce a successful end result. For example, when reaching out to grasp an object such as the handle of an exercise bike, the arm and hand accelerate away from the body but then decelerate at the appropriate time to allow the fingers to open before contact with the object is made. This precise sequence of reach-to-grasp action is often affected by stroke (van Vliet and Sheridan 2007), which can lead to colliding, missing or dropping objects.

IMPROVING PERFORMANCE OF DAILY ACTIVITIES

As mentioned before, exercise programmes should include exercises and activities that directly reflect everyday tasks, while emphasising the development of balance, appropriate limb and trunk alignment and movement sequencing that is as normal as possible. Dynamic balance allows the centre of gravity whilst in motion to remain within the individual's base of support, thus preventing loss of balance.

It is important for the exercise professional to closely observe the correct control of postural alignment, especially when exercises are aimed at symmetrical or alternating movement phases (Fig. 10.9). Asymmetry of posture in this type of exercise is often a clear sign of overworking (or straining) muscles. Overworking to complete an exercise that is too difficult or unsuitable for an individual may cause increased tone, a shift in centre of gravity and thereby

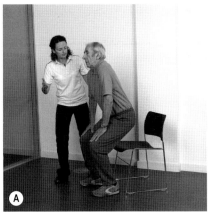
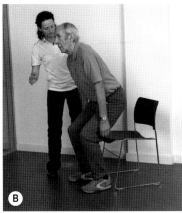

FIG 10.9 (A) Incorrect posture during sit-to-stand. Compare with the correct posture (B) during this task.

reduce the efficiency of movement. This may result in a rigid posture, which makes it more difficult for an individual to adapt to a sudden perturbation (e.g. having to avoid an obstacle), thereby increasing the risk of losing balance.

PROMOTING THE ATTAINMENT OF PERSONAL GOALS

Effective personalised goal setting is crucial if exercise aims are to be achieved and if physical activity is to be maintained in the longer term (chapter 6). Current guidelines recommend that goals be SMART (i.e. specific, measurable, ambitious, relevant and time-limited), although, as explained in chapter 6, there are different interpretations of this acronym (Playford et al. 2009, Wade 2009).

Goal setting also enables progress to be checked to ensure that the exercise programme remains appropriate and relevant for the individual (Fig. 10.10). Box 10.5 gives an example of goal setting for an individual.

As explained in chapter 7, successful communication between the exercise professional and stroke survivor is crucial to ensure that both parties know, understand and work towards the stroke survivor's goals together. For each individual, the exercise professional should have a strategy that enables two-way communication in order to facilitate goal setting, explain exercises and motivate stroke survivors as effectively as possible, especially for those with

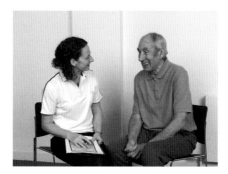

FIG 10.10 Effective individual programming and goal setting rely on good communication skills.

BOX 10.5 An example of goal setting

When setting goals with his exercise professional, Mr R indicated that he wished to walk 1 mile to and back from the leisure centre for his exercise session. However, if he does this, he will be too tired to participate fully in his session and/or in other activities with his family later in the day. Effective goal planning will help Mr R. reach this goal in small increments.

One way to do this could be by Mr R getting a lift to the centre for the first month and then gradually walking some of the way back before he is picked up, until he can manage half of the journey to and from the centre. This way, his progressions are small yet measurable, while still enabling Mr R to realise his goal to engage in physical fitness training and other activities. His progress in this 'out of session' development is important to record, as it directly impacts on his participation in his exercise sessions.

communication or cognitive difficulties. Much of the information on communication support needs should be gleaned from the referral documentation. However, if this is not available, the stroke survivor's speech and language therapist or family may be able to assist in the development of a strategy for enhancing communication with each individual.

ENHANCING SELF-EFFICACY AND SELF-MANAGEMENT OF PHYSICAL ACTIVITY

Stroke survivors in early stages of rehabilitation may have difficulty in decision making, goal setting and self-management. This may be for a variety of reasons, including a lack of knowledge about stroke and difficulty predicting recovery, lack of familiarity with the goal setting process, cognitive, communication and executive difficulties, as well as depression and grief reactions (Laver et al. 2010, Leach et al. 2009; see chapter 6). When designing an exercise programme, it is important to be aware that motivation and the ability of the stroke survivor to determine their own activity levels and select their own pace are likely to enhance their outcomes. A well-designed programme can create opportunities for self-management, including self-monitoring, by providing individualised goal setting, a personal exercise plan and an individualised exercise programme with a record that provides feedback. Integrating these elements into the programme opens the door to a more physically active, healthy lifestyle outside of any formal exercise sessions.

PERSONAL EXERCISE PLAN

The majority of clinical trials on exercise after stroke provided exercise training three times a week. Where this is not possible in a service setting, other ways of increasing weekly activity levels should be explored. The exercise programme might, therefore, be part of a personal exercise plan that includes appropriate physical activity choices outside the Exercise after Stroke sessions.

INDIVIDUALISED EXERCISE PROGRAMME WITH PERSONAL RECORD

In the UK, each stroke survivor will be given an individualised exercise programme, as recommended by SkillsActive in their relevant National Occupational Standard (2010a,b). This will be formulated with reference to: the referral information, the exercise professional's assessment of the stroke survivor and the stroke survivor's personal goals for exercise (Buckley 2008). This exercise programme should indicate how many repetitions the stroke survivor should aim for at each station of the circuit or of each unison exercise. These should be in pictorial as well as written form. Their current level of physical effort should be monitored (and self-monitored where possible) using, for example, the Borg Rate of Perceived Exertion Scale (Borg 1998; Fig. 10.11).

It is recommended that, on the reverse side of this, there should be a place to encourage stroke survivors to record their progress (e.g. number of repetitions, time spent training strength or resistance in unison exercises) and service-specific outcome measures as appropriate (chapter 11). This can be a

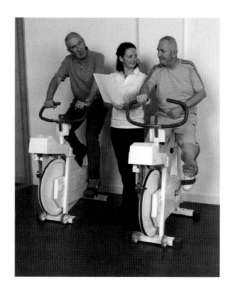

FIG 10.11 Rate of perceived exertion is one way of monitoring intensity for some participants.

useful motivational tool, as it not only reminds individuals of their (often low) starting point, but also captures their fitness improvements – even if they are small. For stroke survivors this is particularly important as other aspects of their recovery may be slow to improve. It also helps to encourage individuals to continue to work at their own pace within a group setting where there may be a tendency to compete, or draw comparison, with peers.

FUNDAMENTAL PRINCIPLES AND VARIABLES OF EXERCISE PROGRAMMING

Programming exercise to improve fitness and function after stroke must first apply the fundamental principles and variables of designing exercise training programmes (ACSM 2010, Dinan et al. 2008, Jones and Rose 2005; Box 10.6).

PRINCIPLES

Specificity

Tailoring exercises to meet individual health and functional goals is essential to a successful fitness training outcome (Wicebloom 2007). Furthermore, it is

---

BOX 10.6 The principles and variables underpinning the design of effective exercise training programmes

Principles	Variables
Specificity	F – Frequency
Progressive overload	I – Intensity
Rest and recovery	T – Time/duration
Individual difference	T – Type
	A – Approach and adherence

ACSM 2010, Dinan et al. 2008, Jones and Rose 2005.

crucial for the exercise professional to be clear that specific exercises lead to specific gains only; it is misguided to assume that any one exercise can lead to generalised benefits. Sports science and motor control research suggests that, when the aim is to improve a specific activity, the training should simulate that activity as closely as possible (Schmidt and Wrisberg 2008). For example, the aim of treadmill training in a harness that partially supports body weight in post-stroke rehabilitation is to allow patients with lower limb paresis, who are unable to walk independently, to practise gait. Using a treadmill helps to normalise the patient's gait pattern in terms of smoothness, symmetry and speed. Evidence for task-specific exercise training after stroke also comes from a Cochrane systematic review (Brazzelli et al. 2011) which showed that cardiorespiratory and mixed training interventions that included walking as an exercise mode improved walking performance. Overall, there is a considerable body of research demonstrating the effectiveness of task-specific training to improve specific motor functions after stroke (French et al. 2007, Langhorne et al. 2009).

This body of evidence means that each exercise within the programme should have a clear purpose, linked to the programme aims and goals for each individual.

Progressive overload

Exercise professionals working with stroke survivors should operate safely and effectively, steadily and cautiously. Therefore, progression is best achieved through small, gradual increases in each component of fitness (e.g. every 2–4 weeks). Programmes should be of a duration that is long enough to allow incremental progressions to ensure that the optimal fitness and functional outcomes can be achieved without causing adverse effects. Although the optimum duration still needs to be established empirically, the current recommendation for best practice is that exercise and fitness training programmes for stroke survivors should be of at least of 12 weeks' duration (Gordon et al. 2004).

Managing progressive overload with stroke survivors presents additional challenges due to the many variations in disability that people may present with, and therefore more diligent, skilled monitoring by the exercise professional may be required than with some other exercise referral groups.

Adverse responses may develop if the incremental increases are not sufficiently cautious and exceed the individual's exercise tolerance. Typical adverse responses are listed in Box 10.7.

BOX 10.7 Adverse responses to excessive overload in stroke survivors

- Abnormal tonal changes (i.e. excessive muscle tension and reflex activity during movement, abnormal trunk and limb posture)
- Increased shortness of breath beyond 'walk and talk' level
- Loss of coordination (e.g. reduced postural alignment, clumsiness)
- Loss of concentration
- Increased fatigue
- Decreased exercise tolerance
- Any new symptom that causes the individual pain/distress/injury

---

Ensuring that every session is a positive experience is perhaps the most important part of the exercise planning process. The importance of achievement and enjoyment during every session cannot be over-emphasised. Gradual increases in the duration or intensity of cardiorespiratory exercises and in the repetitions or resistance of strength exercises, combined with meaningful praise and encouragement about progress can help bring this about. Exercise professionals need to be alert and respond skilfully to any changes in stroke survivors' functional or health status, whether on a weekly or even minute-by-minute basis. They must prioritise and address the needs of each individual as they present on the day, even if the programme at times may only maintain the level of function or fitness. This implies that one tailoring solution for a specific exercise on one occasion might not be an adequate solution on another occasion.

All the potential challenges that the stroke survivor may experience during exercise make it clear that, for this population, progressive overload may need to take second place to the achievement of long-term adherence to the programme, as it is this that helps to promote an active lifestyle and prevent deterioration in fitness and function.

Rest and recovery

All individuals participating in an exercise programme require adequate rest periods within each session, giving an opportunity to enhance the training stimulus, prevent overuse injuries and fatigue-related adverse events, as well as to improve performance and long-term adherence by ensuring that the overall experience remains positive. Stroke survivors may have additional requirements for rest periods. The performance of activities (especially if they are unfamiliar) may need sustained and focused attention, while abnormal movement patterns, hypertonia and poor balance require increased energy expenditure (chapter 4). These are some of the factors contributing to fatigue which, as described in chapter 3, is common after stroke.

Appropriate specific rest and recovery ratios should, therefore, be written into the programme. This will often mean that the rest periods are 'active' rest exercises (e.g. 'marching on the spot') to prevent heart-rate fall below the required training zone, while still working towards the key aim of improving cardiovascular fitness. Therefore, fatigue is likely to be a consideration for the starting point and rate of progression of exercise intensity. Frequent active rests are often required and a very low intensity to start with (e.g. no resistance in any exercise and shorter duration of the core cardio-based exercises, such as 30 seconds per exercise instead of 1–2 minutes). This means that the ratio of active rest to intended exercise will need to be significantly increased, where possible, for each exercise in a cardio circuit over the course of the programme.

Individual difference

The individual difference principle means that exercise design must be person-centred and tailored to each individual (Jones and Rose 2005). Each individual's health, lifestyle, and general disposition is unique, and each has their own preferences, interests, wishes, goals and resources (Wicebloom 2007).

Individual differences are perhaps even more pronounced in relation to people with stroke, as no two stroke survivors present in exactly the same way, due to the complex mix of medical, physiological, pharmacological, functional, fitness, communication, psychosocial, emotional and attitudinal differences, and different expectations and aspirations. Tailoring to individual needs is a central theme in exercise and fitness after stroke and *the* most important skill that exercise professionals must achieve and continue to develop (Dinan et al. 2008). The key to achieving this is by thorough pre-exercise assessment and risk stratification, referral documentation about the individual and goal planning by the exercise professional (Mead et al. 2010). As highlighted in chapter 7, the exercise professional will need to draw on wide-ranging communication skills to understand the unique needs of each individual.

VARIABLES

Table 10.1 provides an explanation of each of the fitness programming variables and demonstrates how the skilful manipulation of each of these enables the professional to apply the principles of training to adapting the programme to stroke survivors (as opposed to low-risk general populations). Examples are longer, more progressive warm up periods and longer rests between activities, with greater emphasis on functional strength and endurance training. The following strategies are recommended to tailor the stroke-adapted STARTER Exercise after Stroke programme according to the specific needs and considerations of individuals (Mead et al. 2007).

Table 10.1 *Programming recommendations: training principles and variables adapted for Exercise after Stroke*

Programme variable	Meaning	Details of recommendations
Frequency	The number of times that the programme is performed, usually per week, but could be per day or per month	Three times per week (or less, but with alternative home programme or activity programme support)
Intensity	The number of repetitions, amount of resistance, rate/speed, range of movement applied to each activity, and also the rest periods between activities	Moderate up to maximum of 70% age-predicted maximum heart rate or adapted Borg Scale level 3–4
Time	The duration of each exercise session and of the programme as a whole	Maximum 60 minutes with active rest incorporated as required; begin with activity and build duration before intensity
Type	The components of fitness included within each exercise session	Simpler, fewer, task-specific exercises, particularly for cardiovascular and strength gains

Continued

Designing and delivering an exercise and fitness training programme

Table 10.1 Programming recommendations: training principles and variables adapted for Exercise after Stroke—cont'd		
Programme variable	**Meaning**	**Details of recommendations**
Approach/adherence	Approach taken to engage each individual to habitually comply with (adhere to) *their* exercise programme in the longer term	Individually tailored exercises to match each individual's goals, impairments and functional status. Adapted motivational strategies and content, as well as exercise location options
Duration of programme	Length of time of exercise programme	A minimum of 12 weeks, but preferably open ended
Content	The type of exercise in each session	Consists of a warm up, endurance exercises, resistance exercises, functional exercises and then a cool down
Progression	The rate of change to render the exercises more challenging	Regular review on an individual basis, e.g. fortnightly/monthly and matched to personal goals and rate of progress
Social interaction	Any opportunity for individuals to benefit from interaction with the exercise professional(s) and/or peers	Create the opportunity for social interaction between the stroke survivors Make the exercise experience fun and rewarding and create a relaxed after-exercise environment (e.g. tea)
Measures	Recordings to show each stroke survivor that they are maintaining or improving activities and/or outcomes	Outcome measures should be documented and included in assessment and feedback of session progress and completion, e.g. goal attainment, Timed up-and-Go (TUAG) and 10-metre walk time (chapter 11)
Programme monitoring	Recordings to demonstrate the extent to which an exercise programme is achieving its aims for its service users	The programme is monitored throughout, including attendance, tolerance of progression, completion of programme, proportion of 'drop out' and outcome measures, expressed as group outcomes

Best et al. 2010, Mead et al. 2007.

After a stroke, some individuals may not be able to attend a supervised session three times per week. To assist with achieving the recommendation of three times per week, self-practice options should be considered. These include those undertaken by the stroke survivor independently, and those supervised by a non-specialist family member/friend/carer, while support from the exercise professional continues to be provided during supervised sessions. Physiotherapists may also include exercise and fitness training in their home-based programmes for stroke survivors. Although a supervised group session is often an hour in duration, self-practice exercise sessions can be as short as 10 minutes initially.

When recommending self-practice, the exercise professional needs to ensure that the stroke survivor/carer is aware of potential risks (e.g. falls) and the actions needed to minimise these, such as temporarily removing rugs and low furniture. Care should be taken in particular to promote familiarity with safe exercise technique. In addition, strategies for developing and maintaining compliance should be considered, e.g. by setting a regular day and time.

EVIDENCE-BASED SESSION CONTENT AND BEST PRACTICE RECOMMENDATIONS

This section of the chapter is based on the STARTER programme (Mead et al. 2007) – an exploratory clinical trial on exercise training for ambulatory stroke survivors, which was outlined in chapter 5. This section describes the content of this programme in more detail.

The exercise training programme in the STARTER trial was based on the best available evidence at the time when the study was designed in 2004, i.e. a Cochrane systematic review on exercise training after stroke (Saunders et al. 2004), exercise designed for vulnerable older people (Dinan 2001), to reduce falls in frailer older people (Skelton et al. 2005), and community exercise sessions designed for the UK charity 'Different Strokes'. The STARTER training programme was also based on current best practice guidance in sport and exercise science from the American College of Sports Medicine (ACSM 1995) and the UK National Health Service National Quality Assurance Framework on Exercise Referral Systems (Department of Health 2001).

This body of evidence and guidelines recommends that all exercise training should be evidence-based, commence with a gradual warm up (circulation, mobility and stretching exercises) and end with a cool down (circulation lowering and flexibility exercises).

The STARTER trial demonstrated that this exercise programme was effective, safe and feasible. As explained in chapter 5, however, on the basis of current evidence it is not yet possible to make any definitive recommendations with respect to the 'FITT' (frequency, intensity, time/duration and type of exercise) principles in the context of exercise and fitness training after stroke. Until further evidence is available, it would be reasonable to use the exercise programme developed for the STARTER trial for community-based services for ambulatory stroke survivors who have completed their usual rehabilitation. Evidence from ongoing trials is likely to evolve and is expected to inform further development of recommendations on exercise after stroke.

Table 10.2 and Figures 10.12–10.27 detail the format and content of the STARTER session. Additionally, this session includes cycling on an upright cycle for cardiorespiratory endurance (Fig. 10.2).

Table 10.2 STARTER session format and exercise content

Element	Exercise	Purpose	Equipment	Examples of stroke-specific adaptations and cautions
Warm-up 15–20 min (extended warm up to enable effective psychological and physiological preparation)	Seated march/arm marching (Figs 10.13, 10.14)	Safe and simple starter exercise using functional activity (walking), involving large muscle groups Enhances upper-body involvement in gait action and postural stability	Appropriate chair for seated exercise with legs that do not protrude laterally from seat base	Commence with legs only to aid introduction of rhythmic arm movement. Focus on posture and symmetry of movement patterns Include element of trunk rotation (often reduced or missing in post-stroke gait)
	Sit-to-stand and transition to back of chair	Sit-to-stand and exercises in standing involve more muscle groups and promote balance for more effective warm up Represents functional activity		Allow as many steps as required, with chair back used as stability aid if required Watch for chair legs protruding especially in those with lower visual field loss or lower limb coordination difficulties. Turn to side with best visual field. Remain 'active' at rest
	Mobility exercises for main joints, e.g. shoulder (Fig. 10.15), ankle, spine (incl. trunk lateral flexion and rotation)	Joint safety		Joint specific, with focus on symmetry of ROM
	Pulse raising activity; marching on spot and side stepping	Functional, large muscle group activities Increases blood flow and simulates gait Actions necessary for developing ability to alter direction and part of anti-falling reactions		Promote rhythmic, continuous activity of very gradually increasing intensity Ensure trunk remains in alignment especially where effort is required to lift legs laterally during side-stepping
	Stretches (Figs 10.6-10.8, 10.16, 10.17)	Encourages larger ranges of movement during main section of session and facilitates neuromuscular recruitment across full ROM		Ensure standing or seated balance is maintained Use non-affected limb to support affected limb
	Transition to circuit area (Fig. 10.19)	Functional activity		Staged transitions, with those requiring assistance or prompting going first and waiting in 'active rest' until those not requiring help have joined them

Cardiovascular endurance component (evidence-based priority)	Cycling (Figs 10.1, 10.2)	Most effective CV activity for many stroke survivors; uses large muscle groups Involves neuromuscular recruitment of large muscle groups through large range of movements	Upright bike	Bike design with option for low step through and adjustable length and seat height. Must have pulse/power resistance. Magnetic/air resistance better than mechanical friction as power output varies in stroke-related weakness through arc of pedal Specific plan is required to ensure safe mount/dismount procedure
Circuit format	Ball lift and lower (standing (against wall if required): lift ball with two hands; Fig. 10.26)	Functional arm activity (lifting)	FitBall/small ball	Avoid taking ball above chest height Ensure appropriate forearm and hand alignment to the ball Seated option or tailored variation for those with difficulties with balance or standing
	Shuttle walking (walk 10 metres between chairs, along wall if required; Fig. 10.18)	Functional and effective CV for many stroke survivors Directly related to walking and turning		Promote optimal gait, reduce pace if necessary Take care especially on turning. A specific direction may be necessary if visual field loss or poor balance to one side Hand rail or other stable objects may be required, placed at regular intervals
	Wall press (press-ups in standing, facing wall; Fig. 10.27)	Active rest for large lower limb muscle groups; encourages awareness of both sides of the body Emphasises work on weaker muscle groups required for stabilisation of posture and movement		Wall/floor must both be matt texture to reduce slip hazard Accommodate hands at different heights, if required Tailored alternative option for those with significant arm weakness or tonal problems and unable to position hand flat against wall
	Sit-to-stand (Figs 10.21, 10.22)	Functional large muscle group activity, repeated with more speed/power than in strengthening section to promote increased cardiac output	Chair	Rigid AFO wearers will need to place affected foot further forward to accommodate lack of ankle ROM and keep foot flat on floor during standing up and sitting down

Continued

10

Table 10.2 STARTER session format and exercise content—cont'd

Element	Exercise	Purpose	Equipment	Examples of stroke-specific adaptations and cautions
	Knee-to-hand (standing (against wall if required): bring opposite knee to hand; Fig. 10.25)	Requires balance and coordination, encourages large range of hip movement, useful for everyday life (e.g. stepping over obstacles)		Encourage upright posture Alternative exercise is required for those unable to balance on one leg and use their upper limb effectively
	Step-up (step-ups alongside wall; Fig. 10.23)	Functional activity related to stair climbing and sit to stand	Step or physio stairs	Must have variety of heights available and be able to position near wall or other upper limb support Contrasting colour surfaces with floor and wall surrounding step is recommended
	Transition to seated area	Gives active rest after standing		Staged transitions for those who need closer supervision or assistance with equipment
Strength component (evidence-based priority)	Pole raise (stand facing chair; lift pole from seat, bring towards body, and return; Fig. 10.5)	Functional lifting activity from lower to higher level and return (simulates functional activity, e.g. moving a tray from kitchen unit to table)	Wooden pole or empty weights bar/ variety of lighter alternatives	Weight must be related to ability of weaker arm to stabilise the object at a specific level during the exercise and also to maintain appropriate palm-up (supination) grip
Unison format	Triceps strengthener (seated: extend elbow, externally rotating shoulder if possible, using resistance band)	Improves postural control and strengthens triceps	Resistance band	Promote elbow extension with external shoulder rotation and 'opening of chest' posture

Upper back strengthener (seated: retract both shoulder blades while externally rotating shoulders, using resistance band; Fig. 10.4)	Improves postural control, scapular control and addresses common muscle imbalance between internal and external rotators at shoulder	Resistance band	Angle of pull should avoid internal rotation/flexion of upper limb Angle of pull must be at lower abdominal level, avoiding being in line with head/face Band should not be wrapped round limb to improve grip for limbs with reduced sensation, but loose end can be bundled into the palm to aid a weak grip
Sit-to-stand	Functional leg exercise, slower than in circuit to promote strength emphasising eccentric control required in functional activities	Chair	As above
Cool down			
Stretches as warm up	Promotes improved posture and symmetry, provides calm end to activity		Standard postures in standing, with seated options where required

Mead et al. (2007).
AFO, ankle-foot orthosis; CV, cardiovascular; ROM, range of movement.

Designing and delivering an exercise and fitness training programme

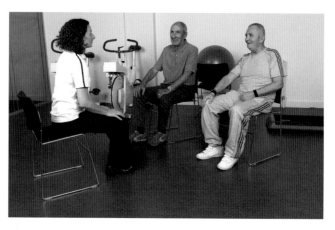

FIG 10.12 A section of the STARTER room plan (Mead et al. 2007).

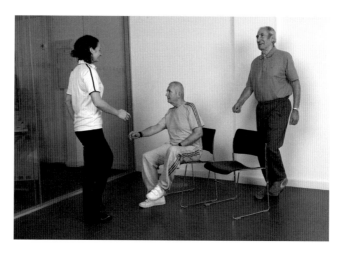

FIG 10.13 Marching on the spot with chair support.

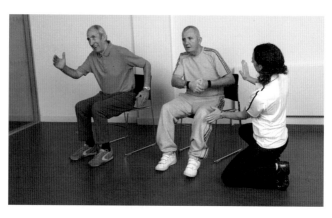

FIG 10.14 Seated arm 'marching'/'pumping' with the affected limb supported (right).

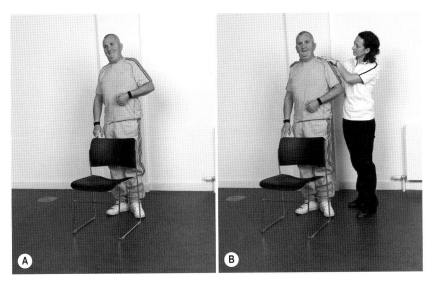

FIG 10.15 Shoulder circles before (A) and after (B) correction.

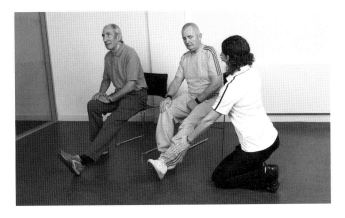

FIG 10.16 Seated hamstring stretch.

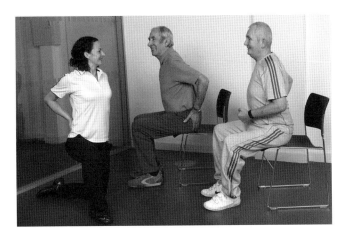

FIG 10.17 Seated chest stretch.

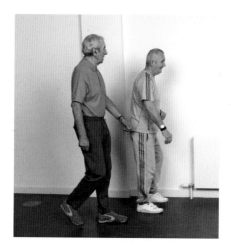

FIG 10.18 Cardiorespiratory endurance: shuttle walk using fartlek training approach.

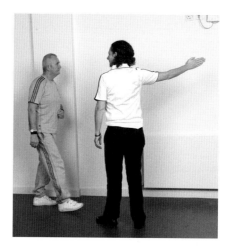

FIG 10.19 Transitions between exercises are indicated by clear visual prompts.

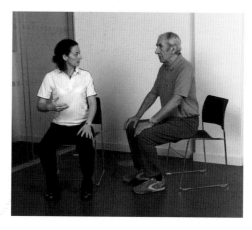

FIG 10.20 Exercises are taught in carefully considered teaching positions to convey key points.

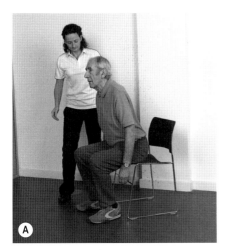

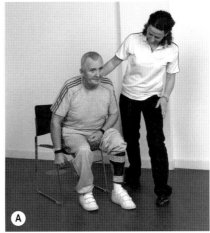

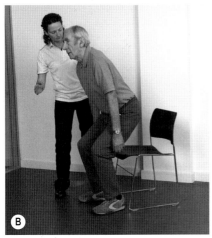

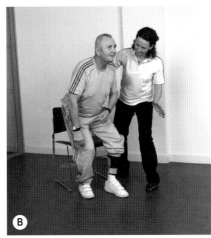

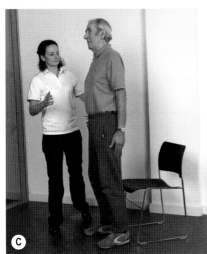

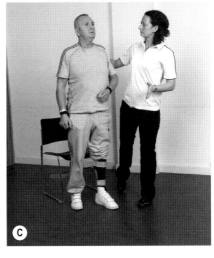

FIG 10.21 Sit to stand: (A) starting, (B) mid and (C) end position with normal stance.

FIG 10.22 Sit to stand: (A) starting, (B) mid and (C) end position with split stance. This adaptation helps to maintain foot flat position and thus improves balance.

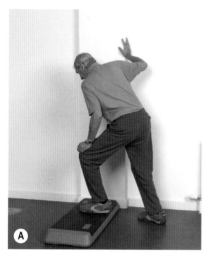
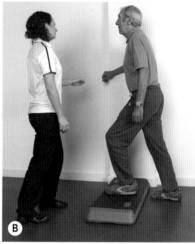

FIG 10.23 Step-up with incorrect posture (A) and correct posture (B).

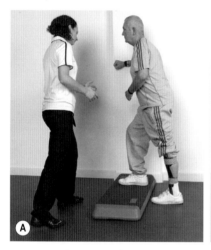
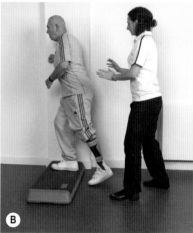

FIG 10.24 Step-up with ankle foot orthosis: stages 1 (A) and 2 (B). Note: less-affected side nearest to wall.

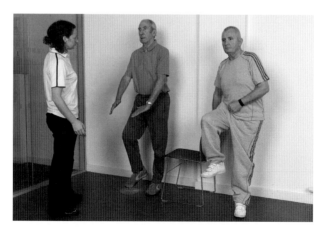

FIG 10.25 'Knee-to-hand'. Note: participants' backs close to wall.

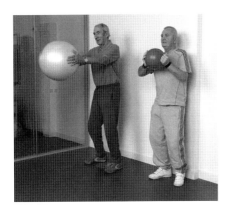

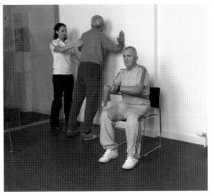

FIG 10.26 Ball lift and lower with tailored option for hand position (right).

FIG 10.27 'Wall press' exercise: correction of postural alignment (left). Note: 'triceps press' as tailored option (right).

SPECIAL CONSIDERATIONS: ADAPTING AND TAILORING EXERCISE FOR STROKE SURVIVORS

There are special considerations associated with stroke survivors that require adaptation in the exercise programme design in general, and tailoring of the specific exercises for each individual in particular, to ensure a beneficial outcome and experience for every stroke survivor. The processes of adapting and tailoring are distinct but closely linked. Skill in their application is necessary when taking account of the diverse and complex post-stroke impairments and activity limitations. This section provides information about how to develop those skills and to adapt and tailor the programme according to the evidence base and individual requirements (see Box 10.8).

BOX 10.8 Definitions of 'adaptation' and 'tailoring' in the context of designing exercise and fitness training programmes for patients, including stroke survivors

Adaptation: the condition-specific modifications to session aims, structure, content, teaching and programming that need to be make to ensure optimal safety and effectiveness for all patients.

Tailoring: the highly individual prescriptive solutions (adjustments, additions and exclusions) that are required to ensure the exercise intervention meets each patient's health, functional and/or psychosocial/emotional needs.

Dinan 2001, Skelton and Dinan 2008

SPECIAL CONSIDERATIONS FOR LOW CARDIOVASCULAR FITNESS

As explained in chapter 4, many stroke survivors have low cardiovascular fitness. Contributing factors include low physical activity levels or health condition prior to the stroke, the direct neurological deficits from the stroke, a lack of physical activity during the immediate rehabilitation post stroke and following discharge (Bernhardt et al. 2007), as well as co-existing disease and/or advanced age. Additional contributing factors may be the psychosocial impact of stroke including low mood and anxiety.

Following the acute stage after stroke, hospital-based rehabilitation initially concentrates on restoring function and specific everyday functional tasks to allow discharge home. Cardiovascular fitness is often not addressed at this time. Taken together, it is likely that, despite rehabilitation input, the stroke survivor will progressively have lost cardiovascular fitness.

Solutions for low cardiovascular fitness

Exercise should be prescribed to commence at a lower physical fitness baseline than for healthy populations.

Adaptations. These should include:

- Selecting cardiovascular training modes that enable a low-moderate or moderate intensity of aerobic activity by utilising the large muscle groups whilst providing activities that are stable (e.g. bike, step-up) that meet functional needs such as stepping and walking.
- A longer and more gradual warm up and cool down (20 minutes in the initial 6–8 weeks, reducing to 15 minutes only as fitness is gained).
- A longer 'build up' and 'cool down' to the aerobic training component to accommodate the slower redistribution of blood to the skeletal muscles and slower increase in coronary supply to meet the increasing demands. This is particularly important in those whose stroke is related to cardiovascular disease.
- Ensuring an interval conditioning endurance training approach with moderate peaks of activity and 'troughs' of lower intensity 'active rest' to achieve a continuous bout of activity that builds gradually to 20–30 minutes or beyond as appropriate.
- Progressing session duration to full period before intensity is increased. Ideally the peaks should involve an effort interval where the work rate is a little harder than 'steady state' or what is comfortable, followed by a moderate recovery interval where activity returns to a comfortable, easily sustained effort level (Brooks 1997). Active rests may take the form of lower intensity aerobic activity (e.g. marching) or light resistance training (e.g. biceps curls with 1 kg x 15 repetitions). Exercise professionals should be aware of the greater effort needed to perform large, coordinated movements of bodyweight against gravity, such as shallow squats, step-ups, etc.
- Aiming at moderate intensity of exercise once the training programme is underway (i.e. low to moderate for the initial 4–6 weeks).
- Monitoring: to establish and maintain a training intensity that is both safe and sufficient to produce beneficial effects, the intensity level of aerobic exercise should be regularly monitored by rating of perceived exertion (RPE) (Borg 1998), the occasional Talk Test (Persinger et al. 2004) at approximately every 15 minutes (Fig. 10.11), and observation.

Tailoring strategies. These could include:

- Incorporating upper limb support or a seated option at each exercise station for those unable to maintain balance when aiming for large muscle group activity.
- Altering approaches to 'grip' of equipment in cases where hand and finger coordination, range of joint motion and/or strength present difficulties.
- Altering the base of support for stroke survivors who wear a rigid style ankle foot orthosis (AFO).
- Changing communication strategies for labelling the exercise stations for stroke survivors with cognitive/communication difficulties.
- Laying out the session exercise stations in a particular order or position to suit those with visual field loss or attention difficulties.
- Using safe methods of mounting/dismounting particular pieces of equipment (e.g. bike or step).
- Emphasising movement in particular patterns where components of movement are shown to be imbalanced.

SPECIAL CONSIDERATIONS FOR HEMIPLEGIA

Hemiplegia often manifests itself as muscle weakness, with associated coordination difficulties that can present major challenges to the stroke survivor as they attempt to perform exercises (chapter 3). Weakness and postural asymmetry often occur in patterns that lead to an imbalance between the flexor and extensor groups of upper and/or lower limb on the affected side of the body, as well as the trunk. The affected patterns of movement can also lead to a reduction in static and dynamic balance. Solutions below indicate the movement patterns that need to be emphasised to address common imbalances between muscle groups that lead to abnormal movement.

Balance has been described as 'the maintenance of equilibrium while stationary or moving' (ACSM 2010, p. 3) and thus comprises static balance (e.g. standing still) as well as dynamic balance (e.g. walking). Walking aids, though designed to improve balance, may also render some activities more complex and hazardous (e.g. climbing stairs, or doing step-ups). Coordinating an impaired gait pattern while safely using a stick demands extra attention and effort. In combination with reduced cardiovascular fitness, using a walking aid often results in a slower gait that may be difficult to sustain for an extended period of time.

Solutions for hemiplegia

Adaptations. These should include:

- Selecting upper limb exercises that concentrate on movement patterns with shoulder external rotation, elbow extension and forearm supination with wrist extension and where possible an open palm (e.g. 'upper back strengthener' or 'ball raise').
- Selecting lower limb exercises involving both flexion patterns at hip and knee with ankle dorsiflexion and gross extension patterns at hip and knee (e.g. 'step-ups').

Tailoring strategies. Such strategies could include:

- Providing seated options for upper limb exercises in cases where standing balance is problematic or where muscle fatigue limits prolonged standing (e.g. 'ball raise').
- Using chair-based cycling (either a mobile pedal unit or recumbent cycle ergometer) if the control of posture and balance on an upright bike is difficult.
- Providing active assisted exercises for the affected upper limb if the stroke survivor is unable to utilise their upper limb (e.g. reach and hold).

Modification of exercises (e.g. lowering the resistance and/or modifying the start position by posture or range of movement) is required if spasticity (e.g. clonus, spasms or associated reactions; chapter 3) or postural malalignment occur during an exercise and the stroke survivor is unable to self-correct even with prompting.

SPECIAL CONSIDERATIONS FOR COGNITIVE AND COMMUNICATION DIFFICULTIES

Post-stroke cognitive and communication difficulties can impact significantly on participation in exercise (see chapters 3 and 9). Impaired memory can make it difficult for a stroke survivor to recall exercise techniques from one week to another, while impaired comprehension can affect the ability to process instructions quickly enough. These impairments can make it difficult for a stroke survivor to keep up, especially in a group setting.

Solutions for cognitive and communication difficulties

Effective communication is an essential skill, especially in group stroke exercise sessions.

Adaptations. Adaptations should include:

- Using visual prompts to assist memory and learning of correct exercises and exercise technique, and also to enhance communication between the exercise professional and stroke survivor.
- Involving the stroke survivor in the planning, delivery and evaluation of the exercise programme wherever possible, using effective communication. This is an important factor in self-management of physical activity after stroke.
- Creating communication opportunities beyond exercise session times (e.g. time to meet before and/or afterwards) to encourage social interaction and communication confidence between the exercise professional and stroke survivors.

Tailoring strategies. These strategies could include:

- Allowing for brief pauses between each instruction and between exercise sections, providing action demonstration and correction prompts, to enable stroke survivors to process information and to enable effective two-way communication.

- Using regular minimal (even single) word prompting and relating all exercises clearly to everyday simple functional tasks to facilitate recall.
- Using gestures purposefully; some gestures with excessive arm movement may distract stroke survivors with concentration difficulties from understanding the intended message.
- Devising a range of mental imagery prompts to help stroke survivors recall their exercises (e.g. based on memories of familiar activities or related to well-known games).
- Using specific positioning by the exercise professional when communicating (Fig. 10.20), tailored to needs of the individual stroke survivor (e.g. visual problems or privacy requirements).

SPECIAL CONSIDERATIONS FOR SENSORY AND PERCEPTUAL DIFFICULTIES

Sensory and perceptual difficulties have the potential to increase risks during an exercise session. Altered midline orientation due to contralateral neglect, which can create uncertainty about the orientation of one's midline, or inability to see and interpret the environment effectively, may make it difficult to carry out exercises safely (see chapter 3). Visual field loss, impaired depth perception and spatial awareness also increase the risk of falls from steps, collisions due to misjudging the speed of equipment or objects (e.g. altered anticipation of doors opening and closing) as well as other people. Deficits in tactile and proprioceptive sensation may also affect stroke survivors' awareness of their affected limbs. To reduce risks (e.g. collisions with apparatus) they may have to look at their limbs to monitor their position and movement.

Solutions for sensory and perceptual difficulties

Care must be taken to ensure that the type and order of exercises minimises risks while setting an appropriate challenge.

Adaptations. Adaptations should include:

- Setting up the circuit over a smaller area than for non-stroke groups, i.e. ensuring minimal distance between stations, unison transitions and same direction of travel around the circuit. These can all help to reduce risk and increase clarity, in addition to helping stroke survivors to hear the exercise professional more clearly.
- Ensuring tightly supervised transitions between exercises where risks are higher and equipment is being carried (e.g. staged transitions in small groups).
- Trying to ensure contrasting surface colours between floor walls and equipment edges to improve object perception.
- Providing assistance/supervision and a specific agreed movement sequence and safety protocol for mounting bikes, etc., where pedals may cause injury if they are out of the stroke survivor's visual field.

Tailoring strategies. Tailoring strategies could include:

- Ensuring there is sufficient space between stroke survivors when there is impaired awareness (e.g. of other people exercising in the vicinity).

- Ensuring appropriate positioning of individuals with visual field loss in seated groups so that the exercise professional can be clearly seen without altering their position, posture and/or exercise technique.

SPECIAL CONSIDERATIONS FOR CO-MORBIDITIES

Consideration needs to be given to any previous or co-existing health condition that may limit tolerance to exercise, e.g. osteoarthritis, diabetes, osteoporosis and pain. Chapter 3 described some of the most common co-morbidities in stroke survivors, and provided generic guidance on the management of these conditions in the context of exercise. Stroke survivors with co-morbidities should be especially encouraged to self-monitor and report any subtle changes in performance or health to the exercise professional. In those where pain is a key problem, using a measure such as a visual analogue scale (chapter 11) before and after exercise may give insight into an individual's exercise tolerance and help to avoid straining vulnerable joints affected by weakness, subluxation, arthritis or other conditions.

SOCIAL SUPPORT

Prior to the exercise session, the exercise professional should be scheduled to be present in the exercise area for 15–20 minutes to assist entry to the premises where necessary. Also, importantly, the exercise professional should ensure contact with each individual prior to the session and facilitate opportunities for socialisation between stroke survivors. After each session social interaction between stroke survivors should be facilitated, e.g. time and a comfortable space to have tea or coffee and a chat. Stroke survivors report benefits from the social aspect of the group (chapter 6).

PROMOTING LIFE-LONG PARTICIPATION IN EXERCISE

Life-long participation in exercise after stroke is recommended in clinical guidelines, (e.g. Scottish Intercollegiate Guidelines Network 2008), although there is little research on how this can best be achieved in practice. Several elements have been identified as contributing to enhanced motivation, enjoyment (Fig. 10.28), long-term adherence and reducing attrition (i.e. drop-out) in other community-based Exercise after Stroke services. These include ensuring that, wherever possible:

- The sessions are at the same (or very similar) time.
- The sessions are in the same venue (or nearby).
- The exercise professional remains the same as in the intake sessions (or is introduced to the stroke survivors and/or is involved in the teaching of the intake phase).
- In-service training is given for all the professionals and support staff involved (including the reception staff). This could include free on-line training (e.g. www.strokecorecompetencies.org).
- Transport is provided for stroke survivors where possible, delivered by dedicated, well-briefed patient transport personnel.

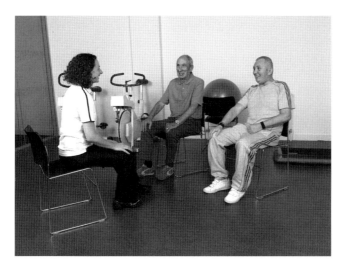

FIG 10.28 Enjoyment is essential for motivation and adherence.

Peer mentor interventions and peer mentor training also appear to be effective in increasing adherence to exercise sessions in both older and patient populations. More research is needed into the effectiveness of peer mentoring interventions in increasing retention to Exercise after Stroke programmes.

FEEDBACK TO REFERRERS

The UK exercise referral guidelines (Department of Health 2001) stipulate that some form of feedback needs to be given to the stroke survivor's referrer (e.g. their GP). This comprises formal feedback at the 'end of term' of an exercise referral period, which may be a 3–12-month period (although this may vary across local health authorities). The guideline recommends that there not only be feedback at the end of this period, but a follow-up after the referral period with each individual at time points agreed by the individual and specified in the service contract (e.g. at 3 and 6 months after the end of the exercise programme). If no follow-up is stated in the service contract, this responsibility should be placed with the referring health professional.

In cases where there is no identified 'end of term', it is important that the links between exercise professionals and referrers be kept open, so that feedback can take place at any time.

SUMMARY POINTS

- This chapter discussed the key principles and variables, as well as special considerations involved in designing and delivering exercise and fitness programmes for stroke survivors. Exercise and fitness training for stroke survivors must be based on current best evidence and best practice guidance to promote safety and effectiveness, while providing a motivating and enjoyable experience with the longer term aim of encouraging a more physically active lifestyle wherever possible.

- In order to design and deliver exercise and fitness programmes for stroke survivors, adaptation and tailoring is required:
  - Adaptation comprises the condition-specific modifications to session aims, structure, content, teaching and programming to ensure optimal safety and effectiveness for all stroke survivors in general.
  - Tailoring refers to the specific solutions (adjustments, additions and exclusions) required to ensure the exercise intervention meets the health, functional and/or psychosocial/emotional needs of each individual stroke survivor.
- The primary aim of exercise and fitness training for stroke survivors is to improve all components of physical fitness, with priority given to cardiovascular endurance and functional muscle strength, power and endurance to achieve optimum health and functional gain. Secondary aims are to improve the performance of specific everyday functional activities, promote attainment of personal goals as well as more general health and functional outcomes, to enhance self-efficacy and self-management in relation to physical activity, and promote psychological and social wellbeing.
- The generic principles of exercise programming are specificity, progressive overload, rest and recovery and individual difference; the variables are the frequency, intensity, type and timing of exercise, approach and adherence. Special considerations for exercise programming for stroke survivors discussed were: low cardiovascular fitness, hemiplegia, cognitive and communication difficulties, sensory and perceptual difficulties as well as co-morbidities. Strategies for adaptation and tailoring that take these special considerations into account were discussed.
- On the basis of current published research literature, it is not possible to make definitive recommendations with respect to the 'FITT' (frequency, intensity, time/duration and type of exercise) principles. On the basis of current evidence it would be reasonable to use the intervention developed for the STARTER trial for community-based services, as it has been shown to be safe, effective and feasible for ambulatory stroke survivors who have completed their usual rehabilitation.
- The recommendations for programme design in this chapter are based on the available published literature and consensus recommendations from experts from stroke rehabilitation and exercise sectors. These include a range of different health professionals, clinical exercise practitioners and clinical exercise scientists with long-standing experience and recognised expertise in the specialist field of physical activity and rehabilitation, as well as stroke survivors themselves.
- Recommendations for the design and delivery of exercise and fitness programmes for stroke survivors will need to be reviewed as new evidence becomes available.

American College of Sports Medicine (ACSM), 1995. Guidelines for exercise testing and prescription, fifth ed. Williams and Wilkins, London.

American College of Sports Medicine (ACSM), 2010. Guidelines for exercise testing and prescription, eighth ed. Lippincott Williams & Wilkins, Philadelphia, PA.

Axelson, H.W., 2005. Signs of muscle thixotrophy during human ballistic wrist joint movements. J. Appl. Physiol. 99, 1922–1929.

Bernhardt, J., Chan, J., Nicola, I., et al., 2007. Little therapy, little physical activity: rehabilitation within the first 14 days of organized stroke unit care. J. Rehabil. Med. 39, 43–48.

Best, C., van Wijck, F., Dinan-Young, S., et al., 2010. Best practice guidance for the development of Exercise after Stroke services in community settings. Edinburgh University, Edinburgh. Available online at: http://www.exerciseafterstroke.org.uk/ (accessed 08.09.2011).

Borg, G., 1998. Borg's perceived exertion and pain scales. Human Kinetics, Champaign, IL.

Brazzelli, M., Saunders, D.H., Greig, C.A., Mead, G.E., 2011. Physical fitness training for stroke patients. Cochrane Database Syst. Rev. 11, CD003316. doi: 10.1002/14651858.

British National Formulary. Available online at: http://www.bnf.org/bnf/ (accessed 27.09.2011).

Brooks, D.S., 1997. Program design for personal trainers. Human Kinetics, Champaign, IL.

Buckley, J.P., 2008. Exercise physiology in special populations. Advances in sport and exercise science. Elsevier, Edinburgh.

Department of Health, 2001. NHS: exercise referral systems: a national quality assurance framework. HMSO, London.

Dinan, S., 2001. Delivering an exercise prescription for vulnerable older patients. In: Young, A., Harries, M. (Eds.), Physical activity for patients: an exercise prescription. Royal College of Physicians, London, pp. 53–70.

Dinan, S., Dennis, J., 2010. In: Mead, G.E., Dennis, J., Paul, S., et al. (Eds.), Exercise after stroke: physical activity and health.

Specialist Exercise Professional Training Course Syllabus. Unpublished Course Syllabus. Queen Margaret University, Edinburgh.

Dinan, S., Skelton, D., Gawler, S., et al., 2008. Exercise for the prevention of falls and injuries. Specialist Professional Training Course Syllabus, third ed. LaterLife Training, Crianlarich.

Duncan, P., Studenski, S., Richards, N., et al., 2003. Randomised clinical trial of therapeutic exercise in subacute stroke. Stroke 34 (9), 2173–2180.

Flansbjer, U.B., Downham, D., Lexell, J., 2006. Knee muscle strength, gait performance, and perceived participation after stroke. Arch. Phys. Med. Rehabil. 87, 974–980.

French, B., Thomas, N.H., Leathley, M.J., 2007. Repetitive task training for improving functional ability after stroke. Cochrane Database Syst. Rev. 4, CD006073. doi:10.1002/14651858.

Gordon, N.F., Gulanick, M., Costa, F., et al., 2004. Physical activity and exercise recommendations for stroke survivors: an American Heart Association Scientific Statement from the Council on Clinical Cardiology, Subcommittee on Exercise, Cardiac Rehabilitation, and Prevention; the Council on Cardiovascular Nursing; the Council on Nutrition, Physical Activity, and Metabolism; and the Stroke Council. Circulation 109, 2031–2041.

Health and Safety Executive, 1981. The Health and Safety (First-Aid) Regulations. Available from http://www.hse.gov.uk/firstaid/program.htm.

Jones, J., Rose, D., 2005. Physical activity instruction of older adults. Human Kinetics, Champaign, IL.

Katalinic, O.M., Harvey, N.A., Herbert, R.D., et al., 2010. Stretch for the treatment and prevention of contractures. Cochrane Database Syst. Rev. 9, CD007455. doi:10.1002/14651858.

Kraemer, W.J., French, D.N., 2005. Resistance training. In: Jones, C.J., Rose, D. (Eds.), Physical activity instruction of older adults. Human Kinetics, Champaign, IL.

Lakie, M., Robson, N., 1988. Thixotrophic changes in human muscle stiffness and

Designing and delivering an exercise and fitness training programme

the effects of fatigue. J. Exp. Physiol. 73, 487–500.

Langhorne, P., Coupar, F., Pollock, A., 2009. Motor recovery after stroke: a systematic review. Lancet Neurol. 8, 741–754.

Laver, K., Rehab, M.C., Halbert, J., et al., 2010. Patient readiness and ability to set recovery goals during the first 6 months after stroke. J. Allied Health 39, e149–e154.

Leach, E., Cornwell, P., Fleming, J., et al., 2009. Patient centered goal-setting in a subacute rehabilitation setting. Disabil. Rehabil. 26, 1–14.

Le Brasseur, N.K., Sayers, S.P., Ouellette, M.M., et al., 2006. Muscle impairments and behavioral factors mediate functional limitations and disability following stroke. Phys. Ther. 86, 1342–1350.

Mead, G., Greig, C.A., Cunningham, I., et al., 2007. STroke: A Randomised Trial of Exercise or Relaxation (STARTER). J. Am. Geriatr. Soc. 55, 892–899.

Mead, G.E., Dennis, J., Paul, S., et al., 2010. 2010 Exercise after stroke: physical activity and health. Specialist Exercise Professional Training Course Syllabus. Unpublished Course Syllabus. Queen Margaret University, Edinburgh.

Nakayama, H., Jorgensen, H.S., Raaschou, H.O., et al., 1994. Recovery of upper extremity function in stroke patients: The Copenhagen Stroke Study. Arch. Phys. Med. Rehabil. 75, 394–398.

Persinger, R., Foster, C., Gibson, M., et al., 2004. Consistency of the talk test for exercise prescription. Med. Sci. Sports Exerc. 36, 1632–1636.

Playford, E.D., Siegert, R., Levack, W., et al., 2009. Areas of consensus and controversy about goal setting in rehabilitation: a conference report. Clin. Rehabil. 23, 334–344.

Saunders, D.H., Greig, C.A., Young, A., et al., 2004. Physical fitness training for stroke patients. Stroke 35, 22–35.

Saunders, D.H., Greig, C.A., Young, A., et al., 2008. Association of activity limitations and lower-limb explosive extensor power in ambulatory people with stroke. Arch. Phys. Med. Rehabil. 89, 677–683.

Saunders, D.H., Greig, C.A., Mead, G.E., et al., 2009. Physical fitness training for stroke patients. Cochrane Database Syst. Rev. 4, CD003316. doi:10.1002/14651858.

Schmidt, R.A., Wrisberg, C.A., 2008. Motor learning and performance. A situation-based learning approach, fourth ed. Human Kinetics, Champaign, IL.

Scottish Intercollegiate Guidelines Network, 2008. Guideline 108. Management of patients with stroke or TIA: assessment, investigation, immediate management and secondary prevention: a national clinical. Scottish Intercollegiate Guidelines Network (SIGN). Edinburgh. Available online at: http://www.sign.ac.uk/guidelines/fulltext/108/index.html (accessed 08.09.2011).

Skelton, D.A., Dinan, S.M., 2008. Ageing and older people. In: Buckley, J.P. (Ed.), Exercise physiology in special populations. Advances in sport and exercise science, Elsevier, Edinburgh, pp. 161–223.

Skelton, D.A., McLaughlin, A.W., 1996. Training functional ability in old age. Physiotherapy 82, 159–167.

Skelton, D.A., Greig, C.A., Davies, J.M., et al., 1994. Strength, power and related functional ability of healthy people aged 65–89 years. Age Ageing 23, 371–377.

Skelton, D.A., Young, A., Greig, C.A., et al., 1995. Effects of resistance training on strength, power and selected functional abilities of women aged 75 and over. J. Am. Geriatr. Soc. 43, 1081–1087.

Skelton, D.A., Dinan, S.M., Campbell, M., et al., 2005. Tailored group exercise (Falls Management Exercise - FaME) reduces falls in community-dwelling older frequent fallers (an RCT). Age Ageing 34, 636–639.

SkillsActive, Level 4 National Occupational Standards for Physical Activity after Stroke, 2010a. D516.1 – Design and agree a physical activity programme with patients/clients after stroke. Available online at: http://www.skillsactive.com/training/standards/level_4/physical_activity_and_health (accessed 09.09.2011).

SkillsActive, Level 4 National Occupational Standards for Physical Activity after Stroke, 2010b. D516.2 – Deliver, review and adapt a physical activity programme with patient/clients after stroke. Available online at: http://www.skillsactive.com/training/standards/level_4/physical_activity_and_health (accessed 09.09.2011).

van Vliet, P.M., Sheridan, M.R., 2007. Coordination between reaching and grasping in patients with hemiparesis and normal subjects. Arch. Phys. Med. Rehabil. 88, 1325–1331.

Vattanslip, W., Ada, N., Crosbie, J., 2000. Contribution of thixotrophy, spasticity and contracture to ankle stiffness after stroke. J. Neurol. Neurosurg. Psychiatry 69, 34–39.

Wade, D.T., 2009. Goal setting in rehabilitation: an overview of what, why and how. Clin. Rehabil. 23, 291–295.

Wicebloom, S., 2007. Training disabled people (fitness professionals). A&C Black, London.

Designing and delivering an exercise and fitness training programme

Evaluating exercise and fitness training after stroke: outcome assessment

Frederike van Wijck

CHAPTER CONTENTS

INTRODUCTION

Previous chapters discussed the preparation, design and delivery of exercise programmes for stroke survivors. In this chapter, we will focus on outcome assessment to determine the impact of such programmes. Some of the measures used in outcome assessment may be similar to those used for screening stroke survivors prior to referral for exercise (chapter 9), but the purpose of using measures for outcome assessment is distinctly different.

213

Outcome assessment is crucial for providing feedback to individual stroke survivors and their families, exercise professionals, referring health-care professionals, service managers and commissioners about the effects and experiences of exercise after stroke. In the current climate of accountability and evidence-based practice, outcome assessment is an integral part of service provision. The purpose of this chapter is to discuss the 'why, what and how' of outcome assessment in the context of exercise after stroke.

DEFINING MEASUREMENT AND ASSESSMENT

First of all, we need to define what we mean by 'assessment' and another term with which it is often used interchangeably, i.e. 'measurement' (Wade 1992). There are many definitions of both terms. Kondraske (1989) proposed the following:

'Measurement refers to the use of a standard (such as a metric ruler) to quantify an observation.'

'Assessment is the process of determining the meaning of a measurement or collective set of measurements in a specific context.'

According to these definitions, 'measurement' is purely about collecting quantitative information, while 'assessment' involves interpreting the *meaning* of this information. In a clinical context, 'assessment' often refers to the application of clinical judgement, which is usually based on clinical signs and symptoms and clinical experience, while it may or may not include formal measures.

Let's take the example of the Timed Up-and-Go (Podsiadlo and Richardson 1991), a test that measures how long it takes to rise from a chair, walk 3 meters, turn round and sit down (see Table 11.1). Determining the time taken to complete the test involves actual measurement, whereas deciding how the result compares with healthy people of the same age and sex involves assessment. Thus, according to the definitions above, the process of assessment involves an additional element of judgement.

ASSESSMENT: WHY?

As mentioned in the Introduction, outcome assessment is undertaken to provide feedback to stroke survivors, exercise professionals, service managers and commissioners, about the impact of the service. Outcome assessment can be considered at different levels of analysis, as illustrated in Figure 11.1:

- At the level of the individual stroke survivor: outcome assessment may involve collecting quantitative information on the effects of exercise. This may include indicators of improved fitness and function, reduced pain or fatigue, the extent to which personal goals have been achieved, and/or qualitative information about their experiences of the service. Information about fitness improvements may well serve to motivate the stroke survivor to continue to exercise and encourage self-management of exercise, as explained in chapter 6.

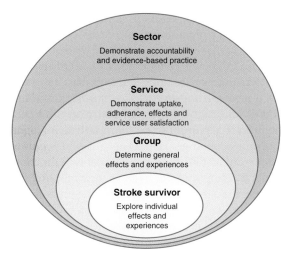

FIG 11.1 Outcome assessment can be undertaken at different levels – from the individual stroke survivor to the service sector as a whole.

- At the level of a group of stroke survivors: data can be compiled from individuals to yield information on changes between the start and end of an exercise programme for a whole cohort.
- At the level of a local exercise service: outcome assessment could comprise information on uptake and adherence, effects and adverse events, stroke survivor satisfaction, as well as data on the costs of running the service. Such information demonstrates the impact of the service and may be crucial in justifying the need for the service and hence for funding.
- At the level of a whole service sector: data from local services could be compiled to yield information about the effectiveness and cost-effectiveness of an entire service sector for a particular region, country or organisation (e.g. national charity organisation) – provided that standardised assessment procedures are used. This information can also be used by the sector to demonstrate accountability and evidence-based practice, and the extent to which the service meets user needs.

ASSESSMENT: WHAT?

Relevance

Before choosing an outcome measure, it is important to clarify what one wants to know. In principle, it is possible to gather a plethora of information, as Table 11.1 suggests, but just collecting data for its own sake is unethical. One should always start by asking 'What do I need to know?', 'What does this information tell me?' and 'What am I going to do with the data?' In other words: What is the question?

If the purpose of outcome assessment is to assess the extent to which an individual stroke survivor has attained their exercise goals, we need to have a clear understanding of what these goals are and how to measure them. Chapter 10 explained that the general aims of health-related exercise and fitness training after stroke are to improve cardiovascular/cardiorespiratory endurance, muscle strength and endurance, as well as flexibility, motor skills and coordination. In addition, the individual stroke survivor is likely to have their own goals. It may be useful to bear in mind that stroke survivors are more likely to formulate their goals in terms of activities of daily living (e.g. wanting to get up from a chair more easily), general function (e.g. wanting to feel less tired when shopping), or even in more general terms (e.g. wanting to get back to normal) than in terms of specific impairments (e.g. muscle weakness or maximum oxygen uptake) (Lawler et al. 1999). The challenge for the exercise professional is to analyse the stroke survivor's goals and judiciously choose one or more outcome measures that reflect these goals, while bearing in mind that the measures also need to be scientifically robust.

The International Classification of Functioning, Disability and Health (ICF) as a framework

How does an exercise professional decide which outcome measure to use? A framework that may help to clarify matters is the World Health Organization's International Classification of Functioning, Disability and Health, or ICF (WHO 2001). The ICF is an international scientific framework that describes and explains different aspects of health and factors that influence health. It can also be used to identify and categorise measures that capture different aspects of a health condition.

Let us use 'stroke' as an example of a health condition to explain the ICF model, which is presented in Figure 11.2.

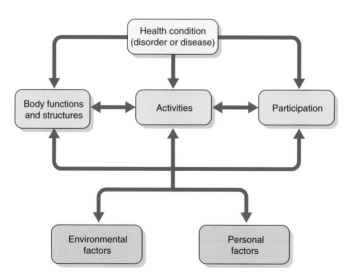

FIG 11.2 Diagrammatic overview of the World Health Organization's International Classification of Functioning, Disability and Health (WHO 2001). See text for details.

Body functions, structures and impairments

Body functions refer to the physiological or psychological functions of body systems, such as the cardiovascular and pulmonary systems, musculoskeletal, visual or attentional systems.

Body structures are anatomical parts of the body such as organs, limbs and their components, such as joints, muscles and nerves. Impairments are defined as problems in body function or structure such as a significant deviation or loss. Chapter 3 described how a stroke can impair a wide range of functions, e.g. muscle activation or sensation of the affected side of the body, visual perception and attention. The corresponding impairments are paresis, reduced sensation, visual agnosia and hemi-inattention, respectively. As described in chapter 4, many stroke survivors also have a number of fitness-related impairments, including reduced cardiovascular and muscle endurance, muscle power and strength.

Activity and activity limitations

Activity is defined as the execution of a task or action by an individual. Activity limitations are difficulties with undertaking activities. Following a stroke, activity limitations may include difficulty with grasping objects, dressing and walking, preparing meals and using equipment for exercise, carrying shopping and using stairs, or difficulties with problem solving and communication.

Participation and participation restrictions

Participation is involvement in a life situation, e.g. holding a job, being engaged in a hobby or looking after a child. Participation restrictions are problems with being involved in life situations, e.g. barriers with return to work after stroke, difficulties engaging in previous leisure activities, or problems with interpersonal relationships.

Environmental and personal factors

Finally, the ICF includes two important factors that influence a health condition, i.e. environmental and personal factors.

Environmental factors make up the physical, social and attitudinal environment in which people live. For example, attitudes towards disability at work are likely to influence a stroke survivor's opportunities for returning to work. Lack of accessible transport may make it difficult for stroke survivors to attend community leisure services (Rimmer et al. 2008).

Personal factors are related to the particular background of an individual's life (e.g. age, race, education, coping styles). For example, one study suggested that greater use of avoidance coping strategies (e.g. sleeping more than usual or refusing to believe that one has had a stroke) early after stroke was predictive of post-stroke depression (King et al. 2002).

Having presented an outline of the ICF, let us explore how this framework may assist in clarifying the domains represented by outcome measures in the context of exercise after stroke. Table 11.1 lists the various fitness components as categorised by the American College of Sports Medicine (ACSM 2010), as well as other constructs that may be relevant for assessing the effects of exercise after stroke. These are tabled alongside examples of possible outcome measures and their corresponding ICF domain(s). It is important to emphasise that this table is not exhaustive but rather an overview of a range of options for outcome assessment. From this, one could choose one or more measures that are relevant and appropriate to the individual(s) and the context in which the assessment is to take place.

Chapter 9 mentioned exercise testing in the context of pre-exercise assessment. Exercise testing with open circuit spirometry may also be used to evaluate fitness outcomes over the course of an exercise programme (Ivey et al. 2011). It is important that the risks involved with exercise testing on a treadmill or bicycle are carefully assessed, as many stroke survivors do not have the required balance or strength for conventional treadmill testing. For an overview of validated protocols for exercise testing, readers are referred to Ivey et al. (2011). Further detailed information about stroke-related outcome measures can be found in Salter et al. (2010) while fitness-related outcome measures are described in the American College of Sports Medicine (ACSM) guidelines (ACSM 2010).

Table 11.1 *Examples of outcome measures for evaluating the effects of exercise and fitness training after stroke and their corresponding ICF domain(s)*

Fitness component	Example of outcome measure	ICF domain
Cardiovascular endurance	(Maximum) cycling work rate Gait economy Maximum VO$_2$ uptake Respiratory exchange ratio	Body structure and function
Body composition	Body mass index Body circumference Skinfold measures	Body structure and function
Muscle strength	Upper limb: grip and pinch force Lower limb: isometric or dynamic ankle, knee and hip flexor and extensor force	Body structure and function
Endurance	6-minute walk test (Eng et al. 2002, Fitts and Guthrie 1995, Guyatt 1985, Steffen 2002, Wade 1992, Willenheimer and Erhardt 2000)	Body structure and function
Flexibility	Passive and/or active joint range of movement	Body structure and function
Agility	Biomechanical gait parameters (e.g. stride length, stance symmetry, contact time, maximum vertical ground reaction force) Timed up-and-go (Podsiadlo and Richardson 1991, Steffen et al. 2002)	Body structure and function
Coordination	Fugl-Meyer test of physical performance after stroke (Fugl-Meyer et al. 1975)	Body structure and function Activity
Balance	Berg Balance Scale (Berg et al. 1989) Tinetti (Tinetti et al. 1986)	Activity
Power	Explosive lower limb extensor power	Body structure and function

Table 11.1 *Examples of outcome measures for evaluating the effects of exercise and fitness training after stroke and their corresponding ICF domain(s)—cont'd*

Fitness component	Example of outcome measure	ICF domain
Reaction time	Dependent on the task: time between a cue to a specific action and the start of the action	Body structure and function Activity
Speed	10-minute walk test (Duncan et al. 2007, Wade 1992)	Body structure and function Activity

Construct	Example of outcome measure	ICF domain
Goal attainment	Canadian Occupational Performance Measure (Law et al. 1998) Goal Attainment Scaling (Turner-Stokes 2009)	Body structure and function Activity Participation, depending on the goal
Independence in self-care and mobility	Barthel Index (Mahoney and Barthel 1965)	Activity
Independence in physical functioning	Functional Independence Measure (Granger et al. 1993), comprising function (i.e. self-care, sphincter control, mobility, locomotion, communication and social cognition) and cognition (i.e. social interaction, problem-solving and memory) Functional Ambulation Category (Collen et al. 1990, Holden et al. 1984, 1986)	Activity Participation
Self-reported stroke impact	Stroke Impact Scale (Duncan et al. 2003a,b), comprising physical strength, hand function, activities of daily living, mobility, mood and control of emotions, thinking and memory, communication, participation, stroke recovery	Body structure and function Activity Participation
Health status	Medical Outcomes Study Short Form SF-36 (Ware and Sherbourne 1992), comprising physical functioning, role limitations – physical, bodily pain, social functioning, general mental health, role limitations – emotional, vitality, and general health perceptions	Body structure and function Activity Participation
Pain	Visual Analogue Scale (Bond and Pilowsky 1996, Price et al. 1999)	Body structure and function Activity Participation, depending on the aspect of pain being examined
Mood: anxiety and depression	Hospital Anxiety and Depression Scale (Zigmond and Snaith 1983)	Personal factor

VO_2, oxygen utilisation.

Table 11.1 might suggest that outcome measures neatly fit into distinct ICF domains. In reality, however, the boundaries between different ICF domains may be blurred. For example, the construct of 'walking' (e.g. crossing the road) can be seen as a functional activity and therefore difficulties with walking could be interpreted as an activity limitation. However, when we measure walking in terms of biomechanical parameters (e.g. joint displacement or muscle activation), are we still measuring an activity or have we shifted to body function and structure? One could argue that each gait parameter represents a specific body function or structure, and that, by focusing on these, we have lost sight of the functional context in which the 'walking' takes place. This example illustrates that there are cases where the same construct may be viewed from different perspectives.

Additionally, some outcome measures comprise items from more than one domain. For example, most items in the Fugl-Meyer test (Fugl-Meyer et al. 1975) evaluate joint movement in specific patterns that have no explicit functional goal, but some items evaluate functional activity (e.g. holding an object). Thus, the majority of the Fugl-Meyer is impairment-orientated, while a small proportion is activity limitation-orientated.

Having decided which measure(s) is/are most relevant, the exercise professional needs to consider all ethical implications (such as safety and data protection), and verify that each method used to gather information is scientifically robust (i.e. valid, reliable, sufficiently sensitive). Finally, practical aspects need to be thought through, such as the complexity and duration of the tests and whether these are appropriate. Instrumentation and training requirements need to be considered, as well as how the results will be interpreted and communicated. Each of these aspects will be discussed in more detail below.

ETHICAL CONSIDERATIONS

Before starting the actual outcome assessment process, the exercise professional must ensure that all ethical requirements have been given due consideration.

Consent

Permission must be sought from the stroke survivor (or their carer if required, e.g. in the case of cognitive impairment) prior to assessment, having explained its purpose, what it involves and how confidentiality will be ensured. It is important that the exercise professional documents that permission has been obtained. When information is to be used for research purposes, investigators must go through the statutory process of ethical approval. This process of obtaining ethical approval will vary between different countries.

Risks of performing outcome assessment

The exercise professional should assess the risks involved in the assessment process, and reduce these as far as is reasonably practicable; for example, the timed up-and-go, an assistant may be required if the stroke survivor is known to have poor balance.

Data protection

All documentation – unless held by the stroke survivor – must comply with usual health service or local authority standards of written/electronic records and security. Any records written, stored and kept by the exercise professional should comply with the regulations pertaining to where they are sited and employed by (or contracted to). This may vary between local authorities, but is standard across the National Health Service in the UK. The Department of Health (2001) in the UK stipulates that records should be filed securely in the exercise setting or, alternatively, stroke survivors could make a personal log book available if they are prepared to do so.

SCIENTIFIC PRINCIPLES OF MEASUREMENT

It is essential to check the scientific properties of any assessment tool prior to considering its use, to make sure it works properly (e.g. one would avoid a broken scale to measure one's weight!). These properties are validity, reliability and sensitivity (or responsiveness) (Durward et al. 1999). Each property will be explained in more detail below.

Validity

The validity of a measure indicates whether it does what it is purported to do. For example, a weighing scale clearly measures weight, but a pain scale in the form of a questionnaire could assess a person's level of pain, their comprehension of using the scale, their ability to express their opinion on the scale, or a mix of all of these factors. Thus, the validity of the pain scale is clearly questionable.

It is important to highlight that any outcome measure, before it is fit for purpose, should have undergone a thorough process of validation. The scientific literature is replete with studies reporting the validity and reliability of a wide range of outcome measures. Such studies are essential, as using a measure with poor validity is simply a waste of time. However, sometimes it is difficult for professionals to find an outcome measure that meets all their requirements (including being relevant and easy to use), and they may resort to 'making up their own'. This may involve changing items on a questionnaire, omitting some and adding others, simplifying the tool or using a different protocol. However, changing an outcome measure corrupts its validity (a bit like bending a ruler!) and as a result it will be impossible to interpret the information properly or compare findings with others. For example, there are numerous versions of the 10-metre walk test, which can create confusion and make comparison with other findings difficult. In other words, when using an outcome measure, it should be a validated one and used according to the published protocol.

There are different types of validity:

- Construct validity: this is the validity of the theoretical construct or phenomenon that is being measured (e.g. temperature). If one does not have a clear definition of a construct (e.g. tiredness) one would not be able to measure it.
- Content validity: this is the extent to which a measure comprehensively represents the construct that is measured. For example, the construct 'mobility' would normally involve both indoor and outdoor mobility and, therefore, a comprehensive assessment of mobility would need to include both elements. However, if 'mobility' is only assessed indoors, the content validity of tests can be considered to be limited (Lord and Rochester 2005).
- Criterion validity: this is the degree to which a measure (e.g. isometric grip force) is associated with other measures (e.g. arm function). There are two types of criterion validity:
  - Concurrent validity involves the extent to which a measure compares with a gold standard (e.g. in the measurement of physical activity, video recordings may be used as a gold standard against which the output of a novel activity monitor can be compared).
  - Predictive validity is the extent to which a measure predicts a future outcome (e.g. the extent to which the Berg Balance Scale at 1 month after stroke predicts independent walking at 6 months post stroke).

Reliability

Reliability indicates to what extent a measure is reproducible, in other words whether the measure gives the same result each time the same quantity is being measured. One challenge in measuring human performance is that this is inherently variable, both between people and within the same person (these sources of variation are known as *inter-subject* and *intra-subject* variability, respectively). An example of intra-subject variability is the fluctuation in balance within the same person; on a 'good day' one may be able to remain standing on one leg for a relatively long period of time, while on a 'bad day' one might lose balance after just a few seconds. After stroke, performance is known to be more variable than in healthy age-matched controls (van Vliet and Sheridan 2007). The inherent fluctuation in human performance is one of the reasons why group studies rather than single case studies are undertaken in research and, where possible and appropriate, the average of multiple rather than single measures (e.g. of the 10-metre walk test) are taken for an individual.

Another factor to consider is the reliability of the *instrument*; for example, measuring body height with a rigid ruler is likely to yield a very similar result each time, whereas a fabric tape measure will yield different results. Furthermore, it is important to note that the reliability of a measure is determined not only by the instrument itself but also by the way in which it is used. For example, if one exercise professional provides encouragement to a stroke survivor during the 10-metre walk test whilst another does not, they are likely to obtain different results. Or if the same exercise professional positions themselves in the middle of the trajectory on one occasion, but at the end of the trajectory at another occasion, this is also likely to affect findings, because the different lines of sight affect the assessor's perception of the end position (a phenomenon known as parallax). These examples highlight the need for *standardised protocols*.

Ideally, Each Exercise after Stroke service should have a core set of standardised outcome measures, together with written protocols in which professionals are trained, to ensure an acceptable level of standardisation. This is to improve the following types of reliability:

- Inter-rater reliability: the consistency between different assessors in measuring the same phenomenon.

- Intra-rater reliability: the consistency within the same assessor in measuring the same phenomenon on more than one occasion.

Sensitivity to change

Sensitivity (also known as responsiveness) is the level of change that an instrument is capable of detecting. On rating scales, a dichotomous scale (e.g. Yes/No) provides limited sensitivity, while a 10-point scale provides a considerably higher level of sensitivity. Working with stroke survivors, it is important to use measures with a sufficient level of sensitivity to detect relevant changes. Changes are unlikely to be fast or dramatic in this population, and more subtle changes may be missed if only crude scales are used. Limitations to responsiveness are:

- A *floor effect*: this means that impairments below a certain threshold cannot be detected reliably. For example, small improvements in active finger movement in severely affected stroke survivors may not show up on the Nine Hole Peg Test (Heller et al. 1987), which requires a high level of dexterity.
- A *ceiling effect*: this means that the scale is incapable of registering any further improvement. For example, the commonly used Barthel Index (Mahoney and Barthel 1965) is unable to record improvements in subtle impairments and activity limitations, and may (wrongly) report that a stroke survivor has fully recovered if they score the maximum possible score (Duncan et al. 2000).

MEASUREMENT ERROR

No matter how sophisticated the instrument, *errors* are inevitable in any form of measurement. There are two sources of error (or variance): systematic and random.

Systematic measurement errors

A *systematic* error is a constant error. An example is a weighing scale that has been poorly calibrated, and always overestimates body weight by a certain amount. Provided that this error is known (i.e. by systematically comparing the readings from the scale with known weights), it is, in principle, relatively simple to deal with: for every measurement, the error should be reduced from the measured quantity to yield the actual quantity.

Random measurement errors

A *random* error fluctuates unpredictably and is therefore more difficult to deal with. Several measurements may be required to obtain an accurate average; but in practice this is clearly problematic, especially when working with stroke survivors in whom fatigue may limit repetitive testing.

In order to reduce error, measurement tools should be properly calibrated, and detailed standard protocols should be used in which assessors have been trained.

Now that these generic scientific principles of measurement have been discussed, let us turn to the more pragmatic aspects of outcome assessment.

PRAGMATIC CONSIDERATIONS

Practicability

Practicability is a generic term to indicate how feasible it is to use a measure in practice. This comprises the amount of information required (e.g. blood pressure requires just a single measure, whereas the Stroke Impact Scale involves numerous questions); the duration and complexity of the process; and the burden of assessment on the stroke survivor as well as the exercise professional. Although there are many excellent outcome measures available – in the sense of their scientific properties – many are unused because they fall down on their practicability. If the process is complex, time consuming, and tiring for the stroke survivor, it is unlikely to be used routinely.

This brings us to the setting in which the outcome assessment takes place, and how this may inform the choice of outcome measures. Clearly, in a routine leisure setting, it is not feasible – or sensible – to use an extensive battery of complex, detailed outcome measures; unless, perhaps, there is a specific audit or research project underway. It may be helpful to imagine a continuum, with 'routine evaluation' at one end and 'research' at the other (Fig. 11.3):

- For routine evaluation of individual participants, UK national clinical guidelines on Exercise after Stroke in community settings (Best et al. 2010) recommend that this comprise an attendance register and at least one outcome measure (e.g. a timed walk test, the timed up-and-go (Podsiadlo and Richardson, 1991), or a measure of personal goal attainment). The register provides information on the number of sessions attended over a particular period of time, while absence may alert the exercise professional to a participant who may require follow-up.
- For service evaluation purposes, a wider range of additional outcomes may be considered, including functional outcomes (see Table 11.1 for examples) and stroke survivors' experiences of the service (see below).

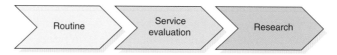

FIG 11.3 A continuum of complexity of outcome assessment, from routine evaluation to research.

- For research purposes, the outcomes selected will depend on the specific research question or hypothesis of the study. The Fugl-Meyer test (Fugl-Meyer et al. 1975) and Stroke Impact Scale (Duncan et al. 1999, 2001, 2003a,b) are examples of detailed tools that are more appropriate for research purposes. Additionally, VO_2 max, considered the criterion measure for cardiorespiratory fitness, requires specialist equipment and trained staff and it, therefore, also tends to be reserved for clinical and research settings (ACSM 2010).

Inclusivity

As we have seen in chapter 3, sensory/perceptual, cognitive and communication difficulties are common amongst stroke survivors. This may mean that a proportion of people with stroke are excluded from the process of outcome assessment, if they are presented in a format (e.g. long questionnaire with complex questions) that the individual is unable to engage with in a meaningful way. It is therefore important that the language, design and format are all suitable given the person's abilities and disabilities. Stroke survivors with communication difficulties may need communication support if they are asked to fill in a questionnaire or report on their experiences.

Communicability

Communicability indicates how easy it is to communicate the information obtained from the outcome assessment to others (e.g. the stroke survivor, colleagues and service managers). Factors to consider include the amount, format and standardisation of information. Blood pressure measurement usually yields two figures, which are easy to report and understand, as there is a standardised format for this information. In contrast, biomechanical gait data tend to be extensive, complex and usually require training to fully understand.

INTERPRETING THE RESULT

After the assessment process is complete, how do we decide what the findings mean? Firstly, error needs to be taken into account to distinguish 'noise' from a 'real' outcome. For example, if one measures dexterity on the Nine Hole Peg Test (a task where the participant places wooden pegs in a board as fast as possible), a change of 0.05 pegs per second is more likely to be 'noise' associated with inconsistent use of a stopwatch than a 'real' improvement.

The interpretation of outcomes also depends on how they compare, for example, to the same individual at an earlier time point (e.g. before starting an exercise programme), to a group of similar individuals (e.g. a whole stroke exercise class), or other data published in the literature, including age-matched, healthy controls (i.e. normative data). For this reason, it is often helpful to choose an outcome measure that is commonly used – provided that it meets the criteria listed in this chapter. Which measures are commonly used in the field of exercise and fitness training after stroke? In the Cochrane systematic review of 24 trials evaluating the effects of exercise and fitness training after stroke (Saunders et al. 2009), the majority of measures concentrated on the activity domain of the ICF, within which most focused on walking. Impairment-orientated measures featured less frequently and comprised gait biomechanics, muscle strength and motor performance. Interestingly, measures of cardiorespiratory fitness were used infrequently, with (maximum) cycling work rate being used in four of the 24 studies, followed by gait economy and maximum VO_2 uptake in two studies each. Respiratory exchange ratio, ten repetition maximum or the step test were only used in one study each. Measures of body composition were entirely absent in this body of literature. Measures reflecting the participation domain of the ICF appear to have been rarely used in these studies with the SF-36 featuring in only four studies, exposing a considerable gap in the evidence.

Finally, to judge whether a difference in outcome represents a change that is meaningful, the term 'minimal clinically important difference' may be a useful concept to consider. Although this is subject to debate, it has been described as a difference considered to be meaningful by the patient (Copay et al. 2007). For example, for the Stroke Impact Scale, a change of between 10% and 15% was considered to constitute a clinically relevant difference (Duncan et al. 1999).

EVALUATING EXERCISE AFTER STROKE: A QUALITATIVE APPROACH

So far, we have taken a predominantly quantitative approach to outcome assessment; however, qualitative information can also be invaluable. Qualitative data (e.g. on participants' experiences of the exercise programme) can help explain findings on attendance rates and the impact of the service on stroke survivors' health and wellbeing. There is currently very little research on how people with stroke experience exercise or fitness training programmes.

The studies that have been published to date (Carin-Levy et al. 2009, Sharma et al. 2011, Wiles et al. 2008) suggest that exercise undertaken in groups of stroke survivors can improve confidence, not just in undertaking exercise, but also in other activities outside the sessions. An evaluation of stroke survivors' perceptions of a community-based exercise and education scheme (Reed et al. 2010) suggested that exercise and goal setting were valued as positive actions in the process of reconstructing life after stroke. Stroke survivors participating in a stroke-specific exercise referral scheme indicated this had been pivotal for their independence and enhanced lifestyle, work and social participation (Sharma et al. 2011). Together, these studies indicate the benefit of obtaining information on the experiences of service users. It is therefore recommended that Exercise after Stroke services seek user views routinely to further inform and improve service delivery.

In collecting service user views, rigorous methods should be employed, such as validated questionnaires, semi-structured interviews or focus groups, to minimise the effects of bias and enhance dependability of the analysis. For further guidance on qualitative research methods, the reader is referred to Richards (2005) and Auerbach and Silverstein (2003).

ADVERSE EVENTS

Information on adverse events should be recorded accurately to enable services to conduct risk–benefit analyses. The greatest risk of adverse events during exercise (for a general population) is from musculoskeletal injuries and cardiac events. Cardiac events are a particular concern for people with stroke because of the significant co-morbidity between stroke and coronary artery disease (see chapter 9).

The Cochrane systematic review of physical fitness training after stroke (Brazzelli et al. 2011, Saunders et al. 2009) examined adverse events reported in studies included in the review. Unfortunately, however, these had not always been reported systematically. This finding was echoed in another Cochrane review of circuit class interventions to improve mobility after stroke, where only two of the six trials reported adverse events during the intervention (English and Hillier 2010). This included more falls in the intervention group and, although these were minor and there were no injuries in these studies, the findings highlight the importance of recording falls. As a minimum, falls and cardiac events should be recorded, as well as hypoglycaemia in people with diabetes. Other events that could be recorded include cardiac events, falls with no injury, falls with an injury, muscle aches, fatigue.

Adverse events should be noted in records specific to the exercise after stroke sessions – not just in the venue's incident and accident book. This is to enable stroke-specific audits to take place, and analyse any trends specific to this population.

SUMMARY POINTS

- Outcome assessment enables stroke survivors and their family, exercise professionals, service managers and commissioners to evaluate the impact of exercise on health, wellbeing and personal goal attainment.
- The World Health Organization International Classification of Health Functioning and Disability (or ICF) (WHO 2001) can provide a framework for identifying the ICF domain(s) that outcome measures represent.
- Fitness-related outcome measures fall predominantly in the body structures/function domain of the ICF.
- Where possible, exercise professionals should consider including outcome measures that represent the exercise goals that have been chosen by the stroke survivor.
- One should begin the process of outcome assessment by asking 'What do I need to know?' Once this has been identified, the process of choosing an outcome measure can begin. The requirements for an appropriate outcome measure are that it be relevant, ethical, valid, reliable and responsive to change, as well as inclusive, practicable and easy to communicate. Interpretation of the meaning of outcomes should take into account the inevitable measurement errors, normative data and minimal clinically important differences, wherever this information is available.
- Information from outcome assessment – whether obtained through qualitative or quantitative methods – is essential for tailoring and improving services to the needs of service users, and demonstrating accountability and evidence-based practice.

American College of Sports Medicine (ACSM), 2010. Guidelines for exercise testing and prescription, eighth ed. Williams and Wilkins, London.

Auerbach, C., Silverstein, L., 2003. Qualitative data: an introduction to coding and analysis. NYU Press, New York.

Berg, K.O., Wood-Dauphinee, S.L., Williams, J.I., et al., 1989. Measuring balance in elderly: preliminary development of an instrument. Physiother. Can. 41, 304–311.

Best, C., van Wijck, F., Dinan-Young, S., et al., 2010. Best practice guidance for the development of Exercise after Stroke services in community settings. Edinburgh University, Edinburgh. Available online at: http://www.exerciseafterstroke.org.uk/ (accessed 08.09.2011).

Bond, M.R., Pilowsky, I., 1966. The subjective assessment of pain and its relationship to the administration of analgesics in patients with advanced cancer. J. Psychosom. Res. 10, 203–208.

Brazzelli, M., Saunders, D.H., Greig, C.A., 2011. Physical fitness training for stroke patients. Cochrane Database Syst. Rev. 11, CD003316.

Carin-Levy, G., Kendall, M., Young, A., et al., 2009. The psychosocial effects of exercise and relaxation classes for persons surviving a stroke. Can. J. Occup. Ther. 76, 73–76.

Collen, F.M., Wade, D.T., Bradshaw, C.M., 1990. Mobility after stroke: reliability of measures of impairment and disability. Int. Disabil. Stud. 12, 6–9.

Copay, A.G., Subach, B.R., Glassman, S.D., et al., 2007. Understanding the minimum clinically important difference: a review of concepts and methods. Spine J. 7, 541–546.

Department of Health, 2001. Exercise referral systems: a national quality assurance framework. Department of Health, London. Available online at: http://www.dh.gov.uk/prod_consum_dh/groups/dh_digitalassets/@dh/@en/documents/digitalasset/dh_4079009.pdf (accessed 09.09.2011).

Durward, B.R., Baer, G.D., Rowe, P.J., 1999. Measurement issues in functional human movement. In: Durward, B.R., Baer, G.D., Rowe, P.J. (Eds.), Functional human movement. Measurement and analysis. Butterworth-Heinemann, Oxford, pp. 1–12.

Duncan, P.W., Wallace, D., Lai, S.M., et al., 1999. The Stroke Impact Scale version 2.0. Evaluation of reliability, validity, and sensitivity to change. Stroke 30, 2131–2140.

Duncan, P.W., Lai, S.M., Keighly, J., 2000. Defining post-stroke recovery: implications for design and interpretation of drug trials. Neuropharmacology 39, 835–841.

Duncan, P.W., Wallace, D., Studenski, S., et al., 2001. Conceptualization of a new stroke-specific outcome measure: the stroke impact scale. Top. Stroke Rehabil. 8, 19–33.

Duncan, P.W., Bode, R.K., Lai, M.S., et al., 2003a. Rasch analysis of a new stroke-specific outcome scale: the Stroke Impact Scale. Arch. Phys. Med. Rehabil. 84, 950–963.

Duncan, P.W., Lai, M.S., Bode, R.K., et al., 2003b. Stroke Impact Scale-16: a brief assessment of physical function. Neurology 60, 291–296.

Duncan, P.W., Sullivan, K.J., Behrman, A.L., et al., 2007. Protocol for the Locomotor Experience Applied Post-stroke (LEAPS) trial: a randomized controlled trial. BMC Neurol. 7, 39.

Eng, J.J., Chu, K.S., Dawson, A.S., et al., 2002. Functional walk tests in individuals with stroke: relation to perceived exertion and myocardial exertion. Stroke 33, 756–761.

English, C., Hillier, S.L., 2010. Circuit class therapy for improving mobility after stroke. Cochrane Database Syst. Rev. 7, CD007513. doi:10.1002/14651858.

Fitts, S.S., Guthrie, M.R., 1995. Six-minute walk by people with chronic renal failure: assessment of effort by perceived exertion. Am. J. Phys. Med. Rehabil. 80, 837–858.

Fugl-Meyer, A.R., Jaasko, K., Leyman, I., et al., 1975. The post-stroke hemiplegic patient. 1. A method for evaluation of physical performance. Scand. J. Rehabil. Med. 7, 13–31.

Granger, C.V., Cotter, A.C., Hamilton, B.B., et al., 1993. Functional Assessment Scales: a study of persons after stroke. Arch. Phys. Med. Rehabil. 74, 133–138.

Guyatt, G.H., Sullivan, M.J., Thompson, P.J., et al., 1985. The 6-minute walk: a new measure of exercise capacity in patients

PRACTICAL APPLICATIONS OF EXERCISE AND FITNESS TRAINING

with chronic heart failure. Can. Med. Assoc. J. 132, 919–923.

Heller, A., Wade, D.T., Wood, V.A., et al., 1987. Arm function after stroke: measurement and recovery over the first three months. J. Neurol. Neurosurg. Psychiatry 50, 714–719.

Holden, M.K., Gill, K.M., Magliozzi, M.R., et al., 1984. Clinical gait assessment in the neurologically impaired. Reliability and meaningfulness. Phys. Ther. 64, 35–40.

Holden, M.K., Gill, K.M., Magliozzi, M.R., 1986. Gait assessment for neurologically impaired patients. Standards for outcome assessment. Phys. Ther. 66, 1530–1539.

Ivey, F.M., Ryan, S.A., Hafer-Macko, C.E., et al., 2011. Stroke. In: Saxton, J.M. (Ed.), Exercise and chronic disease. An evidence-based approach. Taylor & Francis, London, pp. 56–91.

King, R.B., Shade-Zeldow, Y., Carlson, C.E., et al., 2002. Adaptation to stroke: a longitudinal study of depressive symptoms, physical health, and coping process. Top. Stroke Rehabil. 9, 46–66.

Kondraske, G.V., 1989. Measurement science concepts and computerized methodology in the assessment of human performance. In: Munsat, T.L. (Ed.), Quantification of neurologic deficit. Butterworths, Stoneham, pp. 33–48.

Law, M., Baptiste, S., Carswell, A., et al., 1998. Canadian occupational performance measure. CAOT Publications, Ottawa.

Lawler, J., Dowswell, G., Hearn, J., et al., 1999. Recovering from stroke: a qualitative investigation of the role of goal setting in late stroke recovery. J. Adv. Nurs. 30, 401–409.

Lord, S.E., Rochester, L., 2005. Measurement of community ambulation after stroke: current status and future developments. Stroke 36, 1457–1461.

Mahoney, F.I., Barthel, D.W., 1965. Functional evaluation: the Barthel Index. Md. State Med. J. 14, 61–65.

Podsiadlo, D., Richardson, S., 1991. The Timed 'Up & Go': A test of basic functional mobility for frail elderly persons. J. Am. Geriatr. Soc. 39, 142–148.

Price, C.I.M., Curless, R.H., Rodgers, H., 1999. Can stroke patients use visual analogue scales? Stroke 30, 1357–1361.

Reed, M., Harrington, R., Duggan, A., et al., 2010. Meeting stroke survivors' perceived needs: a qualitative study of a community-based exercise and education scheme. Clin. Rehabil. 24, 16–25.

Richards, L., 2005. Handling qualitative data: a practical guide. Sage Publications, London.

Rimmer, J.H., Wang, E., Smith, D., 2008. Barriers associated with exercise and community access for individuals with stroke. J. Rehabil. Res. Dev. 45, 315–322.

Salter, K., Jutai, J., Zettler, L., et al., 2010. Outcome measures. EBRSR: Evidence-Based Review of Stroke Rehabilitation. Available online at: http://www.ebrsr.com/ (accessed 07.09.2011).

Saunders, D.H., Greig, C.A., Mead, G.E., Young, A., 2009. Physical fitness training for stroke patients. Cochrane Database Syst. Rev. 4, CD003316. doi:10.1002/14651858.

Sharma, H., Bulley, C., van Wijck, F., 2011. Experiences of an exercise referral scheme from the perspective of people with chronic stroke: a qualitative study. Physiotherapy doi:org/10.1016/j.physio.2011.05.004.

Steffen, T.M., Hacker, T.A., Mollinger, L., 2002. Age- and gender-related test performance in community-dwelling elderly people: Six-Minute Walk Test, Berg Balance Scale, Timed Up & Go Test, and gait speeds. Phys. Ther. 82, 128–137.

Tinetti, M.E., Williams, T.F., Mayewski, R., 1986. Fall risk index for elderly patients based on number of chronic disabilities. Am. J. Med. 80, 429–434.

Turner-Stokes, L., 2009. Goal attainment scaling (GAS) in rehabilitation: a practical guide. Clin. Rehabil. 23, 362–370.

van Vliet, P.M., Sheridan, M.R., 2007. Coordination between reaching and grasping in patients with hemiparesis and normal subjects. Arch. Phys. Med. Rehabil. 88, 1325–1331.

Wade, D.T., 1992. Measurement in neurological rehabilitation. Oxford University Press, Oxford.

Ware Jr., J.E., Sherbourne, C.D., 1992. The MOS 36-item short-form health survey (SF36) I: Conceptual framework and item selection. Med. Care 30, 473–483.

Wiles, R., Demain, S., Robison, J., et al., 2008. Exercise on prescription schemes for stroke patients post-discharge from physiotherapy. Disabil. Rehabil. 30, 1966–1975.

Willenheimer, R., Erhardt, L., 2000. Value of 6-min-walk test for assessment of severity and prognosis of heart failure. Lancet 355, 515–516.

World Health Organization (WHO), 2001. International Classification of Functioning, Disability and Health. Available online at: http://www3.who.int/icf/intros/ICF-Eng-Intro.pdf (accessed 08.09.2011).

Zigmond, A.S., Snaith, R.P., 1983. The Hospital Anxiety Depression Scale. Acta. Psychiatr. Scand. 67, 361–370.

PART 4
EXERCISE AFTER STROKE: SERVICE DESIGN AND GUIDELINES

PART CONTENTS

Models of Exercise after Stroke service design

Catherine S. Best

CHAPTER CONTENTS

INTRODUCTION

In the previous chapters, we detailed the design, delivery and evaluation of exercise and fitness training programmes for stroke survivors. This final part of the book will take a wider perspective. This chapter will explore the different models currently in existence that provide Exercise after Stroke services, and address key questions regarding the implementation of such services. The next and final chapter will present current best practice guidance for community-based Exercise after Stroke services.

The content of this chapter is based on a survey of existing Exercise after Stroke services in Scotland (Best et al. 2011) which – to our knowledge – is currently the most detailed source of information on models of service design for Exercise after Stroke in the UK. Other relevant international publications will also be discussed, including a survey of fitness facilities in Canada (Fullerton et al. 2008).

EXISTING MODELS OF COMMUNITY EXERCISE AFTER STROKE SERVICES

Our research, which included contact with Exercise after Stroke service providers in the UK (Best et al. 2011), and a review of the international exercise after stroke literature, showed that there are several means by which stroke survivors access exercise:

- Exercise referral schemes.
- Cardiac rehabilitation, adapted cardiac rehabilitation and falls prevention schemes.
- Stroke-specific exercise sessions (run by health services, leisure services, and/or stroke charities).
- Multi-pathology exercise services, i.e. services that provide exercise to groups of people with a variety of different health conditions.
- Other options for aerobic exercise not specifically adapted to stroke, e.g. disability sports groups, disability swimming sessions, over fifties classes, aqua aerobics, personal trainers.
- Other options without an aerobic training component, e.g. Tai Chi, yoga, Pilates and stroke-specific seated exercise.

Each of these options will be discussed in more detail below.

EXERCISE REFERRAL SCHEMES

Exercise referral schemes (also known as physical activity referral schemes or exercise on prescription) are multi-agency services whereby general practitioners (primary care physicians) or other nominated health-care professionals can refer patients for an individually tailored programme of exercise, designed by a suitably qualified exercise professional (Department of Health 2001).

Exercise referral is designed to combat the high levels of physical inactivity and sedentary behaviour within the population as a whole. People referred to exercise referral schemes are those who need more than just advice or recommendation from a health-care professional in order to become more active, e.g. motivational support and a programme of exercise that has been tailored to their needs and preferences.

Exercise referral schemes are a structured link between health and leisure services which ensures that:

- The exercise professional has appropriate qualifications and resources
- The exercise professional receives adequate medical referral information
- The participant has been risk-assessed for exercise by the health professional prior to referral.

In 2001 the UK Department of Health published a quality assurance system for exercise referral schemes to ensure these standards of service delivery.

Exercise referral schemes are organised locally and therefore have different characteristics (e.g. referral pathways, inclusion criteria), depending on local circumstances. For this reason, exercise referral schemes in the UK vary greatly in terms of:

- Their target groups: these can be defined as sedentary individuals, the economically deprived, people with existing health conditions or people at identified risk of future health problems.
- The length of the intervention.
- The location: this includes local leisure centres, swimming pools, or the outdoors.
- The type of intervention: this could be individual gym programmes, group exercise, or walking groups.
- The amount of follow up: that is, whether participants who do not attend a session are contacted to ascertain the reason for non-attendance and/or whether outcome measures are recorded.

We have anecdotal reports that stroke survivors are successfully using these services and achieving good outcomes. It is estimated that around 400–500 stroke survivors per year access the Live Active exercise referral scheme run in the NHS Greater Glasgow and Clyde area of the UK (Forsyth 2009).

Generic exercise referrals schemes (i.e. not targeted at stroke survivors) exist across the world, including Scandinavia (e.g. Leijon et al. 2009) and Europe (e.g. Schmidt et al. 2008), while the principle of referral for exercise is also well developed in the United States (American College of Sports Medicine 2010).

The positive aspects of using exercise referral schemes for stroke survivors are that exercise referral is a highly individualised process where each participant will have a personal activity programme tailored to their preferred mode of exercise, with attention given to individual barriers and motivators to becoming more active. Another positive factor is that generic exercise referral schemes can achieve good community penetration: a recent survey found that 70% of general practitioners in Scotland had access to a generic exercise referral scheme (Jepson et al. 2010).

There are some limitations, however, in using exercise referral as a model for Exercise after Stroke, which pertain to:

- Exercise professional qualifications. Most exercise professionals employed on exercise referral schemes in the UK have a general qualification (in the UK a Register of Exercise Professionals Level 3 qualification) rather than an advanced exercise qualification specific to stroke (in the UK a Register of Exercise Professionals Level 4 qualification). The majority of exercise professionals in exercise referral schemes, therefore, do not have the specialist qualifications required to work with people who have had a stroke. In a qualitative study of stroke survivors, physiotherapists and exercise professionals involved in an exercise referral scheme in the south of England, appropriate knowledge of stroke amongst exercise professionals was considered important by stroke survivors (Wiles et al. 2008), and there were concerns from physiotherapists that, due to the limited knowledge of exercise professionals about stroke, only the least physically impaired patients could be referred to the service.

- The emphasis on individual exercise. Most exercise referral schemes do not include group exercise sessions. Therefore, stroke survivors may miss the social aspects of exercising in a group with other people in a similar situation. The element of social support from fellow exercise participants has been reported to be highly valued in studies of experiences of Exercise after Stroke (e.g. Carin-Levy et al. 2009, Reed et al. 2010, Sharma et al. 2011), as described in chapter 6.
- Time-limited nature of exercise referral schemes. Exercise referral schemes work mainly on an individual basis and therefore capacity issues mean they are often time-limited. Some stroke survivors may not be able to move on to independent or mainstream exercise, so they would either have to continue with one-to-one support indefinitely, which is not cost-effective, or the individual may not be able to continue in structured exercise.

CARDIAC REHABILITATION

Cardiac rehabilitation is *'the process by which patients with cardiac disease, in partnership with a multidisciplinary team of health professionals, are encouraged and supported to achieve and maintain optimal physical and psychosocial health'* (Scottish Intercollegiate Guideline Network Guideline 2002, p. 1).

Cardiac rehabilitation programmes for patients with cardiac disease include supported exercise and lifestyle advice. The process of cardiac rehabilitation is divided into four phases that begin in acute hospital care, and end in long-term maintenance of exercise and healthy lifestyle, in the community. An important component of cardiac rehabilitation is the exercise intervention and this has been shown to have considerable health benefits independent of other aspects of the programme (Jolliffe et al. 2001). Overall, the evidence of the effectiveness of cardiac rehabilitation in improving outcomes for people with cardiac problems is very strong. Cardiac rehabilitation programmes are widespread across the UK and the rest of the developed nations and, although access to long-term maintenance exercise classes in the community is limited in some areas, cardiac rehabilitation community exercise sessions are far more widespread than Exercise after Stroke groups at present.

Adapted cardiac rehabilitation

Tang and colleagues working in Canada argued against developing new community Exercise after Stroke services, suggesting instead that cardiac rehabilitation should be adapted to include stroke survivors (Tang et al. 2009). The arguments for this are as follows:

- There is considerable co-morbidity between stroke and heart disease. It has been estimated that up to 75% of stroke survivors have co-morbid heart disease (Roth 1993) and the two conditions have considerable overlap in modifiable risk factors.
- Cardiac rehabilitation services are already well established, and there are well-developed referral pathways from the health service.

However, in a survey of cardiac rehabilitation services in the Ontario area of Canada, only about 5% of participants in these classes were stroke survivors, even though 60% of cardiac rehabilitation services accepted stroke survivors (Tang et al. 2009). Tang et al. (2010) compared the outcomes of users who had primary stroke diagnosis and cardiac diagnoses, or primary cardiac and stroke, or just a cardiac diagnosis: all three groups had similar benefits from a cardiac rehabilitation programme in improving peak oxygen capacity.

There are two ways in which the cardiac rehabilitation model could be utilised to develop Exercise after Stroke services:

1. By including stroke survivors in existing cardiac rehabilitation services as described above; however, stroke-specific adaptations should be in place, as described in chapter 10.
2. By using cardiac rehabilitation exercise classes as a template, i.e. designing a stroke-specific service based on the phased model of cardiac rehabilitation.

Where cardiac rehabilitation is used as a template for stroke-specific services, there are two key elements of cardiac rehabilitation that could be transferred. The first is that cardiac rehabilitation begins during inpatient stay and the first exposure to exercise is in a clinical environment, supervised by a health-care professional. When the cardiac patient then starts to exercise in the community, they know the duration and intensity of exercise that they can tolerate and will have learnt about their body's response to exercise. The second element is that cardiac rehabilitation includes lifestyle advice and more holistic rehabilitation interventions. Exercise after Stroke services run by several health services in Scotland have taken on some elements of the cardiac rehabilitation model. Although their exercise programmes were specifically adapted for stroke survivors and tailored to the individual, the systems approaches were similar to cardiac rehabilitation in that they:

- Were conducted in a rehabilitation setting
- Were run by health-care professionals (physiotherapists, nurses and assistants)
- Included an educational component
- Were time limited
- Acted as a risk assessment or transition to exercise in community venues.

In this way, these services were very similar to phase 3 cardiac rehabilitation which has '*historically taken the form of a structured exercise programme in a hospital setting with educational and psychological support and advice on risk factors*' (Scottish Intercollegiate Guidelines Network Guideline 57. 2002, p. 1).

It is a very parsimonious solution to replicate models from other health service programmes that have already been implemented effectively. However, we need further research evidence about whether the education component is independently effective in improving outcomes for stroke survivors. Harrington et al. (2010) conducted a randomised controlled trial of a community-based exercise and education intervention for stroke survivors. Their parallel qualitative study (Reed et al. 2010) indicated that participants did not find all of the education sessions useful.

Aerobic training is already recommended as part of rehabilitation for stroke in UK clinical guidelines (Royal College of Physicians 2008) so it would seem that joining up inpatient and community-exercise programmes to an integrated patient pathway would seem an optimum model for future service development (this will be further discussed at the end of the chapter).

FALLS PREVENTION MODEL

In addition to cardiac rehabilitation, another example of existing models of exercise for older people that has been applied to stroke is falls prevention. Stroke survivors are more likely to have falls and fractures than unaffected community-dwelling older people. In an ongoing trial in Australia, Dean et al. (2009) are looking at the effects of a group exercise programme on balance and mobility in stroke survivors. Batchelor et al. (2009) are also looking at the effects of a complex intervention, including exercise, on the rate of falls in stroke survivors in the community. More information will be available on completion of these studies but it seems likely that exercises for falls prevention should be incorporated into Exercise after Stroke sessions, as was done for the STARTER trial (Mead et al. 2007).

STROKE-SPECIFIC EXERCISE SESSIONS

At the time of writing, there was only one published paper on Exercise after Stroke service implementation, describing how a 'real world' service was developed. This paper by Stuart et al. (2008) described the Adaptive Physical Activity programme provided in the Empoli region of Italy. Italy has a very high proportion of older people in the population (22% of the population in the Empoli region are over 65 years of age). The Adaptive Physical Activity programme was developed to serve people with back pain, flexed posture, Parkinson's disease or stroke.

Adaptive Physical Activity programme

Stuart et al. (2008) reported that around 200 people with stroke were accessing 17 stroke Adaptive Physical Activity services in Empoli. The sessions were held in gymnasia throughout the region and run by exercise professionals who were trained by physiotherapists in the principles of the programme. Participants were referred to the programme by their general practitioner. Participants exercised three times a week. The programme, which consisted of three 1-hour exercise sessions per week, was intense in comparison to other community programmes that we are aware of in the UK, which offer sessions only once a week. The Adaptive Physical Activity programme sessions were held during off-peak periods at the gymnasia in order to reduce the costs.

Organisation and delivery of the programme

The Adaptive Physical Activity programme was developed through collaboration between the US National Institutes for Health and their Italian counterpart. It was planned to replicate this service in the Maryland region of the US through a collaboration between the US Veteran's Health Administration and the Administration on Aging. To our knowledge, this was the only large-scale implementation of stroke-specific exercise classes to have been reported. Importantly, this project also included a research component.

Evaluation of the Adaptive Physical Activity programme

Stuart et al. (2009) reported a non-randomised controlled study of the Stroke Adaptive Physical Activity programme. The study included 40 participants in the intervention group and an equivalent number in the control group. At 6 months follow-up, the intervention group improved, whereas the control group declined on measures of walking speed, balance and social participation. There were 15 participants in the intervention group and 13 in the control group who were assessed as depressed on entry to the study (Hamilton rating scale for depression ≥8). Participants in the intervention group who were depressed on study entry improved by follow-up at 6 months (mean improvement of 4.4. points on the Hamilton scale), whereas the controls were unchanged (this difference in change score was significant at $p < 0.03$).

This study is important both because it is an existing programme, i.e. it is real-life implementation, but also because it shows what the potential benefits of long-term attendance might be. Most research interventions last around 12 weeks and it has been noted that, after the end of the intervention, much of the benefit is lost (e.g. Mead et al. 2007). The Adaptive Physical Activity programme was an on-going programme where participants exercised for 6 months. It is very interesting that much of the difference between groups was caused by the control group deteriorating over this time, while the intervention group did not.

EXERCISE AFTER STROKE SERVICE DEVELOPMENT IN OTHER NATIONAL CONTEXTS

The Adaptive Physical Activity programme is the only report of large-scale strategic Exercise after Stroke implementation to date. In the absence of any published evidence from other national contexts (e.g. where there is a lower proportion of older people in the population or no national organisations leading on Exercise after Stroke initiatives), the best available evidence on implementation strategies is to find out how Exercise after Stroke services have evolved at a local level. These services have generally developed in a piecemeal fashion by responding to local circumstances. However, they provide important information on models of stroke-specific exercise that are both feasible and acceptable to stroke survivors in practice.

Surveys of Exercise after Stroke services

To our knowledge, as ascertained through comprehensive searches of the research literature and more general search via internet search engines, there have only been two systematic attempts to identify existing exercise provision for stroke survivors. One was by our research group, when we conducted a survey of Exercise after Stroke services in Scotland UK (Best et al. 2011); the other was by Fullerton et al. (2008) in their survey of fitness training for stroke survivors in the Greater Toronto area, Canada. Both studies found that there was a very low level of Exercise after Stroke service provision. Both studies also found that the majority of exercise sessions for stroke survivors were run by non-profit-making (i.e. charity, or third sector) organisations.

From our survey, we found that the Exercise after Stroke services varied considerably based on the lead organisation, i.e. whether they were run by charities, leisure services or health services. We found no Exercise after Stroke groups run by private organisations. The characteristics of the charity-, leisure- and health service-led Exercise after Stroke services in Scotland are outlined below.

Charity-led Exercise after Stroke services

- Services were not time-limited, i.e. stroke survivors could continue to attend for as long as they wanted; in some instances, stroke survivors had been attending Exercise after Stroke services for over 13 years.
- Emphasis was placed on mutual social support. Service development was driven by the wishes of the members (i.e. members wanted to work on their fitness so the group sought ways to enable this to happen).
- Referral and assessment processes were reduced to a minimum.
- Assessment methods were largely informal, i.e. not using standardised instruments and no outcome measurement. This aligns with the history and aims of these groups, which are primarily about empowering stroke survivors to access exercise.
- Sessions were led by exercise professionals or physiotherapists, either on a voluntary basis (unpaid) or paid on an hourly basis.
- Sessions were located in community halls, colleges or leisure centres.

Leisure centre Exercise after Stroke services in Scotland

- Sessions were led by exercise professionals with an advanced qualification in designing, adapting and delivering exercise for stroke survivors. The exercise professionals were employed by the leisure service.
- Minimal inclusion and exclusion criteria. Participants also underwent only minimal outcome assessment. This aligned with the stated aim of these services to normalise (or 'de-medicalise') exercise for these groups, i.e. to make the experience of stroke survivors exercising at the leisure centre as close to that of other people as possible.
- Services were not time-limited.
- Close working relationships with the local physiotherapy teams. Although physiotherapists were not involved in delivering these sessions, they were highly involved in delivering training and specific advice to the exercise professionals.
- Sessions were located in leisure centres.

Health services providing Exercise after Stroke services in Scotland

- Services were time-limited.
- Sessions were all led by health-care professionals and assistants.
- Clear protocols for pre-exercise screening by a specified health-care professional were in place.
- Standardised assessment measures were used to screen participants before entry and to measure progress.
- Sessions were located in health-care venues.

As can be seen from the comparison above, the lead organisation clearly influences the structure and processes of Exercise after Stroke services.

MULTI-PATHOLOGY SERVICES

Our survey found that two areas in Scotland had comprehensive, functionally tiered, multi-pathology services that had sessions designed to accommodate stroke survivors. The multi-pathology services provided exercise sessions for people with a range of health conditions (e.g. cardiac disease, pulmonary disease, Parkinson's disease, multiple sclerosis and stroke). The exercise sessions were tiered according to level of mobility and cardiovascular fitness rather than the health condition. The multi-pathology services were described as comprehensive, as all the stroke-specific services ran one session per week in one venue, whereas the multi-pathology services were able to offer sessions across a number of venues in their area and on more than one day of the week.

The two multi-pathology services varied quite markedly in their assessment and referral processes. One service aimed to minimise the amount of referral information required and were moving towards a self-referral mechanism based on a modified Physical Activity Readiness Questionnaire (Canadian Society for Exercise Physiology 2002). This was in order to make the process of accessing exercise as similar to the experience of other leisure centre users as possible, and to facilitate access to these services. At the time of writing, participants were not referred to that service, but 'signposted' by their physiotherapist who gave the participant the information on medical and functional status required by the exercise professional in order to tailor the exercise programme to the individual. However, the other service only accepted referrals from acute care health professionals and had a condition-specific referral and assessment process in place.

The reason that these services opted to become 'multi-pathology' was that historically, beginning with cardiac rehabilitation over 15 years ago, leisure centres had been asked to provide condition-specific exercise classes for a growing number of health conditions. They were running separate classes for multiple sclerosis, chronic obstructive pulmonary disease, Parkinson's disease and a number of other conditions. There were three key reasons why condition-specific classes were abandoned in these areas:

- The numbers of people attending some of the condition-specific classes were very small, so the entrance fees were not enough to cover the cost of the exercise professional's time. Within the same area, some of the classes, e.g. the cardiac rehabilitation sessions, were often full to capacity.
- Participants did not come with only one health condition; many had co-morbidities that did not fit the model of condition-specific classes.
- The leisure centres were being asked to provide more condition-specific classes than was feasible.

The solution in these cases was to combine the classes into one single multi-pathology service that served people with a range of health conditions. This involved a partnership between health and leisure services. The stroke-specific services were not jointly funded or managed, although they worked closely with local physiotherapy teams and with members of the Stroke Managed Clinical Network. Managed Clinical Networks are 'linked groups of health professionals and organisations from primary, secondary and tertiary care, working in a coordinated manner, unconstrained by existing professional and [...] boundaries, to ensure equitable provision of high quality clinically effective services' (Department of Health 1999). Both multi-pathology services had jointly funded service coordinator posts.

For both multi-pathology services, devising the content of the sessions was a complex process whereby specialist physiotherapists involved with all the relevant health conditions came together with the exercise professionals and leisure managers to agree on the content of the sessions. This took a period of piloting and revising the interventions. The exercise professionals running these sessions had advanced training in, for example, cardiac rehabilitation or postural stability, and received additional 'bolt on' training from the local physiotherapy team in condition-specific considerations for exercise programming.

Positive aspects of multi-pathology exercise services are that:

- They are pragmatic: i.e. if it is not feasible for leisure centres to run the numbers of condition-specific classes they are being asked to provide, this is a way to ensure Exercise after Stroke services can be provided.
- They are potentially economically sustainable. In one service, participants pay to attend the sessions and the service aims to be economically sustainable by graduating the exercise professional/participant ratio across the tiers. That is, the classes for the less functionally impaired participants have high participant to exercise professional ratios and subsidise the sessions for the more functionally limited participants, which have lower participant/exercise professional ratios.
- Groups with different health conditions are mixed, with the result that stroke survivors do not get defined for the rest of their lives by the fact they have had a stroke. This may happen in condition-specific classes that support long-term attendance.

OTHER OPTIONS FOR AEROBIC EXERCISE NOT SPECIFICALLY ADAPTED TO STROKE

Our Scottish survey found that stroke survivors were accessing other kinds of exercise that had not been specifically adapted to the needs of stroke survivors. Respondents told us that stroke survivors were using 'over fifties' classes, aqua aerobics, disability sports groups and disability swimming sessions. We do not know whether these sessions, which have not been specifically adapted for stroke, lead to improved fitness or are safe in terms of managing post-stroke problems (e.g. increased tone, shoulder subluxation) and further research in this areas is required.

OTHER OPTIONS WITHOUT AN AEROBIC TRAINING COMPONENT

We were also told through our survey that stroke survivors were accessing Tai Chi, yoga and Pilates classes. There is very little research evidence about the application of Tai Chi and yoga to stroke. Some very small studies have found some evidence of potential benefits for Tai Chi (e.g. Hart et al. 2004) and specifically for Tai Chi on balance (e.g. Au-Yeung et al. 2009), but this requires further exploration through larger and more methodologically robust trials.

Model	Exercise professional	Coordinator	Venue	Participant fee
Table 12.1 *Overview of different service models for community-based Exercise after Stroke, as identified through a Scottish survey*				
Charity 1	Voluntary	Existing – charity	Existing – various	No
Charity 2	Service	Voluntary	Existing – LA	Yes
Local authority leisure services	Service	Service/existing – LA	Existing – LA	Yes
Multi-pathology services	Service	Health and LA	Existing – LA	Yes (free for first 10 weeks)
Health service	Existing – health	Existing – health	Existing – health	No

Voluntary, someone working in a voluntary (unpaid) capacity.
Existing, the service uses existing resources.
LA, local authority, local government provides this element.
Health, health services pay for this element.
Service, a new post associated with the Exercise after Stroke service.
Data summarised from Best et al. (2011).

FINANCIAL SUPPORT

Conducting the survey of Exercise after Stroke services involved contacting individuals in health services, local authority leisure services and stroke charities across Scotland. Table 12.1 shows the models of funding currently being employed in Scotland.

A finding worth highlighting was that the Charity type 2 service had been running for over 10 years in two areas of Scotland. This model therefore appears to be sustainable; however, the services are coordinated by stroke survivors working on a voluntary basis and their energy and commitment to these services have been crucial in keeping them running. It is unclear whether this could be replicated in a national service.

KEY QUESTIONS REGARDING THE IMPLEMENTATION OF EXERCISE AFTER STROKE SERVICES

The discussion of different models providing Exercise after Stroke services above highlights some key questions regarding the optimum implementation of Exercise after Stroke. These are:

- Should new models or existing templates be used?
- Should stroke-specific rather than multi-pathology classes be used?
- Is any activity a good thing?
- Which organisations should be involved in developing Exercise after Stroke services?
- How can access, equity, and quality assurance be ensured?

These questions will be addressed in turn below.

NEW MODELS OR EXISTING TEMPLATES?

The question is whether to adapt existing programmes (e.g. cardiac rehabilitation or falls prevention) to stroke, or to develop new stroke-specific programmes. At first glance it makes sense to build on existing infrastructure (e.g. referral routes), procedures (e.g. risk assessment, stratification and management) and experience in both the health and leisure services about running exercise services. Applying some elements of the cardiac rehabilitation template in a stroke-specific service is definitely of benefit, as described earlier in this chapter (e.g. the idea of providing a seamless but graduated service from inpatient to community exercise). However, we recommend that stroke survivors be provided with stroke-specific exercise services for the reasons outlined below.

Firstly, the evidence for exercise after stroke is based on trials that provided an intervention adapted to the specific needs of stroke survivors. It is not known whether a cardiac rehabilitation model of exercise would be effective (though this is being tested in at least one ongoing trial).

Secondly, stroke survivors are often left with a wide range of long-term post-stroke problems, which are very different from those experienced by most people surviving an acute coronary event. As described in chapter 3, these can include multiple complex neurological problems including 'hidden' impairments such as cognitive, executive or sensory impairment, coordination difficulties, as well as pain and joint instability. This has implications for the practical delivery of exercise, including the ratio of exercise professional to participant.

Thirdly, the fitness sector in the UK has developed national occupational standards for the training of exercise professionals working with stroke survivors. This is also a requirement to validate their professional insurance. This qualification is different from that of those working in cardiac rehabilitation.

Finally – and importantly – stroke survivors themselves have indicated that they can gain psychosocial benefits from exercising in a peer group, as described in chapter 6.

However, in the absence of stroke-specific exercise services, it would be reasonable to identify funding for exercise professionals working in cardiac rehabilitation and falls prevention to undertake stroke-specific training, and make use of the existing exercise referral schemes, applying appropriate pre-exercise screening and assessment, as described in chapter 10. We would, however, view this as a temporary measure.

The template of exercise referral used in the UK should also be used selectively. The fact that exercise referral is organised through primary care is a strength as it fits with the UK guidance on exercise referral requiring appropriate health professional assessment (Department of Health 2001). However, exercise referral schemes generally involve an exercise professional developing a tailored programme for the *individual*. This programme would then be carried out by the stroke survivor independently and progress reviewed by the exercise professional after a number of weeks (Wiles et al. 2008). For people who are unable to exercise without supervision, continued one-to-one support would be the only option – which is unlikely to be sustainable for large-scale implementation.

STROKE-SPECIFIC OR MULTI-PATHOLOGY?

Multi-pathology services are designed to include stroke survivors and it is better that stroke survivors have access to these groups than no adapted exercise session at all. However, for the reasons discussed above, the ideal would be that stroke survivors exercise in groups designed specifically around their needs and led by instructors with specialist stroke qualifications.

IS ANY ACTIVITY A GOOD THING?

Some of the options available to stroke survivors are not based on the evidence for Exercise after Stroke, discussed in chapter 4 (e.g. Tai Chi or Pilates). In these cases, we believe that service commissioning and development should be based as closely as possible on current and best quality research evidence and avoid directing stroke survivors to exercise options without evidence of safety or efficacy.

INTERDISCIPLINARY WORKING

Our survey found that most Exercise after Stroke services are run by charitable organisations in Scotland and the same is true in Greater Toronto, Canada. National stroke charities are the lead organisations most likely to be able to provide large-scale stroke-specific services in the UK. Our survey and contact with service providers has highlighted the importance of close interdisciplinary working in delivering Exercise after Stroke services; the ideal model would be a partnership between health, leisure services and stroke charities for optimum implementation.

ENSURING ACCESS, EQUITY, QUALITY AND COST-EFFECTIVENESS

As we have seen in previous chapters, Exercise after Stroke has been shown to have clear physiological, functional and psychosocial benefits and has the potential to reduce long-term health-care costs. At the time of writing, there is increasing interest in developing Exercise after Stroke services in the USA, Canada, Australia and Europe. The inclusion of recommendations for Exercise after Stroke in national policy documents and clinical guidelines (e.g. Royal College of Physicians 2008, Scottish Government 2009, Scottish Intercollegiate Guidelines Network 2008, 2010) is expected to drive forward the development of Exercise after Stroke services across countries (Mead & Bernhardt 2011).

Therefore, a considerable amount of work needs to be undertaken to develop national strategies that ensure that stroke survivors have access to exercise programmes that have been adapted to their needs, that these services are accessible, their number sufficient and their provision equitable, together with quality assurance mechanisms to ensure that these services are safe and based on current best quality evidence.

The discussion of the various Exercise after Stroke service models above leaves many more specific questions open about which direction is best for future service development. Based on our recent survey of existing services and published research evidence, we have developed guidelines for best practice in developing Exercise after Stroke services with a view to address these questions as far as possible, given the state of the art in research and practice. An outline of these guidelines will be given in the next and final chapter of this book.

SUMMARY POINTS

- At present there are very few specialist (i.e. designed and adapted for stroke) community exercise programmes for stroke survivors in the UK, Europe and North America.
- Where specialist programmes are unavailable, stroke survivors currently access other options for exercise, e.g. exercise referral schemes, cardiac rehabilitation exercise sessions, 'over fifties' classes, aqua aerobics, Tai Chi and yoga classes.
- Existing programmes such as cardiac rehabilitation, falls prevention and exercise referral offer important templates for service design; however, there are a number of reasons (including the often hidden cognitive sequalae of a stroke) that necessitate exercise programmes for stroke survivors to be specifically adapted to stroke, tailored to individuals and delivered by an exercise professional with an advanced qualification in this field.
- There is increasing interest in developing Exercise after Stroke services in the USA, Canada, Australia and Europe. Further work is required through research, the development of national strategies and service development in health-care and community settings to ensure that stroke survivors have access to exercise programmes that are safe, quality assured, equitable, accessible and evidence-based.

REFERENCES

American College of Sports Medicine, 2010. Guidelines for exercise testing and prescription, eighth ed. Lippincott Williams & Wilkins, Philadelphia, PA.

Au-Yeung, S.S., Hui-Chan, C.W., Tang, J.C., et al., 2009. Short-form Tai Chi improves standing balance of people with chronic stroke. Neurorehabil. Neural Repair 23, 515–522.

Batchelor, F.A., Hill, K.D., Mackintosh, S.F., et al., 2009. The FLASSH study: protocol for a randomised controlled trial evaluating falls prevention after stroke and two sub-studies. BMC Neurol. 9, 14.

Best, C., van Wijck, F., Dennis, J., et al., 2011. A survey of community exercise programmes for stroke survivors in Scotland. Health & Social Care in the Community. Available online at: http://onlinelibrary.wiley.com/ doi/10.1111/j.1365-2524.2011.01043.x/abstract.

Carin-Levy, G., Kendall, M., Young, A., et al., 2009. The psychosocial effects of exercise and relaxation classes for persons surviving a stroke. Can. J. Occup. Ther. 76, 73–76.

Canadian Society for Exercise Physiology, 2002. Physical activity readiness questionnaire. CSEP, Ontario.

Dean, C.M., Rissel, C., Sharkey, M., et al., 2009. Exercise intervention to prevent falls and enhance mobility in community dwellers after stroke: a protocol for a randomised controlled trial. BMC Neurol. 9, 38.

Department of Health, 1999. Introduction of managed clinical networks within the NHS in Scotland. Scottish Executive,

Edinburgh. Available online at: http://www.sehd.scot.nhs.uk/mels/1999_10.htm (accessed 07.09.2011).

Department of Health, 2001. National quality assurance framework for exercise referral systems. Department of Health, London.

Forsyth, R., 2009. Glasgow Life. Personal communication.

Fullerton, A., Macdonald, M., Brown, A., et al., 2008. Survey of fitness facilities for individuals post-stroke in the Greater Toronto Area. Appl. Physiol. Nutr. Metab. 33, 713–719.

Harrington, R., Taylor, G., Hollinghurst, S., et al., 2010. A community-based exercise and education scheme for stroke survivors: a randomized controlled trial and economic evaluation. Clin. Rehabil. 24, 3–15.

Hart, J., Kanner, H., Gilboa-Mayo, R., et al., 2004. Tai Chi Chuan practice in community-dwelling persons after stroke. Int. J. Rehabil. Res. 27, 303–304.

Jepson, R., Robertson, R., Doi, L., 2010. Audit of exercise referral scheme activity in Scotland. NHS Health Scotland, Edinburgh.

Jolliffe, J., Rees, K., Taylor, R.R.S., et al., 2001. Exercise-based rehabilitation for coronary heart disease. Cochrane Database Syst. Rev. 1, CD001800. doi:10.1002/14651858.

Leijon, M.E., Bendtsen, P., Nilsen, P., et al., 2009. Does a physical activity referral scheme improve the physical activity among routine primary health care patients? Scand. J. Med. Sci. Sports 19, 627–636.

Mead, G.E., Bernhardt, J., 2011. Physical fitness training after stroke: time to implement what we know, but more research is needed. Int. J. Stroke 6, 506–508.

Mead, G., Greig, C.A., Cunningham, I., et al., 2007. STroke: A Randomised Trial of Exercise or Relaxation (STARTER). J. Am. Geriatr. Soc. 55, 892–899.

Reed, M., Harrington, R., Duggan, A., et al., 2010. Meeting stroke survivors' perceived needs: a qualitative study of a community-based exercise and education scheme. Clin. Rehabil. 24, 16–25.

Roth, E.J., 1993. Heart disease in patients with stroke: incidence, impact, and implications for rehabilitation 1. Classification and prevalence. Arch. Phys. Med. Rehabil. 74, 752–760.

Royal College of Physicians, 2008. Intercollegiate Stroke Working Party. National clinical guideline for stroke, third ed. Royal College of Physicians, London. Available online at: http://www.rcplondon.ac.uk/pubs/books/stroke/stroke_guidelines_2ed.pdf.

Schmidt, M., Absalah, S., Stronks, K., 2008. The effectiveness of 'Exercise on Prescription' in stimulating physical activity among women in ethnic minority groups in the Netherlands: protocol for a randomized controlled trial. BMC Public Health 8, 406.

Scottish Government, 2009. Better heart disease and stroke care action plan. Scottish Government, Edinburgh. Available online at: http://www.scotland.gov.uk/Publications/2009/06/29102453/11 (accessed 08.09.2011).

Scottish Intercollegiate Guidelines Network, 2002. Guideline 57: Cardiac rehabilitation. Scottish Intercollegiate Guidelines Network (SIGN), Edinburgh. Available online at: http://www.sign.ac.uk/guidelines/fulltext/57/contents.html (accessed 09.09.2011).

Scottish Intercollegiate Guidelines Network, 2008. Guideline 108: Management of patients with stroke or TIA: assessment, investigation, immediate management and secondary prevention: a national clinical. Scottish Intercollegiate Guidelines Network (SIGN), Edinburgh. Available online at: http://www.sign.ac.uk/guidelines/fulltext/108/index.html (accessed 08.09.2011).

Scottish Intercollegiate Guidelines Network, 2010. Guideline 118: Management of patients with stroke: rehabilitation, prevention and management of complications, and discharge planning: a national clinical guideline. Scottish Intercollegiate Guidelines Network (SIGN), Edinburgh. Available online at: http://www.sign.ac.uk/guidelines/fulltext/118/index.html (accessed 08.09.2011).

Sharma, H., Bulley, C., van Wijck, F., 2011. Experiences of an exercise referral scheme from the perspective of people with chronic stroke: a qualitative study. Physiotherapy. doi:org/10.1016/j.physio.2011.05.004.

Stuart, M., Chard, S., Roettger, S., 2008. Exercise for chronic stroke survivors: a policy perspective. J. Rehabil. Res. Dev. 45, 329–336.

Stuart, M., Benvenuti, F., Macko, R., et al., 2009. Community-based adaptive physical activity program for chronic stroke: feasibility, safety, and efficacy of the Empoli model. Neurorehabil. Neural Repair 23, 726–734.

Tang, A., Closson, V., Marzolini, S., et al., 2009. Cardiac rehabilitation after stroke-need and opportunity. J. Cardiopulm. Rehabil. Prev. 29, 97–104.

Tang, A., Marzolini, S., Oh, P., et al., 2010. Feasibility and effects of adapted cardiac rehabilitation after stroke: a prospective trial. BMC Neurol. 9 (10), 40.

Wiles, R., Demain, S., Robison, J., et al., 2008. Exercise on prescription schemes for stroke patients post-discharge from physiotherapy. Disabil. Rehabil. 30, 1966–1975.

Guidelines for Exercise after Stroke service design

Catherine S. Best • Gillian Mead • John M.A. Dennis

CHAPTER CONTENTS

INTRODUCTION

This chapter will outline best practice guidelines on designing and delivering Exercise after Stroke services. It will build on the previous chapter, which outlined the range of ways in which Exercise after Stroke can potentially be delivered. A clear question arising from the previous chapter is: What is the *best* way to develop Exercise after Stroke services that are safe and effective? This chapter will address this question by outlining best practice guidelines for Exercise after Stroke services.

The growing evidence of the benefits of Exercise after Stroke and its incorporation into UK and international clinical guidelines and policy (e.g. Gordon et al. 2004, Royal College of Physicians 2008, Scottish Government 2009, Scottish Intercollegiate Guidelines Network 2008, 2010) means there is a strong impetus for new Exercise after Stroke service development. For this reason, it is timely to provide some direction as to how service development should progress, based on existing research evidence, clinical and occupational standards and professional experience.

Firstly, we will clarify the scope of the best practice guidance in terms of where the Exercise after Stroke services are placed in the stroke pathway, the range of services covered and the target audience for these guidelines. Then we will outline the key best practice elements of Exercise after Stroke. The best practice guidelines are based on in-depth analysis of the content and organisation of existing services in Scotland (Best et al. 2010a, 2011), current research evidence in this field, plus relevant stroke and exercise guidelines and National Occupational Standards in the UK health and fitness sector (SkillsActive 2010a,b). The full text of the guidelines, full details of the multiprofessional team who wrote the full guidelines and further background details can be found at www.exerciseafterstroke.org.uk.

SCOPE OF THE GUIDELINES

EXERCISE AFTER STROKE SERVICES IN THE PATIENT JOURNEY

There are three key elements of stroke care, as described in chapter 2:

1. Acute treatment: medical care immediately following stroke.
2. Rehabilitation: restoration of function and minimisation of long-term disability after stroke.
3. Secondary prevention: preventing further strokes through medication and lifestyle advice.

Rehabilitation after stroke is very important for maximising quality of life and independence after stroke. Normally, a multidisciplinary team of professionals is involved in providing post-stroke rehabilitation. However, due to resource issues, rehabilitation is generally time-limited, and the majority of patients will eventually come to a stage where the focus of care shifts from professional input to self-management. As highlighted in chapter 5, research has shown that exercise has a vital role to play in improving and maintaining physical fitness and function after stroke (Brazzelli et al. 2011, Saunders et al. 2009, English and Hillier 2010). Exercise is, therefore, an important way in which stroke survivors can continue to improve their own fitness and function after, or in addition to, formal rehabilitation (Mead and van Wijck 2011). Exercise reduces the risk of first-ever stroke and can also potentially play an important role in secondary stroke prevention; although there are no data linking exercise with the risk of recurrent stroke, there is evidence that exercise has important biological effects that are likely to reduce recurrent stroke, e.g. stimulation of endogenous fibrinolysis (Ivey et al. 2003). This chapter describes how to provide services in the *community* that support safe, effective exercise after stroke.

EXERCISE AFTER STROKE SERVICES

The Exercise after Stroke services described here are community services, which means they are for people who are not inpatients in a hospital. Although clinical guidelines recommend that exercise be incorporated into the early management of stroke, there are challenges to engaging inpatients in exercise. For example, medical complications such as infection are common in the early post-stroke period, as is fatigue (Morley et al. 2005). Ongoing research will, however, provide further evidence about the feasibility, safety and effectiveness of exercise training during inpatient rehabilitation. These guidelines focus on delivery of community Exercise after Stroke services that could be accessed by stroke survivors once they are discharged from hospital.

The Exercise after Stroke services we will describe below are positioned at the final stage of the rehabilitation process, i.e. the transition to self-management. They are run by appropriately trained and qualified exercise professionals in community venues such as leisure centres, health clubs, health centres or community halls, or by physiotherapists, stroke nurses and/or therapy assistants in outpatient settings.

The guidelines are aimed at organisations and individuals who currently run Exercise after Stroke services, or may do so in the future, including health services, stroke charities, private health clubs, public sector leisure centres, community centres, exercise professionals, health-care professionals and assistants. It will also be of interest to potential referrers to the service, including general practitioners (GPs), practice nurses, occupational therapists, social care workers and service users.

BEST PRACTICE GUIDELINES FOR EXERCISE AFTER STROKE

Readers are referred to the 'Best practice guidance for the development of Exercise after Stroke services in community settings' (Best et al. 2010b) for the full guidelines. This chapter describes the key requirements for best practice for Exercise after Stroke; these are listed in Box 13.1. Each of these elements will be detailed below.

BOX 13.1 Key requirements for best practice for Exercise after Stroke services

- Service governance and management
  - Multi-sectoral collaboration
- Workforce planning
  - Service coordinator
  - Eight is the maximum number of stroke survivors for each exercise professional
- Referral processes
  - Referral from a health-care professional
  - Procedures for the adequate transfer of necessary medical information
- Exercise professional competencies
  - Specialist instructor qualification in the field of stroke
- Service content, format and delivery
  - Evidence-based
  - Group format
  - Ongoing (i.e. not time-limited)
- Financial support (not included in full guidelines)
  - Dependent on local circumstances

SERVICE GOVERNANCE AND MANAGEMENT

Working group

The guidelines recommend that a local working group consisting of representatives from all relevant local organisations and professional groups should be convened to oversee development of new Exercise after Stroke services.

Although many of the existing Exercise after Stroke services in the UK are led by a single organisation, for optimum delivery all organisations and professional groups involved in delivering stroke services should be involved in the planning of Exercise after Stroke services. In this way, the service would benefit from the perspective of all these different stakeholders (e.g. medical knowledge, experience of delivering as well as participating in community services). Figure 13.1 indicates the possible membership of the working group. The diagram shows the 'core' or minimum membership in the centre circle and the large oval indicating the other professionals that would ideally also be involved, such as these would include all local stakeholders in stroke service provision, including doctors, physiotherapists, specialist stroke and practice nurses, occupational therapists, speech and language therapists, orthotists, podiatrists, exercise professionals, health, leisure and voluntary sector service managers, social services, transport providers and service users, including stroke survivors and carers.

Involvement of the regional stroke networks

Cardiac rehabilitation services and falls prevention services are already integrated as part of the National Health Service in the UK and can provide

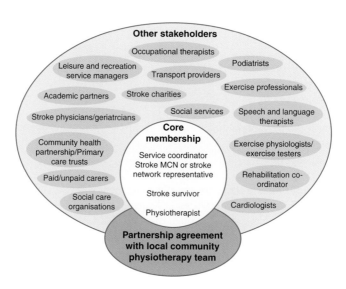

FIG 13.1 Diagram showing membership of the management/working group of an Exercise after Stroke service. MCN, Managed Clinical Network.

a template for service development for Exercise after Stroke, as discussed in chapter 12. These services are part of an integrated care pathway that begins in inpatient care and ends in community maintenance exercise classes. For this reason, our guidelines recommend that the Stroke Managed Clinical Networks (MCNs) in Scotland, the Stroke Care Networks in England or equivalent bodies in other countries should be part of the Working Group planning new Exercise after Stroke services to ensure that the service is integrated and coordinated with the rest of the patient pathway.

Partnership agreement

Importance of local physiotherapy teams

Existing Exercise after Stroke services report how important the positive relationships they have with the local physiotherapy teams are to their services. Many of the Exercise after Stroke services originally began through local physiotherapists providing training to local exercise professionals. This competency-based training enabled exercise professionals to deliver exercise sessions for stroke survivors before nationally accredited training was available. Many existing services say that the ongoing advice and support they receive from local physiotherapists on specific stroke survivor issues is vital to their service. Physiotherapists are also important in referring stroke survivors to Exercise after Stroke services.

Need to formalise links between service provider and local physiotherapists

For this reason, we recommend that, at the inception of a new Exercise after Stroke service, a partnership agreement should be developed between the service provider, where this is a charity or leisure service, and the local physiotherapy team.

Content of the agreement

The structure of the partnership agreement should include:

- Agreed standards and related performance indicators
- Description of roles and responsibilities for all partners
- A quality assurance framework describing how the agreed standards will be monitored.

  Specifically, this agreement should include:

- Ongoing physiotherapy advice and input to the service in terms of workforce development and staff training
- The provision of specific advice from physiotherapists about how to manage co-morbid medical conditions and how to tailor exercises for individuals.

  This agreement is in addition to the Working Group, which provides overall direction to the development and oversees pathways into and out of the service.

Location

In the research literature, lack of transport to venues is cited as a barrier to exercise participation (Rimmer et al. 2008). Therefore, we recommend that when planning a new Exercise after Stroke service, transport and accessibility are central considerations. Services should be provided in accessible venues that have good public transport links.

Stuart et al. (2008, 2009), in their discussion of the Adaptive Physical Activity programme for stroke survivors run in the Empoli region in Italy, state that one of the main attributes of this programme is its wide geographical dispersion. That is, the programme is run in leisure centres right across the region and so participants do not have to travel far to get to a session. The ideal situation would be if Exercise after Stroke groups achieved a high degree of penetration into local communities.

WORKFORCE PLANNING

Exercise after Stroke service coordinator

Existing services told us how important the publicising and promotion of services to potential referrers and participants were to the efficient running of their service. Local community-based health initiatives tend to come and go as funding waxes and wanes. GPs and other community health-care professionals need to be kept up to date on the services available in their area in the face of constant change. Existing Exercise after Stroke services without a service coordinator told us that it was difficult for staff to find the time to visit GP practices, etc. For this reason, we recommend that a dedicated service coordinator should be identified to perform these tasks. This does not need to be a full-time post, but can be included with other responsibilities. However, it does require a clearly designated individual to be the main point of contact and act as the lynch pin and 'champion' for the service. For example, in a number of services identified in Scotland, a senior exercise professional with a job title such as 'Physical Activity Development Officer' or 'Community Health Development Officer' takes on the role of Exercise after Stroke coordinator within a wider remit.

In the research literature, stroke survivors report 'not knowing where to exercise' as being a barrier to exercise participation (Rimmer et al. 2008). Physiotherapists report they are uncertain whether the exercise professionals working with stroke survivors will have sufficient training, knowledge and competence to work with these individuals (Wiles et al. 2008). The role of the Exercise after Stroke service coordinators is to ensure referrers are aware of the service inclusion criteria and the content of the service through provision of clear written materials, personal visits and presentations to potential referrers, e.g. at weekly practice or management meetings. Emphasising the evidence base, the qualifications of the exercise staff, the close, ongoing links with the local physiotherapy teams, the quality assurance and evaluation mechanisms, appear to be effective.

Exercise professional numbers

When developing a new Exercise after Stroke service, the working group will need to estimate how many trained exercise professionals the service will require.

Exercise sessions should have a maximum of eight stroke survivors for each exercise professional initially, although this will depend to some extent on case mix and the length of time participants have been exercising regularly. Ratios should also be agreed with the working group members with reference to the service's inclusion and exclusion criteria.

REFERRAL PROCESSES

Our survey of existing Exercise after Stroke services found that there was a range of referral mechanisms in operation, as described in the previous chapter. In chapter 9, we discussed the reasons why stroke survivors should be formally referred by health-care professionals. The main reason is safety: an appropriately qualified health professional needs to screen the stroke survivor to determine that there are no absolute contraindications for exercise and advise on the management of any relative contraindications and the implications of any medications. For example, the exercise professional needs to know whether the stroke survivor is taking any medications likely to influence their response to exercise. Importantly, the health professional also needs to assess the stroke survivor's functional status so that the exercise professional can tailor the exercise programme to minimise risk and optimise benefit. For example, the exercise professional needs to know whether the stroke survivor has any deficits in grip force that have implications for exercises using an elastic therapy band. Finally, the UK Department of Health's (2001), 'Quality Assurance Framework for Exercise Referral Systems' clearly states that referral from a health-care professional is required. If an exercise professional were to face a charge of professional negligence, this is likely to be the benchmark against which their standard of care would be assessed.

For the reasons listed above, we recommend that a robust referral pathway be established, as detailed in chapter 9 and shown in Figure 9.1.

Exercise professionals have their own responsibility in the risk assessment and management process, which was described in chapter 9. A consultation is currently underway in the UK regarding standards for exercise referral, which comprises the process of risk stratification, including risk assessment and management strategies. It is likely that our recommendations will need to be updated once this document has been published.

EXERCISE PROFESSIONAL COMPETENCIES

The potential for exercise professionals to improve public health through targeted programmes of exercise is becoming more widely appreciated. This has led to increased professionalisation of the health and fitness sector. In the UK, there are a range of qualifications available for exercise professionals. SkillsActive is the Sector Skills Council for Active Leisure, Learning and Well-Being, which sets the National Occupational Standards to ensure that qualifications are comparable across providers. In addition, the Register of Exercise Professionals (2010) is an independent public register that ensures members' qualifications meet agreed National Occupational Standards, abide by a professional code of conduct, have public liability insurance and are committed to a programme of continuing professional development.

In the UK, exercise professionals who work with stroke survivors must have appropriate training in order to be competent in the design, adaptation, tailoring, progression, communication and evaluation of the exercise programme to individuals as well as groups. This should be a nationally recognised and accredited qualification. In the UK, exercise professional qualifications should map fully onto the SkillsActive National Occupational Standard Unit D516 (2010a,b). The qualification must be endorsed by SkillsActive and recognised by the Register of Exercise Professionals at Level 4 (SkillsActive 2010a,b). It is essential to note that this is required for the validation of the instructor's insurance.

SERVICE CONTENT

Evidence-based

The exercise programme should be evidence-based. As discussed in chapters 4 and 5, it should contain a significant proportion of cardiorespiratory walking training, as this has the strongest evidence of improving functional outcomes for stroke survivors (Brazzelli et al. 2011, Saunders et al. 2009, Wevers et al. 2009).

Group format

As chapter 6 explained, participants in qualitative research on Exercise after Stroke reported benefits from the social aspect of the peer group (Carin-Levy et al. 2009, Reed et al. 2010, Sharma et al. 2011).

Group exercise is also likely to be more cost-effective than individual sessions, as indicated by the study of English et al. (2007). Further information will become available on completion of the ongoing trial by van de Port et al. (2009).

We recommend in our guidelines that Exercise after Stroke services deliver group exercise sessions wherever possible.

Ongoing services

The Scottish government's physical activity strategy (2003) recommends that adults in later life *'should be supported and encouraged to stay active in the community for as long as they choose'* (p. 55). Life-long participation in exercise is also recommended in several clinical guidelines, e.g. Scottish Intercollegiate Guidelines Network Guideline 108 (2008). Encouraging life-long engagement in physical activity is especially important for stroke survivors, because evidence shows low retention of cardiovascular training effects after training finishes (e.g. Mead et al. 2007).

Some stroke survivors may be able to move to mainstream exercise provision or maintain fitness by exercising on their own, whilst others may continue to need to participate in Exercise after Stroke services. Thus, Exercise after Stroke services should be ongoing and not time-limited, to enhance a more long-term active lifestyle wherever possible.

FUNDING

There is currently not enough evidence on the cost-effectiveness of the various Exercise after Stroke models, described in chapter 12, to recommend any specific service model. Ideally, health economic analysis of the Exercise after Stroke services should be conducted in the near future to provide information necessary to guide the choice of service design.

The experience from running cardiac rehabilitation and falls prevention services indicates that a service provided by the UK National Health Service that progresses to community-based exercise sessions could be cost-effective in improving patient outcomes. The review conducted by Jolliffe and colleagues in 2000 supports the contribution of exercise sessions to the cost-effectiveness of cardiac rehabilitation.

Any proposal for funding a new Exercise after Stroke service is likely to be based on two key elements:

1. The evidence of effectiveness of exercise and fitness training in improving physical fitness and function, e.g. as shown by the Cochrane systematic review (Brazzelli et al. 2011). Exercise after Stroke services are also likely to save money in the long term, possibly by reducing re-admission to hospital and further morbidity and mortality in stroke survivors through secondary prevention. However, this is a more tentative argument as currently there is a lack of evidence on the health economics of Exercise after Stroke services and further research will be required.
2. Policy documents and clinical guidelines (e.g. Royal College of Physicians 2008, Scottish Government 2009), which recommend that stroke survivors should be accessing exercise and which are based on evidence as referred to above.

The precise mechanisms for obtaining funding for new Exercise after Stroke services will depend on local context and circumstances, and therefore cannot be prescribed universally.

SUMMARY POINTS

- In order to give guidance on best practice for developing new Exercise after Stroke services and to standardise practice in this specialist area across the UK, our multidisciplinary group of experts on Exercise after Stroke have developed a set of best practice guidelines for Exercise after Stroke, which pertain to:
- Service governance and management
- Workforce planning
- Referral processes
- Exercise professional qualifications
- Service content, format and delivery.
- Only a summary of some key elements of the guidelines are given above; readers are referred to www.exerciseafterstroke.org.uk for the full document.

REFERENCES

Best, C.S., van Wijck, F., Dennis, J., et al., 2010a. Models of service delivery for Exercise after Stroke. Cerebrovasc. Dis. 29, S2.

Best, C., van Wijck, F., Dinan-Young, S., et al., 2010b. Best practice guidance for the development of Exercise after Stroke services in community settings.

Edinburgh University, Edinburgh. Available online at: http://www.exerciseafterstroke.org.uk/ (accessed 08.09.2011).

Best, C., van Wijck, F., Dennis, J., et al., 2011. A survey of community exercise programmes for stroke survivors in Scotland. Health & Social Care in the Community. Available at: http://onlinelibrary.wiley.com/doi/10.1111/j.1365-2524.2011.01043.x/abstract.

Brazzelli, M., Saunders, D.H., Greig, C.A., et al., 2011. Physical fitness training for stroke patients. Cochrane Database Syst. Rev 11, CD003316.

Carin-Levy, G., Kendall, M., Young, A., et al., 2009. The psychosocial effects of exercise and relaxation classes for persons surviving a stroke. Can. J. Occup. Ther. 76, 73–76.

Department of Health, 2001. National quality assurance framework for exercise referral systems. Department of Health, London.

English, C.K., Hillier, S.L., Stiller, K.R., Warden-Flood, A., 2007. Circuit class therapy versus individual physiotherapy sessions during inpatient stroke rehabilitation: A controlled trial. Archiv. Phys. Med. Rehab. 88, 955–963.

English, C., Hillier, S.L., 2010. Circuit class therapy for improving mobility after stroke. Cochrane Database Syst. Rev. 7, Art. no.: CD007513. doi:10.1002/14651858.CD007513.pub2.

Gordon, N.F., Gulanick, M., Costa, F., et al., 2004. Physical activity and exercise recommendations for stroke survivors: An American Heart Association Scientific Statement from the Council on Clinical Cardiology, Subcommittee on Exercise, Cardiac Rehabilitation, and Prevention; the Council on Cardiovascular Nursing; the Council on Nutrition, Physical Activity, and Metabolism; and the Stroke Council. Circulation 109, 2031–2041.

Ivey, F.M., Womack, C.J., Kulaputana, O., et al., 2003. A single bout of walking exercise enhances endogenous fibrinolysis in stroke patients. Med. Sci. Sports Exerc. 35, 193–198.

Jolliffe, J., Taylor, R., Ebrahim, S., 2000. A report on the clinical and cost effectiveness of physiotherapy in cardiac rehabilitation. National Service Framework Coronary Heart Disease Evidence-based briefing paper. Chartered Institute of Physiotherapy, London. Available online at: http://www.csp.org.uk/uploads/documents/ebb_cr.pdf (accessed 14.02.2010).

Mead, G.E., van Wijck, F., 2011. Exercise after stroke-time to translate evidence into practice. J. R. Coll. Physicians Edinb. 41, 98–99.

Mead, G., Greig, C.A., Cunningham, I., et al., 2007. STroke: A Randomised Trial of Exercise or Relaxation (STARTER). J. Am. Geriatr. Soc. 55, 892–899.

Morley, W., Jackson, K., Mead, G.E., 2005. Post-stroke fatigue: an important yet neglected symptom. Age Ageing 34, 313.

Reed, M., Harrington, R., Duggan, A., et al., 2010. Meeting stroke survivors' perceived needs: a qualitative study of a community-based exercise and education scheme. Clin. Rehabil. 24, 16–25.

Register of Exercise Professionals (REPs), 2010. Entry qualifications framework. Register of Exercise Professionals, Croydon. Available online at: http://www.exerciseregister.org/REPsQualsFramework2010.html (accessed 09.09.2011).

Rimmer, J.H., Wang, E., Smith, D., 2008. Barriers associated with exercise and community access for individuals with stroke. J. Rehabil. Res. Dev. 45, 315–322.

Royal College of Physicians, 2008. Intercollegiate Stroke Working Party. National Clinical Guideline for Stroke, third ed. Royal College of Physicians, London. Available online at: http://www.rcplondon.ac.uk/pubs/books/stroke/stroke_guidelines_2ed.pdf (accessed 08.09.2011).

Saunders, D.H., Greig, C.A., Mead, G.E., et al., 2009. Physical fitness training for stroke patients. Cochrane Database Syst. Rev. 4, CD003316. doi:10.1002/14651858.

Scottish Government, 2003. Let's make Scotland more active: a strategy for physical activity. Scottish Government, Edinburgh. Retrieved from: http://www.scotland.gov.uk/Publications/2003/02/16324/17895 (accessed 23/1/12).

Scottish Government, 2009. Better heart disease and stroke care action plan. The Scottish Government, Edinburgh. Available online at: http://www.scotland.gov.uk/Publications/2009/06/29102453/11 (accessed 08.09.2011).

Scottish Intercollegiate Guidelines Network, 2008. Guideline 108:

Management of patients with stroke or TIA: assessment, investigation, immediate management and secondary prevention: a national clinical guideline. Scottish Intercollegiate Guidelines Network (SIGN), Edinburgh. Available online at: http://www.sign.ac.uk/guidelines/fulltext/108/index.html (accessed 08.09.2011).

Scottish Intercollegiate Guidelines Network, 2010. Guideline 118: Management of patients with stroke: rehabilitation, prevention and management of complications, and discharge planning: a national clinical guideline. Scottish Intercollegiate Guidelines Network (SIGN), Edinburgh. Available online at: http://www.sign.ac.uk/guidelines/fulltext/118/index.html (accessed 08.09.2011).

Sharma, H., Bulley, C., van Wijck, F., 2011. Experiences of an exercise referral scheme from the perspective of people with chronic stroke: a qualitative study. Physiotherapy. doi:org/10.1016/j.physio.2011.05.004.

SkillsActive, 2010a. D516.1: design and agree a physical activity programme with patients/clients after stroke. Level 4 national occupational standards for physical activity after stroke. SkillsActive, London. Available online at: http://www.skillsactive.com/training/standards/level_4/physical_activity_and_health (accessed 09.09.2011).

SkillsActive, 2010b. D516.2: deliver, review and adapt a physical activity programme with patient/clients after stroke. Level 4 national occupational standards for physical activity after stroke. SkillsActive, London. Available online at: http://www.skillsactive.com/training/standards/level_4/physical_activity_and_health (accessed 09.09.2011).

Stuart, M., Chard, S., Roettger, S., 2008. Exercise for chronic stroke survivors: a policy perspective. J. Rehabil. Res. Dev. 45, 329–336.

Stuart, M., Benvenuti, F., Macko, R., et al., 2009. Community-based adaptive physical activity program for chronic stroke: feasibility, safety, and efficacy of the Empoli model. Neurorehabil. Neural Repair 23, 726–734.

van de Port, I., Wevers, L., Roelse, H., et al., 2009. Cost-effectiveness of a structured progressive task-oriented circuit class training programme to enhance walking competency after stroke: the protocol of the FIT-Stroke trial. BMC Neurol. 9, 43.

Wevers, L., van De Port, I., Vermue, M., et al., 2009. Effects of task-oriented circuit class training on walking competency after stroke a systematic review. Stroke 40, 2450–2459.

Wiles, R., Demain, S., Robison, J., et al., 2008. Exercise on prescription schemes for stroke patients post-discharge from physiotherapy. Disabil. Rehabil. 30, 1966–1975.

Conclusions

Gillian Mead • Frederike van Wijck

This book has focused on physical fitness after stroke, which is often considerably reduced, and exercise and fitness training after stroke. The first part of the book has described the effects of stroke, how stroke is treated, and the long-term consequences of stroke that can interfere with daily life. Some stroke survivors will make a good recovery, whilst for others, life will never be the same again. John Brown has described his own personal journey of recovery from stroke – much of what he has written will resonate with other stroke survivors and those involved in their care. John's contribution to this book is unique as he has so clearly expressed how exercise training can contribute to ongoing recovery after stroke, long after usual stroke care has been completed.

Most stroke survivors will need hospital care, delivered by a multidisciplinary team of health professionals. Acute stroke care has improved substantially over the past few years, and so attention is now turning to how to mitigate the longer term effects of stroke and improve quality of life. There is increasing recognition that the inactivity that often follows (and sometimes precedes) stroke can have profound effects on aerobic fitness, muscle strength, power and endurance. This book has highlighted the extent to which physical fitness tends to be impaired after stroke, and the impact this may have on function, activities of daily living and independence. This evidence clearly indicates that, to facilitate recovery from stroke, attention must be paid to the low levels of physical fitness throughout the stroke survivor's journey.

There is now a strong evidence base that demonstrates that physical fitness training after stroke including aerobic training leads to improvements in physical function – at least for ambulatory stroke survivors. Research on stroke survivors' experiences with community-based exercise groups also suggests that they can benefit in terms of physical and psychological wellbeing and confidence. Although data are currently lacking to make firm recommendations with respect to the 'FITT' principles (frequency, intensity, time/duration and type of exercise) and further research is required to establish the effects of training on disability, there is sufficient evidence to incorporate fitness training into the rehabilitation of stroke survivors. This book has focused on how to deliver evidence-based exercise and fitness training to stroke survivors after they have been discharged from hospital.

We have explained, in detail, our recommendations for the referral of stroke survivors to exercise, highlighting the importance of safety. Thorough and detailed risk assessment prior to exercise is essential. Communication between referring health care professionals and the professionals delivering exercise and fitness training is a requirement for a safe and seamless transition into exercise and fitness training after stroke. We then moved on to the process of designing exercise programmes for stroke survivors, emphasising the need to adapt the principles and variables of exercise programming to the stroke population in general, as well as tailor the training to the individual, taking into account their personal goals and unique constellation of post-stroke problems, possibly in addition to co-morbidities. The specialist skills and competencies involved in adapting and tailoring exercise to stroke survivors require an extensive working knowledge of stroke and its medical and rehabilitation interventions (including drugs and their possible side effects) as well as co-morbidities. The cycle of designing and delivering exercise is completed by outcome assessment, in which the importance of relevance and scientific robustness has been underlined.

We have emphasised throughout this book that our vision is to enable more people after stroke to be more physically active. This requires that exercise professionals fully engage individual stroke survivors in their physical activity programme. Communication skills come into play – and are particularly important when working with people with speech and language impairments – when listening to what individuals wish to achieve, what motivates them and what they see as barriers to becoming more physically active. Motivational interviewing may enable individuals to make decisions about changing their exercise behaviour, while goal setting can be used to identify more specific targets. The ultimate aim is to enable stroke survivors to enjoy a more physically active lifestyle in a way that is safe and meets their personal needs and goals.

We have concluded the book with recommendations on how to develop existing or set up new community-based Exercise after Stroke services, informed by current best-practice guidelines. We have highlighted the importance of teamwork, a sound referral system, exercise professional training and qualification, and evidence-based and person-centred practice.

Exercise after stroke is a topic area that is expanding rapidly, with more and more stroke services seeking to link with leisure services to develop pathways into exercise after stroke. Exercise after stroke is also an exciting area for further research as well as developments in practice and education.

This book is intended as a stepping stone for further developments in the field. It will need to be reviewed as new research emerges, and experience with delivering and participating in exercise and fitness training after stroke – and other forms of physical activity – accumulates. Meanwhile, we are confident that exercise and fitness training after stroke has the potential to make a real contribution to the quality of life of stroke survivors.

GLOSSARY

We gratefully acknowledge the kind permission of Chest Heart & Stroke Scotland for allowing us to base this glossary on its own glossary of stroke terms.

Activity limitations Difficulties with undertaking activities (e.g. difficulty with grasping objects or walking)

Agnosia Difficulty using information from the senses, i.e. touch, sight, hearing, smell and taste, to make sense of objects

Agraphia Difficulty in writing or drawing

Allodynia Disturbed thermal sensation, e.g. the experience of pain when touching normally non-painful stimuli, such as cold metal

Amnesia Loss of memory

Analgesia Medication to reduce pain

Aneurysm Swelling in a blood vessel wall which may burst and cause a stroke

Ankle-foot orthosis (AFO) A splint-like device, covering the foot, ankle and part of the lower leg, to provide external support for the ankle joint

Anticoagulant Blood thinning drug, which inhibits normal blood clotting

Antiplatelet Blood thinning drug, which works by reducing the 'stickiness' of platelets (fragments of blood cells that help the blood to clot)

Aphagia/dysphagia Difficulty with swallowing

Aphasia/dysphasia Difficulty with using language

Apraxia/dyspraxia Difficulty in coordinating functional activities

Aspiration A problem occurring when secretions or foreign material enter the airways in the lungs

Aspirin One of the antiplatelet drugs that is often used in patients with ischaemic stroke to prevent further strokes

Associated reaction A pattern of muscle hyperactivity, often temporary, as a result of effort (e.g. flexion in shoulder, elbow and wrist when a stroke survivor attempts to walk)

Astereognosis Difficulty recognising objects through touch alone (i.e. with eyes closed)

Ataxia Loss of coordination. Ataxic gait is a walking pattern that is uncoordinated ('staggering')

Arteriovenous malformation (AVM) Abnormal structure of arteries and veins in the brain which has a risk of haemorrhage

Atheroma Build up of fatty deposits in the arteries that restricts blood flow and predisposes to the development of blood clots

Atherosclerosis The process of the arteries hardening and narrowing due to the build up of atheroma within them

Atrial fibrillation (AF) Irregular heart rhythm which can be a cause of stroke

Bivariate relationship Statistical expression for a relationship between two variables. Compare with multivariate relationship

Blood pressure (BP) Measurement of the pressure within the arteries

Brain attack A term used for a stroke or transient ischaemic attack, that emphasises the suddenness of onset of symptoms

Brainstem Base of the brain which controls the basic functions of life

Bruit Noise made by a blockage in a carotid artery when examined with a stethoscope

Bursitis An inflammation of a small sac (pocket) of fluid, normally found between different layers of soft tissue in the body (e.g. a muscle and tendon), or bone and soft tissue, which has the function of reducing friction between these layers

Carotid arteries Blood vessels located on both sides of the neck that supply blood to the brain

Carotid Doppler Ultrasound of the arteries in the neck to check for blockages or narrowing

Carotid endarterectomy Surgical procedure to clear blockage from a carotid artery

Cerebral haemorrhage Medical term for a bleed in the brain

Cholesterol Fat which leads to fatty deposits in the arteries

Clonus An involuntary, rhythmic contraction of a muscle that often sustains itself, having been provoked by a fast stretch

Co-morbidity One or more diagnosable medical conditions that exists in addition to the most significant condition (e.g. a stroke survivor who also has diabetes as a co-morbidity)

Contracture A fixed deformity of a joint with a permanent loss of joint range of movement

Constraint-induced movement therapy An intervention for people with stroke where the affected arm is forced to participate in activities while the stronger arm is prevented from being used (e.g. by the hand being placed in a mitt) for a considerable period of time each day

Diplopia Double vision

Dorsiflexors Ankle dorsiflexors are muscles that extend the ankle and lift the forefoot

Drop-foot A drop-foot is noticeable through a lack of heel strike during walking. In some cases the toes are dragged over the ground, increasing the risk of falls. It is often seen as a result of a neurological condition (e.g. stroke) causing weakness of the muscles that extend the ankle and lift the forefoot (i.e. the ankle dorsiflexors)

Dual tasking Undertaking two different tasks at the same time (e.g. walking and talking)

Dysarthria Difficulty in communicating due to weakness or incoordination of the muscles used in speaking

Dysexecutive function See Executive dysfunction

Dyslexia Difficulty with literacy and language-related skills

Dysphagia See Aphagia

Dysphasia See Aphasia

Dysphonia Difficulty in speaking at the desired volume

Dyspraxia See Apraxia

Electroencephalogram (EEG) Record of brain electrical activity

Electrical stimulation (ES)/functional electrical stimulation (FES) A therapeutic method involving an electrical current to stimulate muscles with the aim to encourage contraction. FES is used to stimulate muscles with the aim to elicit functional movement (e.g. opening the fingers to reach and grasp an object, or

lifting the foot to encourage heel strike during walking)

Embolism Blockage in a blood vessel due to a blood clot or very occasionally an air bubble

Executive dysfunction Also known as dysexecutive function or dysexecutive syndrome, this indicates a constellation of problems associated with organising, planning and monitoring one's behaviour

Extensor muscles Muscles that extend a joint (e.g. knee extensors straighten the knee)

Flaccidity Low muscle tone, associated with abnormally low levels of muscle activation, often seen in the acute stage after stroke when the brain is in a state of 'shock'. In some cases, flaccidity persists after the acute stage

Functional electrical stimulation (FES) See Electrical stimulation

Gaze palsy Difficulty controlling eye movements, due to weakness of muscles around the eyes

Goal setting A process whereby targets are identified and agreed between a stroke survivor, their health professional, exercise professional and/or treatment team, towards which they will all work over a specified period of time

Haematoma Blood clot

Haemorrhage Bleeding from a ruptured blood vessel

Hemianopia Blindness in half of the visual field affecting both eyes

Hemiparesis/hemiplegia Weakness (partial paralysis) or loss of movement on one side of the body

Hemiplegia See hemiparesis

Hemisphere Medical term for right or left side of the brain

Homonymous hemianopia A condition whereby the same field (homonymous) of view is obscured in both eyes

Hydrocephalus A build up of fluid on the brain. The excess fluid puts pressure on the brain, which can cause it to be damaged

Hyperglycaemia Higher than normal blood sugar level. The threshold for categorising hyperglycaemia is generally above 7 mmol/litre

Hypertension High blood pressure. The thresholds for diagnosing high blood pressure are generally considered to be systolic blood pressure of more than 140 mmHg and a diastolic blood pressure of more than 80 mmHg (note that there is sometimes slight variation in what is defined as 'high' blood pressure)

Hypertonia Muscle tone reflects the tightness of a muscle or muscle group. Hypertonia is abnormally high tone; hypotonia is abnormally low tone

Hypoglycaemia Low blood sugar level. The level at which a diagnosis is made for different people and in different circumstances may vary; generally considered to be a level of <4 mmol/litre

Impairment A problem in body function or structure (e.g. spasticity, weakness)

Incontinence Loss of bladder or bowel control

Infarct Area of tissue damaged by lack of blood and oxygen

Lacunar stroke syndrome (LACS) Medical classification; a stroke caused by an infarct or haemorrhage in a small, deep area of the brain

Local drugs Drugs that affect a specific location only (e.g. botulinum neurotoxin, injected into specific muscles with spasticity). This is in contrast to systemic drugs, which affect the entire central nervous system (e.g. oral baclofen)

Multivariate relationship Statistical expression for a relationship between more than two variables. Compare with bivariate relationship

Multi-infarct dementia (MID) Dementia caused by several infarcts in the brain that generally occur over a period of time

Minimal clinically important difference (MCID) The difference between scores on an outcome measure that is considered to be meaningful by the person involved

Motivational interviewing A collaborative person-centred form of guiding a person to encourage and strengthen their motivation to change behaviour

Nasogastric (NG) A narrow tube inserted through the nostril into the stomach to provide nutrition

Neuroplasticity The capacity of the nervous system to adapt to change, e.g. by making new connections between nerve cells, or speeding up neural processes, in response to inputs such as exercise, learning a new language or playing a musical instrument

Neglect Also known as unilateral, contra-lateral neglect, visuospatial neglect or hemi-inattention, unilateral neglect is a phenomenon whereby a person fails to attend to, perceive stimuli in, or move towards their affected side

Nystagmus Involuntary jerking of the eyes, which typically occurs in posterior circulation syndrome strokes (POCS)

Paralysis Complete loss of movement in a part of the body

Partial anterior circulation syndrome (PACS) Medical classification; a stroke at the front of the brain

Participation restriction Problem with being involved in life situations (e.g. barriers with return to work after stroke)

Patent foramen ovale (PFO) Hole situated between the right and left sides of the heart; a known risk factor for stroke

Percutaneous endoscopic gastrostomy (PEG) Tube inserted into the wall of the stomach to provide nutrition

Pharynx The part of the throat behind the mouth and the cavity of the nose. It is part of the digestive and respiratory systems and plays a key role in speech

Posterior circulation syndrome (POCS) Medical classification; a stroke at the back of the brain, the cerebellum or in the brainstem

Proprioception A sensory function that provides awareness of the position and movement of one's body in space (without having to look). This is achieved through specific receptors within muscles, tendons and joint capsules, signalling information about posture and movement to the central nervous system

Reliability The extent to which a measure is reproducible; in other words, whether the measure gives the same result each time the same quantity is being measured

Self-efficacy A belief in one's ability to organise and undertake action required to reach a specific goal

Sensitivity Also known as responsiveness, this is the level of change that a measurement instrument is capable of detecting

Shoulder-hand syndrome A complex post-stroke condition whereby the affected limb is painful, swollen and changed in colour

Spasm A short-lived, involuntary muscle contraction, which often produces a pain that is similar to athletic cramping

Spasticity A motor disorder characterised by abnormal muscle activation, which can be felt by both the stroke survivor and the therapist as increased resistance to movement (i.e. 'stiffness') when a muscle is passively stretched

Stance phase This relates to walking (gait); the stance phase is the phase in the gait cycle where the foot is in contact with the ground – in contrast to the swing phase, where the foot is off the ground

Statin Generic name for cholesterol lowering drugs

Stress incontinence Leakage of urine during coughing or sneezing

Stroke Disruption in the blood supply to part of the brain which damages the surrounding brain cells

Subarachnoid haemorrhage (SAH) An uncommon cause of a stroke where blood leaks out of blood vessels over the surface of the brain

Subluxation Partial dislocation of a joint this typically occurs in the shoulder joint after stroke

Systemic drugs Drugs affecting the entire central nervous system (e.g. oral baclofen for spasticity). This is in contrast to local drugs, which affect a specific location only (e.g. botulinum toxin)

Thalamus Part of the brain which deals with sensations

Thixotropy An indication of the stiffness of a substance or tissue (e.g. muscle tissue). Thixotropy is influenced by temperature and movement, thus a warm-up and gentle, repetitive movement can reduce muscle stiffness

Thrombolysis A 'clot busting' drug used to dissolve a blood clot which is causing a stroke

Thrombosis Medical term for a blockage in a blood vessel due to a blood clot

Timed voiding A strategy for stroke survivors who are unaware of the status of their bladder, which involves going to the toilet at specific times

Total anterior circulatory syndrome (TACS) Medical classification; a large stroke at the front of the brain

Transcutaneous electrical nerve stimulation (TENS) A therapeutic intervention that uses a device that can selectively stimulate specific nerves, often used to reduce pain, through electrodes placed on the skin

Transient ischaemic attack (TIA) Medical classification of a mini-stroke; symptoms last less than 24 hours

Validity The validity of a measure indicates whether it does what it is purported to do

Vertigo An abnormal sensation of movement which can cause spinning, dizziness and/ or nausea

Visual inattention See Neglect

Visual field defects Loss of one or more parts of one's field of view

INDEX

NB: Page numbers in *italics* refer to boxes, figures and tables.

INDEX

S

Visual problems *6*, 15, 48–49
Visuospatial neglect 51–52
Vitamin D 62
VO$_2$ peak measures 81–82, *81*, 85, *86*, 100, 225–226
Vocal overflow 57

W

Walking
  aids 203
  cardiovascular endurance *177*
  performance 102–103
  speed 85–87, *86*, *103*
Wall press exercise *201*

Warfarin 25, 34–35, 65
Warning of risk 115–116
Weakness (hemiparesis/hemiplegia) 13, 41, 203
Weight loss 65
Weight training 178
Windows 163
Workforce planning, guidelines 254–255
Working groups 252, *252*
Working memory 56
Written documentation 137

Y

Yoga exercises 146, 242